PRAISE FOR
AN UNLIKELY STRENGTH

What the Tourette community has to say:

An Unlikely Strength is important for people with TS because it lets us know that we are not alone. It gives us ideas of how to better cope with the condition. This book is also important for families of people who have just been diagnosed because so much information out there about the disorder is wrong.

I find this book very relevant to the world today. Bullying, not belonging in society, isolation—these are all themes that cross over way beyond TS. Another thing I have learned from it: there are so many books written by 'experts,' but the true experts are people like us and our families. The people who have to live with and deal with Tourette syndrome day in and day out. Here we are shown as real people with a wide scope of talents.

—Stacy C.

What the medical community has to say:

An Unlikely Strength is such a gift ... so genuine, complicated, humane. The messages within, while in some ways unique to Tourette syndrome, speak to all of us who find ourselves somehow different, who find critical elements in our lives that are beyond our control, find our motivations in question, and our behaviors misunderstood.

This book speaks and informs deeply about TS, but also about the human condition, how we create meaning in our lives, and how much we need to give and receive love and comfort.

An Unlikely Strength is an inspiration and should be required reading for the community of caregivers, including neurologists, pediatricians, psychiatrists, occupational and physical therapists.

—Jo M. Solet, MS, EdM, PhD, OTR/L
Harvard Medical School and Cambridge Health Alliance

What the general public has to say:

A writer tells a story best by finding the person whose voice has not been heard, or not heard enough. Larry Barber's new book, An Unlikely Strength, highlights sixty stories of how a suffering soul can be brought back to life. Larry's skill as an interviewer finds unseen moments that evoke the deep humanity and decency of these brave people. We all struggle, at one time or another; each one of us is wounded in some way. But defeat is not an option. And so it is for the people in this book who are grappling with Tourette syndrome. Their victories, like all victories, take time and care and loving embrace. Reading An Unlikely Strength will change your understanding of Tourette syndrome and of disabilities in general. For many, this book will open the doors to a better life.

—Jack Healey
Director, Human Rights Action Center
Former Executive Director, Amnesty International, USA

June 2016

Julia –

Thank you for opening
your heart to our
community.

AN UNLIKELY STRENGTH

TOURETTE SYNDROME

AND THE SEARCH FOR HAPPINESS IN 60 VOICES

LARRY BARBER

AN UNLIKELY STRENGTH

SQ
PRESS

Published by SQ Presss
Copyright © 2016 by Larry Barber

www.anunlikelystrength.com

Library of Congress Control Number: 2016903400

Paperback Edition ISBN 978-0692652794
Digital Edition available on Kindle

Printed in the United States of America

Author Services by Pedernales Publishing, LLC.
www.pedernalespublishing.com

Cover Design by Rick Jacks

Elsie
mi madre
and
Elena
mi reina

ACKNOWLEDGEMENTS

First and foremost, I want to thank the people who gave me their trust and their stories for this book. Thanks to the indispensable Elena DeVos, my wife and most compassionate, keen-eyed editor. A grateful wish for steady winds and calm seas to Rick Jacks for designing a powerful cover. A hearty *abrazo* to John Kirk for his sharp eye and sharper mind. I'm thankful for publishing guidance and book design to Jose Ramirez and Barbara Rainess at Pedernales Publishing. What would I have done without the generous and enthusiastic support of Raquel Jasso and Javier Lara of iBranit for social media consulting and web design? Thank you also to The Tourette Association of America. And for encouragement and intelligent collaboration, thank you to: Paul Devore, Judit Ungar, Jonathan Estrin, Jo Solet, Jack Healey, Spencer Humphrey, Peter Freedman, Erik Gardner, Loretta and Ronald Staebler, Michael Bamburger, Paul Barber, Lisa Barber, Susan Herrera, Dorothy Wallstein, Dorothy Elchoness, Larry Meyers, Joseph Bobrow, Amalio Madueño, Russell Sharman, Dalton Delan, Bob Renard, Reanne Singer, Jane Bluestein, Susan Fitzell, and Ed Tivnan.

We say, 'I will,' and 'I will not,' and imagine ourselves (though we obey the orders of some prosaic person every day) our own masters, when the truth is that our masters are sleeping. One wakes within us and we are ridden like beasts, though the rider is but some hitherto unguessed part of ourselves.

Gene Wolfe
Shadow of the Torturer

The acceptance of oneself is the essence of the whole moral problem and the epitome of a whole outlook on life. That I feed the hungry, that I forgive an insult, that I love my enemy in the name of Christ—all these are undoubtedly great virtues... But what if I should discover that the least among them all, the poorest of all the beggars, the most impudent of all the offenders, the very enemy himself—that these are within me, and that I myself stand in need of the alms of my own kindness—that I myself am the enemy who must be loved—what then?

Carl Jung
Modern Man in Search of a Soul

TOURETTE SYNDROME

Tourette syndrome (TS, Tourette's) is a genetic neurological disorder with an onset in early childhood or adolescence. It is characterized by tics, or involuntary, "non-volitional" actions. Non-volitional means the individual is caught in the paradoxical position of choosing not to do something and being forced to do it. The individual is therefore not in complete control of mind or body. This is dismaying, as you can imagine, and can pose certain difficulties in forming self-image, gaining social acceptance, and finding happiness and satisfaction in life.

This book is testament to the fact that Touretters can indeed find happiness and a quality of life despite this intrusive and unwelcome illness.

Early Tourette symptoms often are frequent, rapid, repetitive facial or body movements. Vocal tics may occur in addition to motor tics, and can include grunting, throat clearing, shouting, and a host of other noises. The repetitive, and sometimes forceful, nature of tics can cause pain and injury to people with Tourette's.

Tics may also be expressed as coprolalia (swearing or making socially inappropriate statements) or copropraxia (obscene gestures). Despite widespread belief, coprolalia and copropraxia are uncommon with tic disorders.

Tics can change with time, and one person's array of tics is never like another's. Severity of tics ranges from mild and barely noticeable to severe and deeply impairing. The majority of cases are mild. Tics often begin to wane as a child approaches 18-20 years of age.

Tourette syndrome has co-occurring conditions that can complicate living with TS and its treatment. These "comorbid" conditions include ADHD/ADD, impulsivity, obsessive compulsive disorder, oppositional defiant disorder, depression, and behavioral issues such as rage.

Tourette syndrome and other tic disorders occur in all ethnic groups. Males are affected 3 to 4 times more often than females. TS is non-communicable and one person cannot "give" TS to another person. However, the genetic component of Tourette's means a parent *may* pass it to offspring. This is simply biology; it is not cause for blame or self-recrimination.

Many people can suppress tics for a time, but this requires effort and concentration, and is exhausting. Additionally, each tic suppressed is only delayed; it incrementally raises the individual's overall tension and need to express. This pressure invariably releases explosively in bouts of ticcing, which can be painful, and even dangerous.

TABLE OF CONTENTS

The arrangement of interviews is, in some ways, arbitrary. Each individual spoke about many topics.

The Tourette Association of America (tourette.org) is the new name for the organization that provides public awareness, research funds, and support for individuals and families dealing with Tourette syndrome. The Association's name changed while I was conducting these interviews, so most people use the old appellation, Tourette Syndrome Association (TSA).

FOREWORD

Paul Devore

Former Chairman of the Board,
Tourette Association of America

I wasn't diagnosed with Tourette syndrome until after I was forty. Before then, I would make up reasons for the noises I made, or I would pretend it didn't happen. But once I was diagnosed, I became very comfortable saying, "I have Tourette syndrome."

I don't have cancer, I don't have MS, I don't have polio—there are a lot of things I don't have. I'm lucky. I have Tourette syndrome and this is what it does. So be it.

I remember thinking, during the making of the documentary *I Have Tourette's, But Tourette's Doesn't Have Me* that the title describes how I feel. I have Tourette syndrome. I also have some baldness, and I'm short, and I like music and boating. I work a lot. But as far as defining who I truly am, those things are irrelevant.

When I became Chairman of the Tourette Association of America, Sue Levi-Pearl, the liaison with medical and scientific programs, asked me what my vision was for my tenure. And I said, "My vision is to make Tourette syndrome irrelevant."

With Tourette syndrome, we don't know the cause, we don't have a cure. So I, in my life, have tried to make it irrelevant. That's my mission, simply put. To help people who have Tourette's make it irrelevant.

And yet in another way, of course, it's very relevant to my life. I go to a chiropractor twice a month because I've been jerking my neck so long I have terrible problems with it. That's directly related to Tourette syndrome. Self-esteem also has been a problem for me. I was Chairman of the Tourette Association of America. I was Chairman of the Board of PartnersFinancial. These are prestigious positions. I ran Board meetings smoothly, but when we went for cocktails I was in the corner.

I was highly regarded, the Chairman of the Board, and I was standing in the corner while everyone else was socializing. I was afraid because I was always ticcing and huffing and puffing. I felt very uncomfortable in social conversation. One-on-one I was fine, or in a meeting I was fine. Social conversation, I was not fine. And frankly, I'm still not. But I also have many redeeming qualities and these are what I focus on.

I did a lot of public speaking, and had no tics while I was doing that, which is not uncommon for people with TS. After one speech, I heard someone say, "It's amazing how successful Paul is, despite all his handicaps." And I thought, "What handicaps is he talking about? I don't have any handicaps." As time went by, as I became more involved in TAA, I realized some people would say, "I can't do that because I have Tourette's." They would use their Tourette syndrome as a way out.

It bothers me that people use TS, or many other handicaps, as an excuse for lack of achievement. They allow themselves to get lazy and play 'Oh-poor-me-victim,' rather than strive to do the best they can. Maybe you have a handicap, maybe it's going to hold you back, but my gosh, do the best you can.

And that idea goes right back to the documentary, *I Have Tourette's, But Tourette's Doesn't Have Me*. I have Tourette syndrome but it doesn't have me. It's not who I am. I'm me. I'm going to be as successful as hard work will allow. There it is. Striving for and achieving excellence, being the best at what you do.

Viktor Frankl's *Man's Search For Meaning* is a book I think speaks to Tourette syndrome. Okay, we have this. Now how are we going to survive? How are we going to do well *anyway*?

And that's what this book, *An Unlikely Strength*, conveys: people's stories of learning to do well even though they have Tourette syndrome. This collection of interviews gives a wide variety of fascinating and inspiring answers to that most important question—how do we live meaningful lives with Tourette syndrome?

Listen to their voices, these people who share Tourette's, and learn from their courage and creativity.

INTRODUCTION

*A*n *Unlikely Strength* bears witness to the rich variety of successful lives Touretters have made for themselves. Of course, severity of symptoms is a factor in people's ability to adapt. But with that in mind, in your hand you hold the stories of an airline pilot, poet, teacher, musician, cartoonist, business executive, biomedical engineer, choreographer, doctor, painter, composer, and disc jockey who have made happy lives for themselves. Here are a novelist, social worker, graphic designer, dancer, firefighter, high-tech entrepreneur, stand-up comedian, ice hockey goalie, physicist, and many more who have thrived by overcoming limitations. You'll also find parents, whose love and creativity and strength and tears run like sinew through the story of Tourette syndrome.

I collected the narratives here for several reasons. Foremost, I was compelled to write the book in return for my good fortune in the course of my own Tourette syndrome. I also designed it to be a resource for my fellow Touretters and their families, for parents, and for the medical and helping professions. Finally, I hope the general reader will be surprised and enlightened by the book, learning what TS is, and what it *isn't* (notably that coprolalia—swearing—occurs in only about 10% of cases). We all can help diminish the stigma of Tourette syndrome by understanding that its symptoms are not character flaws. We have *formed* character because of Tourette's. This much we do know: the most corrosive results of TS will dissipate only when society changes its response to disability. With acts of compassion we all can become part of the healing process each of us needs and deserves.

It's my desire that the stories collected here are a source of inspiration for those with Tourette syndrome *and* for the general reader, all of whom search for happiness. You will understand the strength it takes to make it through the day with a disability and learn to admire and respect those who do it. The message of successful Touretters is hope and a buoyant spirit. We all seek those qualities, do we not? Our life is our own to make.

Each of us, with or without Tourette syndrome, can learn from the boys and girls, men and women, and family members who live with TS in grace and courage. These stories, told in their own words, detail challenges and the way forward into a meaningful life.

CHAPTER ONE

MY STORY

I write this as *An Unlikely Strength* is a month from publication: a last chance to express gratitude for my life as it is, for my good fortune, and for my ability to offer this work to the Tourette community. My story is unique only in that we all are unique. But the heart of this book is what I share with Touretters the world over; and with a wider point of view, what Touretters share with all people. Yes, society needs to change its perception of disability. Yes, we need more effective medicines and alternative treatments for tics and comorbid conditions. But as Carl Jung so cogently observes, we all stand in need of the alms of our own kindness.

Learning to forgive myself, respect myself, and love myself has been my brilliant creative act. I wish this for all people.

In the spring of 1956, I found myself standing at the parapet of a roof overlooking a low, dirty-white mountain city. The smell of wood cook fires, corn smoke, and damp stone rose to me. The sky was spread with gray clouds that, out beyond the city, were punctured by the rising cone of the volcano. Above me black wings ranged, and as they spiraled down to stumbling rooftop landings, I saw impossibly large birds—*xopilotes*. Hunched and scalp-naked, the vultures peered down with patient attention at a mongrel dog limping along a side street. This was my exile. I was eight years old.

I was in the bosom of my extended family, taken (or more accurately, removed from home for a time) by my mother to Guatemala City. I was guilty of what seemed to be possession by spirits. In less scientific ages, my malady would have confined me to an insane asylum or worse, a fiery stake. So much depends on culture. In other times and places I might well have been revered as a holy man, a seer, a tribal leader.

Still and all, a rational place like Garden City, Long Island, required an explanation for the twitches and jerks of my face, my head, my arms. There was no reason I could give other than I was compelled to do it. It was a difficult sell to adults who believed in free will. My pleas of helplessness collapsed entirely when the vocalizations began—grunts, sniffs, barks—and ultimately my hard, uncontrollable Anglo Saxon profanity. I was banished from elementary school. And more.

Rocking side by side on my backyard swings, dragging the toe of his sneaker in the dirt, a friend confessed he wasn't allowed to play with me anymore. I don't remember, but can imagine the pain on my mother's face, as timid as she was, as I jerked my arm again and again in a supermarket line, or grimaced extravagantly in a bank, or barked in a pharmacy, or spat out *fuckshit!* in the quiet confines of a doctor's waiting room. The sudden turn of faces to glare at me, then at her; the movement away from us, people repulsed, frightened, disbelieving, even angry, depending on my outburst. "Take charge," the faces demanded. "Control him," they admonished. "Be a good mother," they scolded. Fiercely protective and utterly dedicated to me, my mother could do nothing but hold me tighter and find the next doctor, who invariably, like his predecessors, had no answers, or worse, blamed her for what plagued me.

Although I vaguely remembered a time when I wasn't out of control, it had become normal. My life as an observer of my life. Believe me, at first I was no bystander. I fought hard against this intrusive beast. But failure after failure brought me to a bewildering reality: I could not control my mind; I could not direct my body as I chose. I was captive to the mechanism inhabiting my mind, an implacable conveyor belt that rose through layers of increasing tension, hauling me unwillingly to the crest and dropping me into an explosive body movement or embarrassing vocalization.

As things went, in 1956 I was a stand-out freak.

The Maya

In Guatemala I found the first reflection of my own suffering and understood I was not alone. My *compañeros* were the Maya people. Fully grown, they were about my 8-year old size, with cinnamon skin and deep black hair, the women's braided long, sometimes twined with bright ribbons. I was captivated by the patterns and brilliant colors of their tribal garments; the bouncing-pebble rhythm of their many ancient languages; and their eyes, which saw the world from a vast distance.

All these qualities drew me to them, but my heart connection with the Maya came from the weight they carried. Women balancing large jugs on their heads; children carrying children; men bent under towering stacks of firewood held by a tumpline, or nearly disappearing under 100-pound bags of coffee beans loaded on their backs. These were my tribe. Like me, they were burdened. Like me, they were excluded. The Maya were my first vision of suffering outside myself. I loved them because we suffered together.

Rage and compassion

I have very few clear memories of my childhood with Tourette's. I remember standing on our couch, facing the wall, as my grandmother asked me why I made those sounds. I answered, "I don't know," even as I felt the urges crawling around inside me. There is a black-and-white photo of me, perhaps six years old, in my parents' bed flanked by my brother and sister, four years my junior. We've always loved this picture because the three of us are laughing riotously. It was only some years ago that my father told me we were laughing because as he took the photo I ticced, jerking my arm and hurling a toy I held across the room.

I also remember being left overnight in a hospital for testing, and how I stood in the crib wailing in fear and despair as my mother and father left me in the ward. How it must have pierced their hearts.

Two other Garden City memories are more complex.

Gym class with a crowd of elementary school kids hustling up and down the basketball court. The PE teacher yelling and blowing his whistle. I remember the motion, the drum and squeak of sneakers on wood, and running near me a gangly kid, someone who also was teased, another outsider. When he passed me, as a purely emotional response to my life, I stuck out my leg and tripped him. He went down hard. I denied it, of course, when my parents and I were called to the principal's office. But I knew what I did. I understood I let my pain reach out to hurt someone else, someone like me, another isolated, picked-upon, sorry-ass kid. My feelings captured me, but unlike my Tourette's, for this I had a choice. To my shame, I chose to be a bully.

Another day, leaving school ticcing, a kid came up beside me and said something cruel. Next I remember he was flat on his back with me straddling his chest, my fist cocked, ready to bring it down on his face. In that poised moment, I realized two things: I wanted to hurt him because I hated him; and if I hit him, I would inflict suffering on this boy, which seemed terribly wrong. Rage and compassion shared that instant before I smashed him in the face. I walked home weeping for myself, for my tormentor, for my impossible predicament.

Rodent

My father wanted to work internationally, so when I was ten, the family moved from Garden City to Mexico City. Here again I found small, indigenous people with their dignity mysteriously intact. I couldn't grasp how they managed it. I attended Greengates, a British school, where my persecutors, with a different accent, repeated my Stateside ridicule. At recess, three older boys daily backed me into the same corner and, at their leisure, insulted me. They named me "Rodent." That is who, or what, I became. I believed I was subhuman. This created the distance I ultimately would have to travel to reclaim myself.

And then, somehow, I was blessed by what, to this day, remains a mystery. By the time I was thirteen, when we moved to Puerto Rico, my florid symptoms disappeared completely. No more vocalizations—none.

No more body tics—none. I began anew. No more teasing. No more forced isolation. My life became normal and eventually filled with friends and accomplishments. I became senior-class President and yearbook editor. I had beautiful, intelligent girlfriends. I surfed in the Caribbean and baked on the beach. I danced, learned to drive, joked and drank beer with my pals, watching hookers and drag queens parade past La Concha Hotel. My life was good.

But inside, I remained the Rodent.

The nickel dropped

I attended Washington and Lee University, in Virginia, on scholarship. This was the first time in many years I had been in the United States and I found it a completely foreign country. And I was foreign to those rich, white boys at W&L (White & Loaded, was another breakdown of the initials). I was again outcast. I had two close friends, outsiders as well, who gave me a fond nickname: they called me "Spic." I was a stranger to the university culture and lost within myself. Yet again I felt I didn't belong. My presence seemed provisional. I desperately needed to prove I wasn't an interloper in the life around me.

My family lived at this time in Costa Rica, too far to return for Spring Break. Instead I visited a friend from Puerto Rico attending Georgetown University. I was thrilled and intimidated when we went to hear Thelonius Monk, whom I admired greatly. We found a small table in the brick-lined jazz cellar and I struggled to feel at ease in the crowd. I desperately needed to show that I belonged. It was smoky and dark and as I turned to take in the room, I was startled to see Monk standing just behind me, an unmistakable silhouette. A red light on the wall behind him glowed through his beard.

Monk's trio began to play. We were right up front but my attention was divided between the music and the crowd. I felt exposed. To me, every one of these people, despite the dark room, knew I was an outsider. To prove them wrong, I tapped my glass with a swizzle stick in time to the music. Tap, tap, tap, tap. I'm not trespassing. Ting, ting, ting. I'm hip. About halfway into the third number, Monk abruptly stopped playing, stood up, said, "Drum solo," and walked off. So the drummer plays, Monk doesn't come back. I'm incensed. We pay all this money to hear him and he walks off!

Perhaps ten years later I lay in bed letting thoughts come and go, when suddenly the nickel dropped. My body gushed perspiration. I couldn't breathe. My mind burned with the realization that I drove Monk off stage with my tapping. *Drum* solo! Thank all the Gods that, at that time, my self-consciousness was so complete it never occurred to me that I, and the shadow of Tourette's, were the culprits behind Monk's exit.

I had created my own isolation. I didn't belong as a child. I still didn't belong.

All things French

In the 1970s, my mother was reading *The Los Angeles Times* when she came across an article about a French physician named Georges Gilles de la Tourette. My mother was an admirer of all things French: literature, philosophy, music, revolutionary history. She loved the sound of the language, and would sometimes affect a French accent, pretend to hold a cigarette in a casual manner, and walk as if she were the height of chic before she collapsed into self-conscious laughter. So, French doctor—she read the article and wept. Here at last was the answer to our questions about my absurd and frightening behaviors as a child. She called my grandmother, told her, and together they wept. When she told me, I was moved by her emotion. But her discovery of the Tourette Syndrome Association (now Tourette Association of America, tourette.org) was less important to me at the time than the urgent work I was doing to find my way out of despair.

Body armor

Deeply unhappy, in my mid-20's I learned meditation when I lived in Laguna Beach, California. I also began intensive bodywork, like deep tissue massage, Rolfing, and Feldenkrais. It seemed logical that Tourette's had affected my body as well as my mind. Though my tics had virtually disappeared, I still battled OCD, with its checking and counting and that intolerable noise in my head. I couldn't identify it then, but I also suffered from crippling depression.

What good fortune to be in Laguna. Glowing sunshine, temperate days and nights, lush hills, my beach a secluded cove reached by descending a staircase through a grove of eucalyptus and sycamore trees. But I remained isolated. For the bicentennial Fourth of July, lacking an invitation to festivities, I climbed a telephone pole and from there, in the dark, watched fireworks rising from Main Beach.

As I meditated, I discovered groups of muscles that held tension. A shoulder blade would clamp and I'd let it grip tighter and tighter, twisting me until I walked around my apartment like a hunchback. I allowed each muscle group to reach a climax of rigidity, shudder with fatigue, shrug off the tension and relax completely. Another area of muscular tension would reveal itself and I would go deeper. I followed the clenched muscles where they led. I learned this was called body armor, emotional trauma fixed in muscle groups. My face, arms, hands, legs, and feet followed a slow-motion series of extreme contortions. Meditating to keep my mind quiet, I'd wait for another muscle group to present itself. I gave my body complete control.

Occasionally, released tension would toss up a significant memory, although I'd forgotten it until that moment. I relived the episodes and knew each to be true. This work was important. I understood that I was deconstructing myself. This was my path to freedom. At one moment during meditation, I was startled to hear two voices, each an identity. A new self-image, unformed, potential, clearly said to my old idea of myself, "You must die." And to my surprise and relief, my old self said, "I know." What a mistake not to have someone help me through these radical changes I was precipitating in myself. Without guidance from a spiritual teacher or a therapist, I inadvertently proceeded to undertake a killing.

I had to cross this gap

I was obsessed with this self-taught meditation and muscle-memory work. I labored at it five, six hours a day. I exhausted myself until I crawled across the floor to climb into bed. I shook and sweated and gasped, all the while using meditation to hold on to a center of calm. Foolishly, I did this alone for several months. Then, one day, sitting quietly picking out a melody on the piano, I broke. I realized two things simultaneously: I must have human intimacy immediately; and such intimacy was impossible—there was no one. I felt my mind split down the middle.

Suddenly the world had a different sheen. I felt insubstantial. I had the need to touch things to confirm their existence. Crows cawing in the palm trees spoke to me, warning me not to leave the house at night. Before

I slept, I left on the radio so I could find my way back from dreams. I understood individual words of a spoken sentence, but couldn't hold them together to make meaning. I saw myself sitting on a ledge, feet dangling over a black void, back resting against a wall that rose out of sight. I was safe enough, but I was trapped.

On the fourth day after my break, walking along the tide pools at the beach, I stopped to watch ocean water sluice in and out where the jagged rock had cracked wide. I came to the conclusion that, to save myself, I had to cross this gap. It was far enough that I wasn't sure I could make it. The surf wasn't high, but if I missed I'd be swept out among the rocks and sea swell—something of a tight spot. Convinced there were no choices behind me, I jumped. My chest collided with the far side. I cut my hands and arms clinging to the sharp rock, water sweeping my legs seaward, and painfully brought myself up over the edge. How satisfying, that impenetrable, bloody reality of sharp rock and cold ocean water.

Later that day I confessed to someone, "I don't know what's wrong, but I need help." With those words, I came down off the ledge. I had destroyed Rodent, but I did it roughshod, and had nothing left to replace him.

It was a year before I recovered my mental and physical well-being. I began therapy, to good effect. Ultimately, to challenge myself, I took an Outward Bound course in the Colorado wilderness, and at the end of three weeks I stood on the peak of a 12,000-foot mountain I had climbed. I felt like I was back from the dead.

All these years I had been a business writer. I was afraid to try something new, even though I hated the work. When I came down from the mountain, I quit my job. That inspired act opened my life to other possibilities. I taught myself how to write a TV show.

Though my outward Tourette's symptoms had vanished long ago, TS rarely arrives unaccompanied. "Co-morbid" conditions is the medical term for the array of secondary symptoms that afflict us, a term that, to me, always held a macabre ring. And so, Obsessive-Compulsive Disorder and depression held me tightly. I was still in the grip of severe bouts of depression, which would snap open like a trapdoor under my feet and plunge me into an agonizing darkness. And the OCD was cacophonous, like multiple radio stations playing at the same time. In order to write a script, I had to expend half my energy holding the noise at bay, and use the remaining attention to teach myself the craft. It was exhausting. At the same time, I believe OCD helped me remain in my chair and stare at the blank page until I gained confidence that I could fill it.

The inexplicable quality of courage

Eventually, with my brother, Paul, I spent 20 years in Hollywood writing and producing television. I was helped greatly by medication that lessened my OCD and eliminated the depression that had routinely cast me into despair. Paul and I used the TV medium to bring 4,000 new members to Amnesty International by writing two episodes of *21 Jump Street* about the civil war in El Salvador. For a time, we wrote movie scripts for Warner Bros., and had adventures researching stories in Panama and Thailand. Francis Coppola, Quincy Jones, Michael Mann, Oliver Stone—I admired these individuals and found myself working alongside them.

Had I been ticcing, I *never* would have had this career. Not ever. Hollywood is driven by greed and fear. There is a kind of apprehensive lock-step that separates those In from those Out. It takes very little to make someone uncomfortable, and discomfort means "No" to whatever you're pitching. If I'd been sipping Evian and telling a story punctuated with jerks and grunts, facial grimacing and maybe a *fuckshit!*, it would only happen once. Word travels fast.

In all those years, I'm most grateful for my trip to El Salvador in 1990, during the war. It was a direct result of the work I did, and the people I met, writing the *21 Jump Street* episodes. I travelled with a group of North Americans to promote human rights. We hoped to generate international attention to bring some measure of safety to civic organizations under attack. Women's clinics destroyed, labor unions bombed, villages obliterated by Salvadoran military and death squads, trained and equipped by the U.S. military.

Late one afternoon, hot and humid, we met the new director of the NGO[1] human rights office. She spoke quietly as she described the murderous conditions for civilians. As the room dimmed with twilight, she stood and switched on the lights. On the wall hung photographs of her four predecessors, men and women, all dead or disappeared at the hands of death squads. I still wonder, faced with the choice, could I have occupied her chair? I understood something more of the inexplicable

---

1   Non-Governmental Organization.

quality of courage. How did she see herself? Could she choose not to accept that office, and be compelled by her conscience to do it anyway? Fascinating that the non-volitional action of a tic is mirrored in the moral dimension of human behavior.

Little Buddha

I married, I divorced. And Hollywood stopped calling. In an industry obsessed with youth, the Writers Guild of America considers filing ageism suits on behalf of members beginning at age 45. I made it ten years past that.

I lost my marriage, my house, and my career in one stroke.

Rage and bitterness were my daily companions walking through the park on the bluffs overlooking the Pacific Ocean in Santa Monica. Every day I walked and walked, working on my breathing, trying to regain a modicum of composure. I did walking meditation, repeating to myself, "Each footstep is life, each footstep is peace."

One day I was struck by that familiar memory: me as a five-year-old child, standing in a hospital crib, gripping the rail, wailing in fear and grief as my parents left me overnight for testing. But on this day it changed. Abruptly that child became a little Buddha, sitting lotus in the crib, serene. The instantaneous transformation took my breath.

I understood that, to escape my funk, I needed a challenge. I took two. The first was to live and study at the Zen Center of Los Angeles, where I stayed for two and a half years. It was a most healing place.

The second challenge was to face my fear of Tourette syndrome. Like others in this book whose symptoms have diminished, I felt a superstitious chill up my spine even thinking about Tourette's. I shared their portentous fear—if I draw too close, my tics might return. Better not think about it at all.

I resolved not only to think about it, but to immerse myself in it. You hold the result of that decision in your hands.

An enclave of ticcers with hardly any tics

Heading up into the Angeles National Forest to attend my first Tourette syndrome camp, to conduct my first interviews for this book, was a white-knuckle drive. I loosed my grip on the wheel only to dry my sweating palms on my pants. Prior to this, I'd sat in on a few sparsely attended TSA meetings, trying out the idea of writing the book. I didn't ask for interviews because the parents seemed distraught or preoccupied. There were no children.

The Kenneth Michael Staebler Tourette Spectrum Camp was an annual weekend shebang for kids and parents. Organized and run for years by Loretta and Ronald Staebler and many dedicated volunteers, it was their way of honoring their son, Kenneth, who had TS and passed away at 29 from cardiomyopathy. Making a camp for Tourette kids was how they turned suffering into wisdom.

The fears I had about my first contact with Tourette syndrome were eased by the healing qualities of the camp. Throughout that lovely, boisterous weekend the children's energy went into running and chasing, climbing and swinging, making art, making noise, and making friends. It was an enclave of ticcers with hardly any tics. Every boy and girl felt at ease and unstressed. Many were meeting kids like themselves for the first time. Imagine the relief of understanding that you are not alone in the world. The result was happier kids and fewer tics. How beautiful to feel the deep, therapeutic effect of these camps. I attended two of them and got about eight interviews. But by then the Staeblers were getting older and decided to put the camp on hold. I ran out of people to interview.

Each person striving to find happiness

The book languished for seven years. Then in 2014, I visited San Miguel de Allende, Mexico, with my wife, Elena (splendid the deliverance of second chances). Walking the cobblestones, speaking of what we'd do when we returned to the States, I lamented that I couldn't find people to interview for the Tourette project. Elena replied, "Have you tried Facebook?" Of course I hadn't.

Within a week of posting my first request on Facebook TS groups, I had forty people lined up. My method, as before, was to record each conversation, which were sometimes conducted in person, occasionally via Skype, but mostly by telephone. I transcribed each interview word-for-word, and then edited them for clarity, organization, and length. Everyone had final say over content and level of anonymity. I wanted each person to be pleased with the way they were represented and assured that their message was heard.

Filled with enthusiasm, I scheduled two, sometimes three interviews a day, and soon found myself emotionally exhausted. Each story was fraught with suffering and the heroic, often successful, effort to overcome suffering. After a conversation I might feel exhilarated, and immediately after another I might weep. The stories... the people... how sad... how beautiful... what strength... what courage. Each person striving to find happiness in a body that betrayed them and a world that so often abhorred them. So many with a teetering self-image. So many struggling to focus their deep compassion for others onto themselves.

Throughout it all, taught by their honesty and generosity, I was learning about myself.

The trap of conviction

During an interview a woman related that she sometimes feels like a pretender, even among her loving family. I heard her with a shock of recognition because I occasionally struggle with the need to explain myself. Not simply to account for my actions. I sometimes wrestle with the vile belief that I must justify my presence among human company. Why am I here at all when so clearly I don't belong? There are so many ways in which we Touretters isolate ourselves.

Conversations with the folks in this book helped me scrutinize details of my own life. Long ago I found that Buddhism resonated with my feelings about the world. As a Zen Buddhist, I'm fascinated by self-image: how we form it, maintain it, and how inaccurate and illusory it is. Buddhism teaches that my idea of myself is a shadow that directs my life. My ego is merely a point of view, useful to integrate the changing aspects of who I am. But the ultimate truth is this: my ego is insubstantial. It's an opinion. I realized I was Rodent only while I fed that identity with my belief.

Follow your bliss

The search for happiness has little to do with the material world. "Follow your bliss," said mythologist Joseph Campbell. The people in this book have repeatedly confirmed this maxim. And what holds true for Touretters holds true for everyone. Each person has some flaw, some fear, some incapacity. And each of us can find happiness despite it.

To me, what is heartbreaking about Tourette syndrome is its childhood onset, a corruption of innocence. A child looks to the world for responses and forms a self-image. I saw myself in others' eyes and believed I was monstrous. I was Rodent and unable to see contrary evidence.

Bullying, physical abuse, discrimination won't vanish by disbelieving them. They exist, they hurt, they damage, and you fight them. What I'm saying is, it's not personal. Hold yourself responsible for your actions, certainly, but don't use another's opinion to inform and form your own image.

As Touretters, we forgive ourselves for being 'out of the norm' by realizing that the norm is an illusion. St. Augustine said, "The reward of patience is patience." Patiently practice compassion. Find the courage to look beyond fears and sorrows. Respond to social blindness with loving-kindness. Understand that, by ridiculing you, people reveal their own unhappiness. Tourette syndrome gives you the power of compassion and resilience. Your strength, and its unlikely source, is yours to use.

It's how we live within our own hearts that matters. As Touretters, as humans, we stand in need of the alms of our own kindness.

CHAPTER TWO

ROMANCE

L et's start with a love story.

Should it begin, "Once upon a time...?"

Or perhaps, "In a faraway land...?"

No. This story is not far away in time or in distance. It's as near as Oregon, it's happening now.

Love stories are mythic. There is healing when two minds and hearts meet. Love stories help the rest of us feel joined in our humanity. As Touretters, this is what we need from society—understanding, acceptance, and the creature-comforts that arise from a sense of shared destinies.

This story echoes what many in this book said: that the love of a good man or woman improved their relationship with Tourette's and with themselves. Understanding, acceptance, creature-comforts.

So meet Annie and Oreya. Hear their story and, along with me, wish them well.

I interviewed Annie and Oreya via Skype video. They had cups of steaming coffee for our early morning talk, and sat nestled together so they'd both fit into the camera frame. They are young, they smile a lot, and their conversation is animated. I liked them right away. They've suffered, in one instance unimaginably so, and I'm grateful they've found relief and comfort with each other. They had a baby girl named Elsa in August, 2015.

ANNIE AND OREYA
she is 31 years old and he is 35 years old

Drive you mad a little

Annie: We met on the Tourette syndrome group on Facebook. And you wrote a lot of run-on sentences all bunched together in one big paragraph, and I liked that.

Oreya: Yeah. I tend to write novels in Comments.

Annie: It was very deep, very personal. A lot of pain, a lot of poetry. I would just *get* it. It was like an instant buddy I connected with. We started Skyping, and we'd been talking on the phone once in a while for about a year or two. And he sang…

Oreya: "Come a Little Closer."

Annie: *That* one. [*She sings a few lines*] I couldn't. He was in Maine and I was in Oregon [*she laughs*]. Drive you mad a little.

Oreya: Three thousand plus miles away.

Annie: At some point, after some boyfriend argument, I was talking to him and he let me know that he wouldn't mind dating me.

Oreya: I've adored her for some time. It started with her intelligence, it started with her mind and how it works. It moved on to the heart of who she is, her character, and what she's about.

Annie: He stalked me [*they laugh*]. He's always very sweet. We try to come off hard. We have a reputation to uphold [*they laugh again*]. And our Tourette's is surprisingly similar.

Stigma

Oreya: I've developed an uncanny ability to suppress, which is detrimental because it creates physical distress. My Tourette's has always more so been physical. Ever since I've been off meds I do have coprolalia-related tics.

As a child I had to learn to control my tics just for self-preservation. But since I've been with Annie, she's helped me start undoing the process I did out of absolute necessity. I didn't know which was harder—to relax enough to release, or to suppress. I'm learning to release tics without fear of retaliation or judgment.

Whenever we go out in public it seems to want to manifest a *lot* more. We get frowned upon a lot. If I'm thinking about my tics, ultimately I'm going to do them. Trying *not* to think about my tics, I'm still thinking about my tics so I'm going to do them. I try to keep concentration on something I may be interested in. But it's mentally draining, which leads to emotional fatigue, which leads to physical fatigue and more tics. At the end of the day I get very ticcety.

Annie: I'm not ashamed of Tourette's so I don't really have any problem. Other than that people don't understand I'm not on drugs, I'm not crazy, I don't hear voices. I would like to remove the public's—

Oreya: Stigma.

Annie: Ignorance. And I think that would remove the stigma. Because there would be an educated public. You know, kids don't mind me. Kids are the best. People expect a certain behavior in public and when they don't see it, they tend to react negatively. Which can make us react more negatively because we're scared [*she laughs*].

I would say I'm scared of a lot of people, yeah. The mob mentality. It's very frightening. Out at the Fair or the grocery store. In crowded places. I've been followed by mall security while shopping for shoes for my son. I've had people ask me what was wrong—people who look afraid, like security guards.

They wouldn't look at me like I was me

Annie: I had a traumatic incident that overloaded my circuits a couple of years ago. [*She pauses.*] Suffice it to say, I sent somebody to prison for twenty years. It was a depraved event... a violent assault. That person was finally put away.

I walked back into work and I could not stop the tics. It was a completely different world. I'm saying uncontrollable, high volume tics. I'd always been able to go into the bathroom and sing a little song or bounce on my toes or do whatever. I never had any problem concealing it.

I thought I was keeping it together, but it was like people didn't recognize me. I trained future nurses to do basic care, I taught CPR. I was well liked and busy. Little Miss Bubble Sunshine. All of a sudden I was having to say, "It's a neurological condition, blah, blah, blah." They wouldn't look at me like I was me. They looked at me like I was a problem. I was very isolated.

So yeah, the brain trauma was... yeah. I kept having to go on disability. I kept missing work. At some point my son also started getting sick, mentally and emotionally. So I had to tell my boss, "You guys have been wonderful, but my doctor says I need to let my brain heal."

I'm a lot better now. I'm voluntarily on an anti-depressant. It's been over a year. So my plans are to heal my brain and do something less stressful.

I have a second chance at life

Oreya: I was diagnosed at age eleven, but it was apparent at age two. My family life, up until I was thirteen, wasn't very good. I was adopted by my mother's third husband. The guy was absolutely horrible. Unfortunately, my mother and I had to literally escape.

I went through all kinds of traumatic things as far as any kid would be concerned, let alone a kid with the diagnosis I have. I have multiple co-occurrings. I have to say that my life's experiences, they have definitely made me a very hard individual, but also a very fragile-in-psyche individual.

There were constant med changes. I'd go to a doctor and they'd ask, "How is this medication working?" And I'd say, "It's working pretty good." And they would change it. Or it wasn't working well and they wouldn't change it. I feel I haven't got proper health care. I am off meds now. I control everything on my own to the best of my ability.

Annie: He controls his tics, I don't. I can't [*she laughs*]. I won't. If I sense

I'm going to smack my head against a wall, I'll find a way to not do that. I have a 'Do No Harm' mantra, so I try not to let it go beyond that. I do try to shift words that I don't think might be appropriate, however that doesn't happen all the time.

My ability to control disappeared. I haven't been able to ground myself. It feels nearly impossible. And I'm more comfortable when I don't. I used to do deep, deep meditation. It would take hours and I would have to let it all out through that. It allowed me to cope. Something I might start doing again, now that I'm feeing better.

Oreya: For me it was my youth. I was labeled a problem child, AKA 'The Devil's Child.' My diagnosis was never accepted. I was overruled and under people's thumbs. Got my ass, pardon my language, I got my ass beat a lot. Got picked on in school a lot.

Annie: He was physically assaulted in high school in a very dangerous way.

Oreya: Age thirteen I couldn't have been more than ninety-five pounds. I took beatings like a man from an almost three hundred-pound man. That was my adopted father. That was one of the reasons my mother said, the one morning, "Pack what you need. We're leaving." We kinda had to do it in covert and then we had to fear for our lives, literally.

Annie: They lived in a women's shelter.

Oreya: Yeah. My mother was strict but she was very liberal at the same time. She was my rock in my youth. I grew up—I'm gonna classify it a tough-love sort of thing. "You have this, but don't let it stop you." That's kind of the way I look at it now. But I think if my diagnosis would've been more accepted, I might not have had to go through the things I've had to go through.

Actually I have a second chance at life at this moment. I feel I've come to the right choice. I wouldn't be sitting here with someone I consider my best friend.

[They look at each other, smile. Then a silence rises that seems to encompass them. I sense Annie's troubled. Something large remains unsaid. Oreya looks at her tenderly, and after a moment, she speaks about her son, Ryan.]

Annie: The court gave Ryan's father temporary custody because I was unable to care for him, due to life circumstance. It's been going on for over a year and hopefully we'll do shared custody. He's eight now. He's beautiful. Always. Very smart little boy.

The issue I'm having mostly with his father is that he doesn't believe

Ryan could even have Tourette's. I have video of him ticcing from two months. Yeah. People tell him not to tic and people tell him not to act like me. Because they reacted poorly when I wasn't able to hide it anymore. [*She pauses*] They say I'm crazy.

I still need him to be evaluated. I wanted to start when he was four and all the grandparents were telling me, "You're trying to find something wrong with him." Ryan hasn't been diagnosed with Tourette's but he has PTSD from the event in 2012.

[*She pauses*] He was involved. It was Ryan, actually. I was hurt by proxy, so you can imagine… yeah. Yeah. Not enough. Prison for twenty years, not enough. It took two years for the goddamn courts to finally sentence him. My mom's husband. He's gone. And my mom's gone. My brother's gone. Everybody's gone.

[*There's silence. Then Oreya's words revive Annie.*]

Oreya: Annie kinda went incognito for a while there. I was very worried for her and that is when I realized how deep my feelings had rooted for her as a human being.

Annie: Absence makes the heart grow fonder. Or panic [*she laughs*].

Oreya: I always did my damndest to be sure she had some way of being in touch with me, so she knew I was all right.

Oreya: It was that time in each of our lives…

Annie: We were going through some very delicate changes that required a lot of support and care. And we didn't have any.

Oreya: We only had our own selves. We were always a support for each other.

Annie: Oreya came out because I wasn't sure if I was going to… well, he came out because he wanted to. We started talking and it was just, a kind of… I don't know. What happened? [*They laugh*]

Oreya: Well, from my end, I have always cared very deeply for Annie. I knew she was going through a rough time—

Annie: I told him not to come out, too. I mean, it sounded really good on paper, but I had a lot of stuff going on. I've never been that depressed before. It turned out I was able to, super rapidly, with somebody who was good, to feel like myself again. It's amazing.

Oreya: I felt for her.

Annie: I didn't want him to get stranded or just…

Oreya: I didn't want her to fall again.

Annie: And I knew he was in a delicate space emotionally.

If it wasn't for Tourette's we wouldn't know each other

Oreya: I had been displaced for about a year. I had checked myself into a psychiatric hospital because I felt I couldn't do it anymore. For the first time in my life I was absolutely ready to give up. I hit rock bottom and the rock bounced on top of me [*he laughs*]. I try to humorously look at it.

Annie: And I didn't want to cause any harm to him. Or not be able to help him because I could not help myself. I was very, very doubtful.

Oreya: One of the biggest lessons in my life I've learned—absolutely no fear. I've let fear in my life overrule everything.

Annie: When I saw him get off the train, he was very underfed. My phone rang as I got out of the car, and he goes, "I'm here." And I look over and see a guy with a bunch of bags and he's on the phone and I said, "Hey—look right [*she laughs*]." He ran up to me and I picked him up. Light. Very light. It made me feel… burly. The first thing I did was feed him.

Oreya: She loves to cook. Loves to bake.

Annie: That was fun. He's been healthy and balanced ever since he got here. He's had a couple of kinks to let out. But he's wonderful. My spirit has been growing and growing. It's been a long time since I've cared about a person who cared back. It is really nice to have somebody who is your best friend with you. I'm very tuned in to him and he's very tuned in to me.

Oreya: April 8. That's when I came. It's been a couple of months now.

Annie: Yeah, we're pretty new. But we feel pretty old.

Oreya: [*He laughs*] I feel if it wasn't for Tourette's we wouldn't know each other. I wouldn't know one of the greatest people I've ever met.

Annie: Yes.

Oreya: And one of the best people for me.

Annie: As much as I love my best friends, and how unique and different each one of them is, the one I connect to the most, the one I feel really understands me *all* the way through, that's you.

Oreya: Yeah.

CHAPTER THREE

MOTHERS AND CHILDREN

The brunt of dealing with Tourette syndrome falls naturally to mothers, married or single. They deal with doctors and meds, more doctors and meds, and yet more doctors and meds. They work with or wrestle with schools and teachers to get educational accommodations for their children. They pick up them up from school when the kids are having a bad tic day. They deal with the incomprehension, judgment, and even hostility of the public. They arbitrate between siblings to keep peace. And often a mother is first to see tears and disillusionment on their child's face. Add the pressures of maintaining a relationship and a home, often working a job, and it's small wonder that one mother described herself as a frayed net, sustaining the family even as she struggled to hold herself together. Dipping into a deep well of love and hope, each mother here finds a way to embrace her entire family.

In this chapter you'll find female voices (some alongside their children) speaking of home and husbands, creative solutions to problems, the guilt, grief, and joys of helping their children thrive with Tourette syndrome.

When I first met Laura and Nevin, his TS diagnosis was very new and Laura couldn't talk about it. Perhaps a year later we met again, drank fresh Medjool date milk shakes, and spoke under palm trees. Laura had come to see her role, as so many mothers have, as the binding that holds her family together. Going to a Tourette camp gave them tools and techniques, and helped Nevin understand he wasn't alone. And Laura finds strength and meaning as she helps other mothers deal with their children's diagnoses.

LAURA AND HER SON NEVIN (14 YEARS OLD)

It was happening to other people

Nevin: I don't remember much about when it started.
Laura: You remember.
Nevin: Like ten or eleven, my behavior was getting a little worse, or bad, I guess. Eye blinking, twitching, that type of stuff.
Laura: Excessive hand washing when he was in kindergarten. Very talkative in the car, very creative, but jumping from subject to subject. Socks that didn't have the right texture, shirts—he couldn't wear them. I don't know [*she laughs*], I was just going with it. He was behaving, doing his schoolwork, doing his chores. He was diagnosed when he was ten. Tourette's was the main disorder, along with…
Nevin: OCD, ADHD, I believe.
Laura: It was a breath of fresh air. This is happening to other people. Now we had an answer and we could go forward. Because the unknown in many things in life is difficult.
Nevin: She read a lot of books about it. A lot.
Laura: We backed off a little, let him behave the way he did. At the beginning, anyways, when it was minimal. Then it began to change.

An earthquake

Nevin: I started doing those things. Very violent… like swearing a lot, that type of stuff. I controlled it at school, but let it out at home.
Laura: It was like an earthquake. At the beginning, at fifth grade, he'd

bring home schoolwork and I'd try to help him. He would just yell, "I can't! Don't make me do this!" He would yell *at* me. He wasn't just yelling, he was yelling *at* me. It was overwhelming. We would argue back and forth. Months later he got physical with me, and would push me. He was violent. And he was highly distracted. The movements of his face, his body language, like he was there but not really. It was difficult.

Nevin: [*Softly*] Yep.

Laura: What brought relief was him going to school, so I didn't have to be around him. When he went to school I didn't have to hear him, or fear him. [*She cries softly*] He suppressed his tics and behaviors at school. Home was a safe place. He knew I would love him either way. So I got it all. But I'd rather he do it at home than at school. Because I've seen other kids who were bad and everybody in the office, all the teachers, know their names. I didn't want that for Nevin. But it's hard even talking about it.

Is it true? Will it last?

Laura: I think we've finally found the right medications. I was one, at the beginning, that didn't want to put him on medication because his body was still growing. But I knew we couldn't keep living that way. It was a difficult choice.

Nevin: I remember in sixth grade my medicine was so strong I'd sleep through, like, three classes.

Laura: Kids would throw paper or pencils at him. And he gained a lot of weight. We were seeing a neurologist, who said, "This is it. There's no cure for it. You just have to be strong and get in support groups. Hopefully, he'll grow out of it when he's eighteen."

Nevin: It was seventh grade, I believe, when we found the right balance for the medicine.

Laura: He's on four now. It took about a year to find the balance with his body, and his severity of the disorders. So his behaviors came down a lot.

Nevin: It worked.

Laura: It was a relief, but at the same time you think, "Is it true? Will it last?" It's one of those things you don't want to hold on to because it might change.

Nevin: I'm a lot better.

As I read it, I cried

Laura: His teachers are very helpful. We came up with Nevin shouldn't do homework at home. Because he goes all day to school, and doing schoolwork at home put him over the edge. It makes home not a relaxing place.

Nevin: I had a seventh grade teacher who wouldn't budge. Because of my IEP[2] I can have extra time, but she wouldn't budge on that.

Laura: When he got extra time he would get an A. So we kept working with the teachers and counselors. I've learned to advocate for us, and I'm teaching Nevin to be an advocate for himself.

Nevin: In fifth grade we talked to my class. I said briefly what I have and showed the video[3] and then we had cupcakes. I told them here are some symptoms, that type of stuff. The class asked questions and I answered them. That seemed to make a difference.

Laura: We found some websites that told how to describe it. I wrote it down and then at home Nevin stood up and read the paper, like he was going to read it to the class. We did that a few times so he'd be comfortable with it. In class he was nervous, so he sat down and I read it, and as I read it I cried. If you teach people, they'll be more willing, I guess, to…

Nevin: To accept it.

Laura: To accept it and not be a bully.

Nevin: I wasn't teased at school. I moved my arm a little bit. Sometimes I blink a lot. I count numbers. It helps you with math [*he chuckles*].

Laura: He's always had IEPs. Parents can get pretty much what they want in their kid's education. I usually have Nevin there, to express what he needs. We go over each subject with teachers to see how he's doing, what he can improve on, and what is a goal. We talk about his homework, and that's when we came up with no schoolwork at home. Too I asked that they don't put all his hard classes together. Make every other one a mellow class, or lunch. Break up his schedule so he'll still be able to focus at one o'clock in the afternoon.

---

2   Individualized Education Program. See tourette.org for details.

3   *I Have Tourette's, But Tourette's Doesn't Have Me.* See tourette.org for details.

Take each step at a time

Laura: And we had a service through the County. They have a person who observes us in the home. Then he addresses it with us as parents and with Nevin, and gives us language in what works. When I would say something, he'd see how Nevin reacted, and then correct me to re-word it so he reacted properly.

Nevin: That worked.

Laura: That was a lifesaver. With Nevin, you can't just tell him, "In fifteen minutes we're leaving." He needs time to process that. For us it was important that he learn to do chores at home. We're raising him to be a responsible adult so he'll have a nice home and respect things.

Nevin: That's how a lot of kids in my school are. They get whatever they want and they don't have to pay for it.

Laura: So that was a big one. Not to overload Nevin with chores. Say one chore and have him repeat it back, or explain it if he wasn't sure. Or if it was a new chore, to break it down. And when he came back from doing his chores, to be excited, like a cheerleader almost. Have a list or chart and have him cross it off, so he can see he accomplished something. Then have him do the next one.

Nevin: Take each step at a time.

Whisper it

Laura: Same with these loud episodes. You know it's going to happen. It's how you're going to react to it. You don't need to say a word. Children can read your face.

Nevin: Your expressions.

Laura: You can step into a room and by the expression on your face your child already knows how you're going to react. So I've learned, even though I feel like I've been through a war, I need to not show it as strongly.

The whole family needs to learn. All our feelings are important. You tell yourself you can get through it. For me, finding support groups, that's a big one. You hear somebody else's story and you share ideas. You find out what works and what doesn't, and you can try it with your family.

Like when your child is behaving aggressively, instead of yelling, whisper in your child's ear. That you love them, or, "Can you go pick up those toys and put them in the toy box." Whisper it. And the kid will go, "What did you say?" And you talk quietly, so they're changing their focus from the behavior to what you're whispering in their ear.

As a mother, we hold the family together

Laura: The County guy taught me while my husband was at work, then I'd teach my husband. It's difficult because Nevin is more explosive with his dad. His dad wants to give him ideas or strategies, and a lot of times Nevin goes right to being defiant. Usually when we're in public, I take Nevin and my husband takes his brother, and we basically walk apart. Just recently we're walking together because Nevin's mellowing out. If he's ticcing in public, he has an idea it's coming up.

Nevin: There's usually a warning. I get a lot of energy in my mind.

Laura: So he will quietly rub my arm or cuss in my ear. He has a different look on his face, like he can't hold it in. And he'll say, "I need to tic." And I'll say, "Well, let it out." And he moves to do it to me and I say, "No, just let it out. In the air." He worries people will stare and I tell him, "You're never going to see these people again [*she chuckles*]."

As mothers, we hold the family together. I think prayer and our religion has kept me strong, and knowing that it's okay to ask for help. I feel okay to say, "I'm done with this one. Let's move on to the next challenge [*she laughs*]." I've learned to say, "Please give me something different." I see the future brighter than when things were so difficult because I'm educated about Tourette's and OCD. It is what it is, and you try to make the best of it.

I talked to a mother whose son has behavior similar to Nevin's, and she said I'm giving her hope because I shared that Nevin's mellowing out. That encouraged her to keep going forward. She's where I was a couple of years ago, so she can look at us, and say, "Oh. It is going to end."

I'm going to take control of my life

Nevin: We learned a lot at camp.

Laura: We went twice to the Kenneth Staebler TS camp, and Nevin remembered the kids from the first time and hung out with them the second time. Just had a good time. They wanted to eat together at the tables.

Nevin: It's actually really good food.

Laura: That was the first time we were in a group of people who had TS. Adults too. Again, it was a breath of fresh air. Look how this kid is ticcing so loud, and he's still having conversations with people, he's still finishing his project, he's still unloading the van. Just normal, everyday functions.

Nevin: Just with a challenge.

Laura: It helped Nevin, seeing these kids, when he went back to school.

Nevin: Yeah. Knowing I could hang out with them. And other people have TS, not just me. And that it's not going to control my life. I'm going to take control of my life.

Laura: It's just something you have, like you have glasses, you have freckles.

Nevin: It's part of me.

Laura: It's part of me, but it's not who I am.

Nevin: You just work on it. I got used to it. I'm not going to get rid of it, so why not get used to it? Deal with it.

For a parent, the progression of Tourette syndrome can become very dark indeed. Tics become debilitating, behavior becomes destructive to the child and others. What to do? It's a question that burns like a hot coal in the throat. For Kathy, and other parents, sometimes there are no good choices. She learned that, paradoxically, gaining control begins with relinquishing it. The natural response is to blame yourself. Kathy's happiness, and her son Matt's success, depended on her not doing that. She trusted her instincts, her love for her family, and Matt's ability to find what inspired him.

KATHY, ABOUT HER SON MATT (33 YEARS OLD)

I gave up that concept of having control

Take every day as it is. That was hard for me. Living the highs and lows, I just… it was brutal hoping that things would improve. That some medicine was going to work, and then the crash, recognizing it wasn't going to. I needed to get off that ride. I finally came to a place where I listened to my therapist, who told me, "You need to live in the moment. Enjoy what is right now."

When you're going through the really difficult, painful moments, know that it's going to change. We all do the best we can at any given moment. That helped me get past the blame and the shame that everybody was pouring on me. I knew I was doing absolutely the best I could. Even in those moments when I was not Mother of the Year, I was doing the best I could.

My therapist said, "You can't handle it if it's not your fault. Because if it's *not* your fault, you have no control. And that scares you to death." I was angry when she said that [*she laughs*]. But I knew she was right. I wanted some control because my son's life, and my family's life, was pretty awful. And if I didn't have control over it, that meant I couldn't change it. But once I gave up that concept of having control, yeah, it was like a weight lifted off. I could enjoy my son a lot more and I could be present with my family. It took away that panic. You know? The panic and the stress of, "I've gotta fix this." I *couldn't* fix it. And once I accepted that, life was so much better. Because once you get past trying to control it, it opens you up to more creative strategies.

It's so easy to think you're a bad parent

We were brought up in a time when punishment was the answer. And it became very clear very quickly that punishment was not the answer for Matthew. It doesn't work. I try to get that across in my work with the Tourette Association. Once you get past the punishment/reward cycle, you can be more creative. Once you see a kid as *having* a problem and not *being* the problem, you're much more interested in finding a creative and positive solution.

Unfortunately it's hard for people to get there. Our culture supports punishment, not creative, positive solutions. A lot of times, when parents go out into the community, they're embarrassed by what's happening with their child, particularly when the child becomes disrespectful to them. When I talk to parents I get asked, "How did you deal with that?" And that was another light bulb moment. I don't know how I got there, I just know that I didn't care. I thought, "That's their problem, not mine. I've got enough problems." It's so easy to think you're a bad parent. I hung on to that. I *wanted* it to be my fault. Back to what my therapist told me, "You can't handle it if it's not your fault."

What was my choice?

The best way I can describe it, I felt like the sail on my sailboat was ripped to shreds. And taking care of myself, working in the garden, going to the therapist, it didn't fix my sail, but it patched it enough so I could get through another week. I don't know what I would have done if I hadn't been able to patch my sail. I was afraid for my family. Unfortunately, I think the majority of the times it's the mother who holds the family together. It's just a very, very exhausting, difficult job. What was my choice? People said to me, "I couldn't do what you did. It's so wonderful." No—I didn't have a choice.

Not that there weren't times I wanted to escape [*she chuckles*]. But I knew I wasn't going to do that. I needed to find little escapes. I started turning bowls on a wood lathe. The humming was very, very calming for me. Plus when you're doing a wood bowl, you need to have all your attention on that because it could be very dangerous. That helped me escape too. We all need to find something.

You need to take care of yourself and the marriage

Learning not to blame yourself, that's huge for everybody involved. 'Cause you're gonna get thrown blame all over the place. I see families that are not financially well off getting blamed more. I see people who aren't Caucasian being blamed more. People are going to blame you, whether you're the person with Tourette's or the parents of the kid with Tourette's. And to let that blame bounce off you is important. Are people blamed for having cancer? Are parents blamed for children that have leukemia? It's the mental health stuff where we've got a long way to go. A friend of mine said the first time her son with TS was ever treated well in the grocery store was when he had trichotillomania and was pulling his hair out. People assumed he had cancer. Everybody bent over backwards to be nice to him.

My husband, Tony, and I, we didn't blame each other. I'm not saying it was a happy time. I'm not saying it was a time when our marriage was even good, because it was tough. But we didn't blame each other and I think that's important. I see too many people blame their spouse. "It's from your side of the family." Well, who cares? You need to take care of yourself *and* the marriage, which I think is even harder.

Picture, pictures, pictures

Probably my only regret is not spending more time with my other two kids. Especially my other son—you know, he's the perfect middle child. I regret not spending more alone time with him [*she sighs*]. When Matthew wasn't living at home, I didn't want to do things as a family because there was somebody missing. You look at my photo albums and you see pictures, pictures, pictures, then there's this huge gap when Matthew wasn't at home. There was a hole in our family. If I spent time as a family unit without Matthew, it was just so obvious to me that he wasn't home. And I... I should've overcome that [*she sighs again*]. You know, again, you do the best you can. I wish somebody had told me, or if they did tell me, I ignored it [*she chuckles*].

Matthew had just turned eight when he entered the RPC[4]. We live on a hill in the country, so we see the moon rise over the horizon. I remember before we dropped Matt off at the RPC, that night it was a most beautiful moon. So I took Matt out on the porch and I said, "Even though we're apart, we'll always be together. And I promise you I'll find out what time your bedtime is and at that time I will go out and look at the moon. And even if you can't see the moon from where you are, know that I'm looking at the moon and the moon's where you are too. And we'll be together." I wanted him to know I wasn't deserting him. That was *huge*. I don't think I mentioned in my book[5] that my mother left me when I was four years old. So being deserted was a huge scab, and I wanted Matthew to know definitely he was not being deserted.

It kept him safe

I have a friend who's a minister and she said, "Can you give me an example of a situation where there's no good choice?" And I shared that story, Matt going to RPC. That was not a good choice, but there was *no* good choice. That was horrific. But it kept him safe. It kept him safe from hurting us, which was good for him. If he had damaged us, he never would have been able to live with himself.

I didn't like the foster home contract. I went to an attorney and we put in an amendment. Throughout the contract it said the foster providers—first of all, they called them foster-mother and father, which I told them never, ever. He *has* a mother and a father. So they kept talking about the foster providers bringing him to the doctors, the foster providers going to school meetings. I knew my son's medical history. So the amendment was that I would bring him to the doctors, I would go to school meetings. I would pick him up every Saturday to bring him to his drum lessons with the Community Program at the Eastman School of Music[6].

It's paramount for parents of kids with Tourette's to trust their instincts. We can't rely on what professionals say because they may not know. I think there are many doctors and therapists who don't understand

---

4   Residential Psychiatric Center.

5   *A Family's Quest for Rhythm: Living with Tourette, ADD, OCD & Challenging Behaviors* by Kathy Giordano and Matt Giordano. Available at afamilysquest. com and on amazon.com.

6   The Eastman School is one of the top graduate music programs in the United States.

that TS is a neurological disorder, and see the child as taking advantage of their Tourette's. But then, I do see therapists and doctors who get it. Ross Greene[7] is phenomenal. But unfortunately there still are doctors who simplify the symptoms and put it back on bad parenting.

Kicking holes in the walls and breaking windows

Because I used to be a teacher, I went to the local Tourette chapter[8] and said I'd like to start doing presentations at schools. They agreed and I started doing that. All of a sudden, the Tourette Association asked if I would present at the national conference. I said, "Yeah, I can do that." When I was on the plane heading into Washington, I saw all the national monuments and all of a sudden it was, "Oh my God, oh my God, I can't do this. This is craziness [*she laughs*]." But I did it and people thanked me.

I began working for TAA as the Advocate Specialist. I trained people how to better advocate for parents or for their own children. And it morphed into Education Specialist, which I am now. I contribute to the website[9]—we have an education page. I talk to people on the phone—parents, educators. Anything with education, I do.

There are some positives to media coverage of Tourette's, but I think there's more negative. I think the media portrays the most significantly impacted people. It's amazing to me people still believe you don't have Tourette's if you don't swear. Another disservice is, even the positive depictions of Tourette's don't talk a lot about children who have behavioral issues. I think that's covered up too much. Because people think, "Yeah, people have kids with Tourette's, but their kids aren't kicking holes in the walls and breaking windows." Yeah, there's a significant percentage of kids that do.

They're all feeling isolated

I talk to a lot of people and they're all feeling isolated. That's why I wrote our book. I think there continues to be a lot of blame and shame, and people don't talk about it. So there are people in small communities who think their kids—especially kids who have more severe issues—that he or

7   Dr. Ross Greene, author of *The Explosive Child*.
8   The Tourette Association of America has chapters in many states. See tourette.org.
9   tourette.org.

she is the only one in the world, and they're the only family experiencing this. I think that is a shame.

I don't think anybody understands unless you've been through it. And people with Tourette's, they self-isolate, and that's unfortunate. I feel blessed that my son doesn't do that. That he's a drummer is extremely helpful, 'cause he can go to a city where he knows no one, go to an open mike, start drumming, and he makes friends. I'm very proud of him. He likes to do presentations for students[10], like anti-bullying presentations. Number one, he's a drummer, so automatically he's cool. And his charm and personality come across and the kids listen to him, whereas somebody else talking about bullying, they might not listen.

Support the child's strengths

One of the strongest suggestions I would make is to support the child's strengths. Supporting Matthew's drumming, I don't know where we'd be if we hadn't done that. It wasn't a revelation, "Oh, I'm going to do this so he'll be successful as an adult." We did it because it was such a positive in his life. And why would I not allow him to do that? I wish families would support whatever the child has a strong interest in. It gives hope. It made it so that Matthew was not a one-dimensional person. He has many dimensions. Tourette's is not all of him. Other people saw him as a drummer, he saw himself as a drummer. Going to Eastman School of Music, that was so important to him. And that's important for self-esteem and self-awareness and the non-blaming.

A lot of kids with Tourette syndrome have some kind of creative talent. I see many kids who are creative in music, in art, in writing—it's astounding to me. I hope parents allow that to happen and support it. Don't listen to the professionals who say, "If he's not good, he can't go to his lessons." I was talking to a mother recently, who said, "My son likes drumming and he used to take lessons, but he never practiced, so I couldn't support it." And I said, "My son never practiced, but look at him now." Matthew didn't practice, but he *played*. And when he gives drum lessons, he's not invested in the child practicing. If he learns to read music, that's fine. But if he wants to learn to play from his heart, that's good too.

---

10   drumechoes.org.

———————————— ❧ ————————————

Rock-hard reality, that's what Rosemarie feels like to me. New England accent that could crack a quahog. I like her tough-love approach to living with Tourette's and how she handles her daughter, Jeanne's, similar plight. Rosemarie suffered nightmarish doctoring as a child, illustrating what many in this book have said: a good physician treats patients from a foundation of compassion and respect.

ROSEMARIE
45 years old

You can't feel this

In the beginning, my life with Tourette's was not good 'cause they didn't know what they were dealing with. In the late 70's they just kind of threw medicine at me and did horrible tests to me. I was nine.

I went to the hospital and the neurologist had me do all these nutty tests. None of it had anything to do with Tourette's. Everything was coming out negative. And then the pills and all the medications and all the side effects from them. And then the medicines to counteract the side effects.

I had spinal taps. It was bad. The first time they supposedly numbed me up. I was on my stomach, and I remember turning my head, and the doctor had this long, long needle. I remember thinking, "That's a joke needle." It wasn't. And the worst part was, he tapped my lower back and said, "You can't feel this." I remember saying, "Yes I can." And he wouldn't listen. I felt all of that test.

So I remember being in the hospital room and my mom was with me, and he came back in, almost like it was a nuisance, and he said, "We have to do it again because she was moving around too much." My mom said, "I'm going in this time." The few times she's brought this up, she actually cries. She talked me through it and was rubbing my forehead. And of course, that test came out normal too.

She saw a commercial of a boy

They had all these medicines they were giving me that had nothing to do with Tourette's. Every day they had to test my blood levels. Both my arms were purple-black because they had to test two times a day. Once that happened, they had to take it from my thighs and my neck. And I was just tapped out. I am so fearful of needles now.

When I think about those things, it sickens me because none of it had to be done. So one night I was supposed to be kept up all night for a test, and my mom was watching television and she saw a commercial of a boy. All I remember was it was a teenage boy, it was in black and white, and the boy was sitting on a chair and he was jumping a little bit and hiccoughing. It said something about if you have a child who does this, it could be Tourette's. And my mom brought it up with the doctors and then there was a diagnosis.

From there they sent me to a hospital that had a day school. Tourette's was new to them. I went to school with children who had serious brain injuries, and they just throw you all in and lump you all together. I could do work a lot of these kids would never do in their life. I was... you know, regular. Except for Tourette's. I said to one teacher, "I did this in first grade," but that was all they had for me. I was there almost two years.

When I spoke to my mother about it years later, I said, "Why did you leave me there?" and she said, "Rosemarie, we thought you were going to be there for a few days and they wouldn't let us take you." And I was so mad because, you know, I just remember feeling abandoned.

They called me monster

I was teased in school. It was awful. I took the bus with all the kids I had always gone to school with, and all of a sudden they're like strangers to me. And there were a couple that were really, really mean. They called me a monster. I think it affected my self-image because I had all these questions and feelings. I didn't know what was wrong, I didn't know how to explain it. You're in school, having fun and having the same friends, and then you're all of a sudden by yourself. I think that does something to you.

I didn't go out, but my mother made me [*she chuckles*]. If we were going to the science museum or to a pool or the beach, it was, "All right, we're going here today so come on, get dressed." You know, like it wasn't an option. I think that was the best thing for me. I probably would have hid in the house. But she didn't let that happen.

C'mon, let's breathe now

I've been married twenty years in August. I had my three children. With Jeanne's Tourette's, at first she kind of hinted about it, and I said, "So how long has this been going on?" And I'm thinking, like, eleven. And she says, "Since I was eight." And I'm like, "No. Eight?!" 'Cause we're really close, I'm always there and I notice everything, and I did not see this whatsoever. I cried. I cried. And I felt very guilty. I was hysterical for two days 'cause I felt so bad. I blamed myself. I was just horrified. I kept saying, "You don't know what it's going to be like for her."

There are things I can tell Jeanne to help her counteract people's ignorance. It doesn't always work. There have been a few times when she's been physically challenged and she'll call me. A few years ago she was at some Homecoming thing and her arms were really going. So I jokingly said, "You're at Homecoming. Grab a flag and you'll fit right in [*she laughs*]."

There've been a few times where we've gone out and it's almost gotten dangerous. Like, "Jeanne, drop the fork. Jeanne, drop the knife. Just open your hand and let it go." There's a good chance someone's going to get hurt because some of her muscle spasms are pretty bad. She tells me her neck has been hurting for weeks, or her jaw. And she's been slamming her fist down on her thigh—she's got all these bruises. She thought she broke her arm the other day. Then she gets herself all upset, and I say, "C'mon, let's breathe now."

What helps me relax is I do a lot of crocheting. I taught myself when I was seven. I was painting yesterday. I also taught myself some origami, so I do that from time to time. And I do a lot of deep breathing. That usually helps. So I tell Jeanne.

This is going to be interesting

I would like to meet another person with Tourette's. I've been telling Jeanne for a while I want to go to Niagara Falls, I want to do something, me and her. She mentioned it in the Facebook group, just chatting, and now we have a group going up in October to meet up with a Canadian group. And it's getting bigger and bigger, so I don't know how many people we're going to end up going with.

It's weird because now I'm thinking, "Oh, God, I've never been with anybody else but Jeanne." I don't know how I'm gonna… be. Because I've never met anybody else, let alone spent a weekend with maybe forty people that all have Tourette's and all different variations of it and different kind of tics. I'm a little nervous [*a sigh*]. This is going to be interesting.

And then my daughter, the other one, is like, "I want to go." And it was so funny because this is the first time in my life when I said, "You won't fit in [*she laughs*]."

I hear a lot from people, "I don't like my Tourette's." Well, no one says you have to like it, but you might as well accept it.

It's important not to be a victim. I didn't treat Jeanne any different. If anything, I think I was tougher on her. I have asked her to do things I would never do. They had a variety show in high school, and there was supposed to be four of them but the other three kids, they got cold feet. So Jeanne got up in front of a student body of four hundred, she got up on stage, everybody's quiet, they know she has Tourette's, and she sang *a cappella*. And I remember, just before she went up, she said, "It's gonna be so quiet and they're all gonna be watching me." And I said, "Just remember we're sitting up at the top of the dark, so look up there." And she did it fine. But that's how she is. She's exceeded everything. She's not afraid to do anything or say anything.

Everybody has their 'I want to feel sorry for me' days. And Jeanne was having one—this is a long time ago—and I remember saying, "Are you going to sit on your little pity pot? Well, when you're ready to put on your big girl undies, then come on." She cried and I said, "Keep crying. That's fine. You can cry all you want, but it's not going to change anything. When you're done crying you're still going to have Tourette's."

You know, you can dope yourself up, you can drink yourself up, but at the end you are still going to have it. And this isn't the worst that you could have. There's the little boy who didn't have shoes but then the boy next to him didn't have feet. It could be worse and you have to think of that. Whatever you do, don't be a victim.

If you don't like something then change it. And if you're not going to change it then shut up. I hear a lot from people, "I don't like my Tourette's." Well, no one says you have to like it, but you might as well accept it. It's the one thing you can't change. It's not the end of the world. You will make whatever you want out of your life or not. You are in control of your destiny. If you're going to sit and let things pass you by, and opportunities, if you're okay with that, I guess that's fine. But if you want to aspire to something or be something, then I think you should.

There's always something you can change. You can change your view of the world. You can change your attitude and put your priorities straight. Everybody's so busy with being perfect and having more, they don't realize what they have. For me, most of the things in life that are important aren't things.

Fluttery and breathless, that's Rosemarie's daughter, Jeanne. As she grows more emotional, she talks faster and faster, until I ask her to slow down so I can pick out individual words from the rushing stream. She's her mother's child, displaying a loving heart, resilience, and humor. The children she teaches accept her tics unconditionally. To me, this is proof that our culture often teaches intolerance and an emphasis on differences. Jeanne and her students focus on our common humanity.

JEANNE
21 years old

I want to be just like you

I teach preschoolers. They have their moments [*she laughs*]. When they like to listen. My earliest memories of working with children are with my mom. We had an at-home day care growing up. I would wake up and go downstairs and start playing with the kids. I'd say, "Oh, mom, this is what I'm going to do when I grow up. I want to be just like you." I love what I do. It's hard, but it's really rewarding.

I had a very bad tic today in school where I kept hitting my leg and one of my kids started copying me. I've noticed two kids who I think have tics. One, he repeatedly blinks his eyes. So I brought it to the mom's attention and they're going to have it looked at. And one of my kids, her brother is in second grade, and whenever he would come with his mom to pick her up, I noticed he kept blinking his eyes and doing something with his neck. I talked to the mom and gave her the name of my neurologist.

It's just the way God made me

Me and my mom have a close relationship. My friends always tell me, "You talk to your mom too much." All I can say is, "But we're so close. I need to tell her everything."

The first memory I have of Tourette's, I remember playing baseball with my younger brother and my friend, Beca. And I remember thinking, "Why do I want to move my neck?" I had no idea, so I tried to ignore it. As I got older, I noticed I couldn't take a deep breath. It's really hard for me to breathe sometimes. That is one of the tics I constantly do. I feel I can't take that full breath. I'll clutch a table and do deep breathing.

I don't remember how my mom told me about Tourette's. I mean, I knew something was wrong with her, she'd always do those involuntary movements, those involuntary voices, but I don't remember her sitting down with me and telling me, "I have Tourette's." It's more like something I grew up with. It was always there. My mom told me, "It's just the way God made me."

My earliest memories of my mom are sitting on her bed and her going [*makes a repetitive noise*]. I remember she didn't do it for like thirty seconds and I thought, "My mom doesn't have Tourette's anymore!" Then she did it again. In the grocery store, whenever I would lose her, my first instinct would be, "Okay, I have to be quiet and listen." 'Cause if my brother and I listened, we could hear mom and find her [*she laughs*]. Like a lighthouse.

You taught me to be understanding

My tics didn't get so bad until, I would say, middle schoolish. I got diagnosed when I was sixteen. What I remember distinctly about public school is I was doing a facial tic. I needed to open my eyes as wide as I could. Or clench my eyes. Everyone started asking, "Why are you doing that?" I said,

"I have Tourette's." It was no big deal because my mom is so confident about it and doesn't let anybody else affect her. But people started bullying me.

You know, kids are cruel. I grew up with my mom telling me that. As much as I didn't want to believe it, it is very, very true. It's just really… [*she sighs*]. Sometimes it's hard to accept.

When I was a sophomore I did a project on Tourette's. The teacher only gave me a B and I was like, "Really? Are you kidding me? [*she laughs*]" And there was one teacher who was really, really nice about it. One time I was taking a test and the file cabinet was next to my desk and he was bent over. And one of my tics was I would throw out my arm. And [*she chuckles*] it's dead quiet, right? And I slap his butt as hard as I can and he stands up and says, "Hey!" I'm just like, "Sorry!" And we look at each other and start laughing. He's one of the teachers who really helped me get through high school.

When I graduated, my teacher said, "Jeanne, I never heard of Tourette's before I met you, and you taught me to be understanding and not quick to judge people." It was nice to know I could touch someone like that, just being myself.

They love me regardless

I think it was about April or March of my senior year in high school and I got a job at a day care. I didn't tell them about my TS until after they hired me. But my boss was real understanding. She helped me write a letter to all the parents, explaining that I have Tourette syndrome. It was nice to know they were okay with it.

I can't really explain it to my kids, but I say, "My brain is the boss of my body and she tells me to do things sometimes that I can't control. She has little messengers and they say this and that." They're little kids, they laugh about it. It's great to know they love me regardless of whether I tic or not. It's still a little uncomfortable for me because it's hard to control my tics and still be able to do what I'm doing.

My uncle had given me a guitar and the music teacher at work taught me some chords. When I play the guitar it's so relaxing, no tics happen. It's just me and the music, and I'm singing. Tourette's doesn't interfere at all. Music has helped me through so much. Kinda like there's no room for me to tic.

Count backwards from ten

I do find it's different between school and out of school. In high school, they're more direct about it. They'd look at me and say things. But in public, I see people looking at me so I give them dirty looks back. If they keep looking I say, "I have Tourette's. I can tell you about it."

If there was a bigger supporter than my mom, it would be my boyfriend because he pushes me to be myself and not care who's looking. He'll get my mind off it. And it makes me happy that I have someone who loves me so much he takes my punches too [*she laughs*]. We have a joke that we're in a semi-abusive relationship because I'm always hitting him [*she laughs again*]. You know, without meaning to.

My mom was always a hundred, hundred, hundred percent support-ive. I would come home crying, and to help me get control she'd ask me about something else. If it persists she'd say, "Okay, let's count backwards from ten." Which is actually helpful. She taught me to where I can do that now. That's enough of a distraction to quiet the tics.

We would lie in bed and she would... she just... she *knows*. She knows I'm having a bad tic day. More than anyone else, she knows what I'm going through 'cause she went through it herself. She had a way differ-ent upbringing with her Tourette's versus me. So as much as she told me about herself, it really helped.

We would just sit there in silence

I've never been the kind of person to consistently take medication. I feel it doesn't help me, so I stop taking it. I'm not taking anything for depression. It's still there, but it's held up a lot since I'm not in high school. That had a lot to do with it. Now I'm my own individual. No one really looks down on me like that anymore.

I had really bad depression in high school. If it wasn't for my mom I wouldn't be here. With me going through depression and trying to accept TS, I was in a very, very dark place. And... [*she pauses*] I tried to kill myself twice. She would try as hard as she could to know what was going on, but I would push people away and wouldn't tell them what was going on. Like I said, a lot of my friends turned on me, and my aunt died, my mom's health was horrible, and I had all these things happening that I couldn't control. And it was just really hard [*she stifles tears*].

So the second time that happened, mom and I had a really long talk. I started telling her everything and everything. And then, like... oh gosh... [*she cries softly*]. It doesn't matter what will be bothering me, we would just sit there in silence. Just knowing that she would be there to hear me.

Mom always told me, "Don't let anyone bother you."

At one point she did help me get help. Learning how to be okay with myself, having different techniques for stress. I remember the first time I did try to kill myself, and someone told her, I came home and she said, "Oh, let's get in the car and go for a ride." And the next thing I knew we were in front of the hospital, and that's one of the moments I understood she wasn't against me. She was trying to help me. So she really helped me pull through in the end.

Mom always told me, "Don't let anyone bother you." And that's exactly what she would show me. I love my mother to death. The TS connection makes us stronger together. Me being able to have a role model is very inspiring. With all the stuff she's been through, I think it's amazing that she lets nothing get to her. She's been through hell and back. And knowing that Mom can get through life—if she can do it, I can do anything.

As the buffer between a Tourette child and the rest of society, parents are subject to unfair judgments—a form of soft bullying. Tori's strong message is to resist falling prey to this guilt trip. There is a learning curve for parents and they should give themselves time to travel it. Advocacy can be useful and empowering. Learn and teach coping skills. Put your situation in perspective. And most important of all, accept what is—Tourette syndrome.

TORI, ABOUT HER SON IAN (25 YEARS OLD)

Socially he was pretty rejected

Ian's Tourette symptoms began at eleven. But he had earlier problems. There was some question whether he was going to develop language when he was in kindergarten. Later that was all attributed to autism.

In early elementary school, he was very sensitive to touch and would only wear certain clothing. He had a lot of anxiety. He'd say he had to go to the bathroom, but it was just that he had to get out of the classroom and be by himself. I picked him up early from school and brought him home because it would get too stressful for him. He had a lot of trouble communicating with other kids. Socially he was pretty rejected.

Back then he didn't have tics specifically, although he did have a lot of repetitive behaviors, which are in autism too. When he was a kid he didn't play with toys, it was just a vacuum cleaner that he'd play with every day. He was on Ritalin to help him function in the classroom. He was being mainstreamed in regular Ed with a pull-out for help with math and language.

You don't have to feel bad if your kid has these problems

At about eleven, Ian started developing throat clearing and sticking his two fingers in the corners of his eyes repetitively. I thought it was the Ritalin, so we took him off it, but that didn't make any difference. He was taken out of school for a while because he had trouble coping. Also, he would have impulsivity problems, like wanting to touch people of the opposite sex.

Another tic, that he had for years, was lifting up his t-shirt and digging his finger in his navel. He was going to Sunday school and his teacher told him he could not do it. At that time, I was just learning about Tourette's and it was a lot for me to deal with. I was working, and I didn't know how to advocate for him. I didn't know to say, "Here's some information about Tourette's. There are things you need to know." That's the kind of thing I do now.

Coming to the Tourette syndrome camp, going to conferences and seminars, and reading books was important. Learning about it and realizing you don't have to feel bad if your kid has these problems. Other people can be expected to accommodate them. So by the time Ian was in middle school, I was asking for him to be in a placement where they could accommodate him.

The guilt trip that gets laid on parents

Advocating for your child means realizing people are allowed to be different. It doesn't mean you're a bad parent or your kid's a bad kid and you need to fix them and bring them back to school when they're better. That's the guilt trip that gets laid on parents when they have a kid with a problem and all the other parents talk about you and look at you like [she whispers in a gossipy way].

It's very alienating to be a parent with a kid who doesn't fit in. And it wasn't only Tourette's. Ian was just different. He was slower to mature and didn't fit in with other kids. They didn't want to hang around with him. If a kid is relatively normal, does well in sports, does okay academically, and has friends, when that kid comes out with tics, sometimes their friends will be there for them. But Ian didn't. He grew up not being able to communicate well and he was kind of outcast, wandering the hallways by himself in elementary school. So when he starts acting weird they think, "This kid's off the deep end," and they stay away from him.

I'd have a birthday party and invite all the kids, but he'd never get invited to anybody's house. Or when he would get invited, he'd act weird and the dad would call and say "Come pick your kid up, he did such-and-such."

So as a parent you feel pretty alienated too. It gets to the point where you're looking for other kids with disabilities for your kid to hang out with, so he can be comfortable, and you can be comfortable with the family.

That's how I dealt with it, rather than educating all the other parents. I became involved with Tourette's and autism and the developmentally disabled, and got him a new set of friends. By the time Ian got into middle school he was gravitating to kids in wheelchairs on the Special Ed buses and kids with Down Syndrome. They don't care.

What's hard is how to make their life better so it's not causing pain. People can be cruel. People can be very judgmental. I think the majority of people have a tendency to want to be superior because *inside* they feel inferior. That's their problem, you know?

A certain amount of jealousy

His sister is three years older and it was difficult for her because he got all the attention once he started having problems. It's not easy growing up with a sibling with problems. As a parent, you tend to let them off the hook when you shouldn't. His sister didn't feel it was fair, and it wasn't. So there's a certain amount of jealousy there. And then they get upset with me [*she laughs*].

I would do a lot of things differently. I would've divvied out the attention between my kids more evenly. And I think it's important not to compensate and baby a kid who's got problems. You give them love and support, but you don't ever let them use it as an excuse. You pay attention and make sure that people are not making fun of them, or that their environment is reasonable and comfortable. Go in and educate their peers, educate the classroom and the teachers. I wish I would've known to do more of that.

Teach him how to cope

The big issue in high school was how much of it is the disability and how much of it is Ian taking advantage of his disability? That was always a big question. My husband had a lot of trouble with that. He felt guilt. He did things for Ian rather than allow him to be independent and gain confidence in his ability to take care of himself.

The therapist's response was, "His disability doesn't make any difference. You treat it the same. Teach him how to cope. Give him support, but let him take care of himself. Encourage him to be independent and self-sufficient and have pride in his abilities."

The kid wants to be normal, and sometimes special treatment makes it worse. They sense you're compensating and that makes them feel like they're abnormal. That encourages them to take advantage of you too. And *that* makes them feel bad. For a kid, it's very tempting. "Just buy me a new video game, since someone teased me today." [*She laughs*] Yeah—don't do that. That's not good.

The main thing is to just accept it

Kids pick up on what you're feeling. When we'd go out, I wouldn't say, "Try not to do that arm thing." I never tried to get Ian to suppress his tics in public. I knew it was involuntary. And it wasn't his problem, it was other people's perception of it. I didn't have any trouble with that and don't have any regrets. And one of the core symptoms of autism is that they assume everybody is thinking the same thing they're thinking. So if Ian thinks it's okay, he assumes everybody else thinks it's okay. He never worried what other people think.

The main thing is to just accept it. This is what is. Because when you're fighting against something, that's when it creates a lot of conflict in yourself and in your family. But you know, it's not that big of a deal. And it often is not a lifelong, severely disabling condition, so don't expect the worst. Believe it's all going to be okay and this is just the way it is right now.

Keep the family calm. The house. Nobody get upset. The parents feel guilty, get upset with each other about how each is responding to things. "You're making it worse" or "You're not doing enough." That just creates tension for the kid, especially if he thinks it has anything to do with him. The parents need to get along, calmly.

You can be glad it's not that

Ian's Tourette's was more in your face. The autism was more subtle. You could think, "All he needs is a good friend and he'll socially integrate." Being a parent, being in denial, you could think maybe he was going to outgrow it. But Tourette's is so physically apparent, and makes him stand out so much, that you think he's never going to fit in.

When Ian was in elementary school, I still had hope that by the time he was in high school he was going to be normal, grow up, and have a family. Then, with Tourette's, I had to worry that his kids would have Tourette's. We had a lot of concern involving that, but then I just accepted it.

Life isn't perfect, you know? We all have crosses we have to bear and things we have to deal with. Some kids get leukemia, and you can be glad it's not that. Everybody has problems they cope with. It's not the worst thing. There's always somebody with a worse problem.

As I spoke with Yvonndy and Richard in their home, Richard's little brother played at pounding pegs into holes. She laughed, said "No more building for today," and held him in her lap as we continued. This was a loving family. Some days after our interview, Yvonndy told me Richard's demeanor had changed. He held his head higher, he spoke with new assurance in school, proudly telling his classmates he was going to be in a book. Acknowledgement can make such a difference in self-esteem and confidence.

YVONNDY AND HER SON, RICHARD (19 YEARS OLD)

God made you

Yvonndy: Symptoms appeared when Richard was in kindergarten. We were stationed in San Diego because his father was a Marine. His teacher's saying, "I see behavioral problems. Maybe you should hold him back." His father was like, "Oh, no, he's going forward." And I said, "I want him to have extra help." So we decided to keep him back.

His father got into some military trouble, so we had to pack up and leave for the desert. When school started here, his teacher said, "I think he has Tourette's." And I was like, "What the heck is that?" So we got the specialist who confirmed that he had Tourette's, ADD and ADHD.

I basically was okay with the diagnosis. My son has Tourette's and now we have to move forward. Try to make everything as best for him as possible. I told him there's going to be kids out there who are going to be very cruel. I know it's hard, but you have to turn the other way and keep on keeping on and be who you are. God made you and there's a reason for everything. When you grow up and become who you are, you'll be like, "Oh, I get it now."

Richard: Now I can control it more, but when I was little it was *a lot*. Sometimes I'll find a sound, something I heard. It's weird.

Yvonndy: One summer…

Richard: When I was in fourth grade…

Yvonndy: He would imitate, you know when your smoke detector needs a new battery?

Richard: [*He laughs*] Yeah.

Yvonndy: I thought we were going to lose it [*she laughs*]. We're like, "Please! Stop it!"

Richard: I thought it was annoying too.

High fructose corn syrup

Yvonndy: At first they bombarded me with medicine, but he would lay on the couch sick as a dog. He couldn't go to school, and he'd be crying.

Richard: I threw up.

Yvonndy: He didn't want to take it. So I said, "It's better if you don't put all those chemicals in your body."

Richard: Our aunt found out food coloring and different kind of syrups inside junk food would trigger me.

Yvonndy: So I took a lot of his stuff away. The high fructose corn syrup.

Richard: But I would still eat it.

Yvonndy: Now that he's older, he sneaks. That's his thing.

Richard: [*He chuckles*] Yeah.

Yvonndy: He wants to try medication again.

Richard: I was thinking since I'm older, maybe my body can deal with it more, 'cause I was little at the time.

And he finally cried

Yvonndy: He has IEPs[11] twice a year, in the beginning, and near the end they reevaluate.

Richard: The only thing I struggle in is math and English. I'm fine in my economics class, and art class, stuff like that.

---

11   Individualized Educational Program. See tourette.org.

Yvonndy: In the middle of sophomore year they decided to put him in Special Ed.

Richard: I was teased in school for my Tourette's. I told one kid, and next period everyone started making fun of me. I guess he told them.

Yvonndy: He explained to us what he's going through with girls not wanting to date him.

Richard: This one girl told me, 'cause I asked her to the movies, and she's like, "I don't mind you have Tourette's. I just don't want people making fun of *me* for going with someone who has it." I guess she doesn't want to be called names. Like my mom tells me, there's somebody for everybody.

Yvonndy: Being able to pray, it helps a lot. Trusting that, "Okay Jesus, I'm going to send him out into this world. Protect him, cover him, don't let them be so harsh to him." I know he hides a lot. My heart does hurt for him [*she fights tears*]. He tries to act like none of it hurts. And I know it does because it hurts me. And he finally cried. He doesn't release stuff. And when his father passed away… he committed suicide. I had just barely gotten re-married, there were six new step-brothers and sisters. Richard was handling it well. I give him credit, and the other kids too, because they had a lot thrown at them.

What kind of teacher are you?

Richard: All that stuff I said was happening, it's been happening since sixth grade. Being made fun of. I just kept that in. One time I told my parents and they talked to a counselor and said, "Suspend those kids." They stopped for a week, then they started making fun of me again.

Yvonndy: His elementary school was the best. Teachers were compassionate. Whatever you need, if you want to sit in class, we'll accommodate you.

Richard: I remember the teacher explained Tourette's to the class every year. Until middle school, when everyone starts growing up a little bit. To make fun of people.

Yvonndy: In middle school I was in the principal's every other day because teachers didn't want to put up with him. And I'm like, "What kind of teacher are you? I understand you're frustrated. I have him at home. But you have to have a heart." And it got better. Then high school came and he's *a lot* better. He gets into trouble, but his grades are good. He's A's and B's and C's now.

Richard: It's better, but just this year my Tourette's started to come back more. I've been studying a lot. That wasn't my thing before. I started to read more and do better with comprehension. Sometimes the Tourette's interferes. ADHD too. I can't sit still, but I just try to relax and do my work.

Zip it!

Yvonndy: Now Richard has a step-dad who's having to learn. Because Richard told his sister, "I'm going to kill you." It freaks everybody out. I don't fear... he would never do something like that. He just has no filter whatsoever.

Richard: I don't feel that way. I was just... saying it out of anger. I would say, "Sorry." At first they were like, "Oh, all right." Until I started saying it more or in a meaner way. Then they started feeling sad, I guess. They wouldn't talk to me. I would get aggravated when I said, "I'm sorry," and they'd ignore me. That would set me off. My symptoms were better, but then I started noticing they're getting worse. There's been stress a lot.

Yvonndy: He's trying to graduate.

Richard: I'd be in a lot of fights. I'd get kicked out of classrooms for talking too much, and I didn't know how to stop.

Yvonndy: He always has to have the last word. Even if I'm like, "Zip it!" he *has* to have the last word [*she laughs*]. And finally it clicks, "Oh, yes." So I just let him.

Richard: She used to say, "I have the last word," and I'd go [*softly into his shirt*], "All right."

Yvonndy: [*Big laugh*] Yeah! I'm like, "What did I just say!"

Richard: I wouldn't say it sassy, she'd just say, "No more talking," and I'd go [*quietly into his shirt*] "Okay."

I have a mother's heart

Yvonndy: My husband tells me you can't keep blaming it on Tourette's, the ADD and ADHD. I do have a hard time telling what's what. He's like, "When he gets into trouble he has to have his consequences." And then I feel bad. It's a new marriage. We're still working it out. My husband says, "He's a man now, he should be acting like a man." But not necessarily. We don't know what's going on in his mind, and we have to cut him some slack.

Richard: He's kinda getting used to it, but it took him a while.

Yvonndy: This past one, where my husband said Richard has to leave the house…

Richard: I couldn't live here anymore.

Yvonndy: Because my husband was scared for the girls.

Yvonndy: So Richard was at my mom's. I didn't know what to do, but I'm not going to give up on my child. His therapist says she honestly didn't think he was going to harm people, it's the Tourette's. She was able to calm my husband and Richard came back. Then he did research and got more understanding of Richard's world. With my husband, it's hard, but we talk a lot. That's a good thing. I tell him my feelings. "I would not endanger my children, your children." I have a mother's heart, but I don't have a blinded eye, either [*she stifles tears*]. Deep in my heart I know Richard is a good boy. He just has so much going on in there.

I still have it, anger

Richard: I'm starting to go to a men's group, young adults.

Yvonndy: Who have been abused. Physically, emotionally, his father… yeah. So a lot of the anger could be from his father, too. He did Mourning Star[12] when his father passed away. This is for kids who lost a loved one and this is where they talked about the abuse. I didn't know. Because I'd rarely leave them alone with him. His father was an alcoholic, he abused drugs, he abused prescription medications.

We knew there were incidences, but Richard never came out and said what's going on with his dad. I was always with the kids because he was deployed, or he was a drill instructor. I think that's why our marriage lasted so long, because he was never around [*she laughs*]. When he got thrown out of the military, and served time in military prison, I said, "I can't do this anymore." He was going downhill and was gonna take us with him.

Richard: I still have it, anger. When I was little it was worse, but it's gotten better.

---

12   A grief counseling program for children, teens, and families.

I'd like to be working, living on my own

Richard: There's a program I'm in, it's called TPP[13], and it helps kids with learning disabilities. Whatever you want to be, what you want to do after high school. It helps you how to live. You stay in there for like four years. I got in because I'm in Special Ed. It's just seniors who can get it.

Yvonndy: But the last thing is, you *have* to graduate. I tell him he has to work hard.

Richard: Yeah. I'd like to be working, living on my own. That's what I look forward to.

Yvonndy: But now I try to keep structure with him because he's chaos.

Richard: It's hard for me to go to sleep.

Yvonndy: When he gets enough sleep he's not as agitated. Eating too. He skips meals and I'm saying, "Don't do that, because you can totally tell in your aggressiveness." It's not good. When he was younger I brought him his own snacks because teachers would hand out candy. If you don't want those problems you're telling me he has, don't give him that stuff. Don't let him have school lunches, don't let him have other people's food. They were good about helping me.

I suggest you keep walking

Yvonndy: In public, people stare because he does the vocal, like *haw haw haw*.

Richard: Yeah.

Yvonndy: When he was younger and more rambunctious, people would be like, "Get a hold of your child." One lady told me something and I said, "You don't understand half of what's going on with my child, so I suggest you keep walking, because I'm trying to be a nice person [*she laughs*]. Don't make me be ugly." People stare at us. If somebody asks me I tell them, this is what he has.

Richard: Yeah, at PetSmart this lady was like, "Why did you do that?" And I said I had Tourette's and she was like, "Oh, I never knew that."

Yvonndy: He's been trying to get a job at Petco and PetSmart.

Richard: I did this Workability[14] thing, it gives you work experience.

---

13   Transition Partnership Program of Riverside County, CA.
14   See thehelpgroup.org.

He tamed them

Yvonndy: Research is a good thing. To get from other people who have gone through it. Also I found a good support group at church. You need support. My family too. When I've had enough, I can call and say, "Can you please come get him?" So he can have a break, I can have a break. I'd say to him, "Find a hobby and see if that helps."

Richard: My hobby is my lizards.

Yvonndy: They calm him down a lot.

Richard: In fourth grade I had a leopard gecko.

Yvonndy: He got it for Christmas.

Richard: At first I was scared of it and never held it, until I saw stuff on YouTube. And I got interested. I looked into different lizards and started liking them. Right now I've got a Pac-Man frog, a chameleon, and a Chinese water dragon. At first they would bite me and hiss at me and whip their tail, until I started holding them.

Yvonndy: He tamed them [*she laughs*].

Richard: Yeah. I'll put my hand in my tank and my chameleon will crawl on me. And my Chinese water dragon sits in my room and walks around. It doesn't act squirmish or anything. Just calm. That calms me.

Yvonndy: I have quiet time in my room, like I'll take a bath. I'll read or listen to articles on my phone. I do a lot of journaling. That helps me release. I write about the day, what my struggles have been. What were my weaknesses that day? Did I do something to overcome it or did I make the matter worse? I try to evaluate.

It scares you

Yvonndy: Part of me feels I made a mistake with Richard with the medication. Being so adamant about not doing it, because he feels like, if he'd had the medication maybe he would be different. I did my part, parentwise, the best I could. And if he wants to try it, then okay. The wise choice I made was eating habits. That helped us a lot, kind of a breather. And I monitored what he watched—TV, no killing video games. Then, MTV had a documentary on kids with Tourette's and they were really bad.

Richard: One girl would always swear and get crazy.

Yvonndy: Flinging her arms everywhere. I said, "Thank you, Jesus, for giving me what I can handle [*she laughs*]." I tell him, "Somebody always has it worse than you. That girl has to deal with people laughing at her and she comes home crying daily."

Richard: Yeah. Even though I have it, I know someone probably has it way worse.

Yvonndy: When you're dealt the hand you're dealt, you choose to make something good out of it, or you make yourself a victim. I'm praying he's learned this. And now that he's saying he wants medicine…

Richard: It scares you.

Yvonndy: I'm having to put my faith in God that this boy has learned everything and he'll make the correct choices.

Rosie personifies the unending strength and hope parents display as they grapple with Tourette's effects on their children. Her story is intimate to us all, as a nation struggling to face the truth about police response to people of color. No other parent in this book has endured the sorrows and fears Rosie has, and still she raises her head, opens her heart, and moves on with her life. Her voice has a plaintive quality that belies her courage. She reminds us that, whatever our tribulations, we always have the stars.

ROSIE, ABOUT HER SON JAVIER (23 YEARS OLD)

I hate Tourette's

I love it up here where I am. I was married for twenty-two years, then I got a divorce, so it was a decision—do I pay rent for the rest of my life or get my own house? And I found this tranquility. I get to see the stars every night. The air is so nice and clear. It's just beautiful. I even love the dirt [*she laughs*].

My son, Javier, he has the Tourette's, the really bad one. He has tics, he has coprolalia, he has OCD, ADHD, depression. I first noticed when he was little, and he wasn't diagnosed until he was eleven. I'm an LVN[15]

---

15   Licensed Vocational Nurse.

and it took me three days to accept the diagnosis. I was sobbing and crying out. But I realized this was something we were going to have to deal with for the rest of our lives.

He is still in denial. I told him to join a Tourette group on Facebook, he would feel better knowing other people. He yells out, "I hate Tourette's. My life is miserable because of Tourette syndrome." It's tough. Oh, my God, it breaks my heart.

He was in Special Ed with accommodations. He dealt better with it because he was stable on medication. But when he came out of high school and he decided to stop the medication, the symptoms came out. He decided he was no longer going to be bullied. And he decided the answer was to hang out with the tough guys. [*A long pause*] He's hanging out with gang members. They accept him and he can be himself.

In a way, I was asking for help

Yeah. So Javier decided to go off the medication. Then the divorce. Then my youngest son, Jesse, was killed. And after that Javier just went into a rage.

Jesse was killed by the Los Angeles Sheriff's Department in Whittier, California. He was sixteen. After the divorce, Jesse's father had custody of him. But it was better that he be with me, because his father didn't keep track of him. Jesse was gone this last time for three days, so I filed a missing-child report. When the judge gave me custody, I had to bring Jesse to court, to cancel the missing-child report. But Jesse didn't want to go.

So I called the police. In a way, I was asking for help, you know, to the ... [*she sighs*] the law, the system. I thought they would help me bring him to court. When the police came, he resisted. Things got out of control very quickly and they tasered him and arrested him and the judge sent him to Juvenile Hall for one year. Why would a judge do that? After about four months, for good behavior, they sent Jesse to a foster home.

When he ran away from the foster home he came back to me, but he was very scared. I knew he had an arrest warrant. *Tenia mucho miedo de volver al*[16] Juvenile Hall. He told me they put him in 'The Hole.' He felt unsafe because my address was registered with the court. This is when he put on all his tattoos, like he was trying to hide, to disguise himself.

And one day the Humane Society came looking for stray animals.

---

16   He was very afraid of returning to Juvenile Hall.

They have blue uniforms and Jesse thought they were cops and he ran, and that's when they killed him. Had he stayed in the foster home, his release day was gonna be January 10, which was the day he was killed.

What's going on?

What happened was there was a robbery and one of the suspects had a gun. From the description, an officer spotted Jesse, who was walking with a friend. The officer told Jesse to stop. Because of the foster home, he ran.

The policeman shot him and Jesse was limping away, wounded. And then he was caught in a cul-de-sac. So they came in and the whole street was lined up with police with their guns drawn. They asked him to stop and surrender. Jesse kept limping away backwards.

They felt threatened for some reason. They say in the report that a knife was found. I know from a lady that saw what happened, she said what was on the news wasn't the truth. That Jesse was like, asking with his arms, "What's going on?"

So that's what happened. I went back to the scene and talked to some of the neighbors, because their windows were shattered. And one of them said the officer who went to gather the shells… it was over fifty-four. Jesse was hit by seventeen bullets. [*Softly*] Yeah.

Me remueve el dolor[17]. When my lawyer got the police report, my first question was, "Did Jesse use drugs? Was there anything in his system?" The lawyer said, "No."

I'm afraid I'm going to lose him as well

These are things I haven't told Javier because of his Tourette syndrome. I don't know how he's going to take it, having Tourette syndrome and having coprolalia. *Y tengo miedo que le afecte de una forma que el no puede controlar sus[18]* rage outbursts. I'm afraid I'm going to lose him as well. Because he's got this rage towards me, for the divorce, for what happened to Jesse. Yeah.

Javier loaned his car to a friend and the friend was stopped by the

---

17   Grief overwhelms me.
18   And I'm afraid it will affect him in a way that he can't control his rage outbursts.

police and ran away. They researched the car and found it was Javier's. So at three in the morning cops come to my door and ask me questions about Javier.

That brought the memories back. I asked the policeman, can you please come into the other room? I have to show you something. And then I showed him my Jesse's ashes, my sixteen-year-old. I said, "You see this? This is my Jesse's ashes. He was killed by the Sheriff's Department in Whittier. I need to know if you guys killed Javier too." He said, "I don't know, ma'am."

At that time my daughter comes out of the bedroom and he reaches for his gun. It was a very tense, horrible night. And he asks, "Is Javier violent?" And I said, "Javier has Tourette's syndrome. He has coprolalia. Do you know what that is?" And he goes, "No."

So from three to four-thirty in the morning I was almost sure Javier was dead. Then he calls and tells me what happened. I was just so glad he was alive. Yeah. Being the mother of a Tourette syndrome person with coprolalia is very, very stressful, *es muy preocupante. Especialmente me preocupo por su futuro*[19]. While I'm alive I can help him, but with his coprolalia, his tics, everyone thinks he's a drug addict. He doesn't last in jobs. He's a good worker, but his coprolalia, his OCD don't let him perform a hundred percent.

My strength comes from God and my love for my kids

Gracias a Dios, I landed up here. It's an ideal place. It's three thousand feet up, closer to the stars. Closer to calm, closer to peace. I do break down. I cry and cry and cry until there's no more tears. Then I rest and I'm ready for the next day. Just put that on the side and pray for my son, *por Javier*, and keep going. Another day.

Last night I was out looking at the stars until two in the morning and there was a lot of shooting stars out there. One of them was so long. I think it was meant for me... [*she weeps*] ...*como para calmarme*[20]. Like a sign from God. Any comfort I can get from the stars, it's always welcome. If I'm broken down and torn apart, crying away, there are stars that always... *eso siempre me consuela*[21].

You learn to deal with it and it strengthens you. [*A sigh*] Yeah. My

---

19   It's very worrisome. I especially worry about his future.
20   As if to calm me.
21   It always consoles me.

strength comes from God and my love for my kids. I want to protect them. Every time something happens, I just rise, because I want to strengthen them to be independent, productive, and kind human beings.

A tight, supporting hug

Right now Javier's taking a machinist class. He says, "Mom, I just need a certificate and I'll be set." I see him do his homework, blinking and ticcing away. He's trying to read the book while he's blinking and trying to hold his neck still[22].

I think what he hates is that he can't deal with everything happening in his life, especially that he's not accepted. He says, "Mom, I don't have anything in common with anybody. Only my friends down the hill. They don't care that I tic or that I cuss." He tells me he cusses and they laugh. Of course, they're laughing *at* him.

Society needs to be educated big time. I know there's a lot of Tourette kids all over the world who haven't survived the stereotyping. These TS kids are out there and they're part of society too. They need to be understood. Like before, when they didn't understand mental illness and they burned them. That's how they are sacrificing our children who have Tourette syndrome. Society is sacrificing them.

For other mothers… oh, my God, I have no words. Just a deep sadness. We need a support group. Hardly anybody understands this position, being a mother of a Tourette syndrome child. I basically feel alone. [*She weeps, then composes herself.*]

I'm feeling better these days. Yeah. I'm beginning to feel hopeful and a little bit stronger. My strength is with God. If I didn't have that, how could I do it? Being out here, under the sky, looking at the stars, it's relaxation. To build up the strength to keep going. I would just send all the mothers a tight, supporting hug and understanding. I don't know. Keep trying. Keep doing the best we can.

---

22   Javier earned his machinist certificate and is working.

Once Jen found a workable perspective about Jacob's Tourette's and her role as a mother, she was able to relax, stop blaming herself, and take better care of her son. They've had good luck with teachers and supportive schools, but she's also been proactive with her advocacy. Jake's a good example of someone who internalized CBIT²³ techniques and uses them successfully and reflexively.

JEN, ABOUT HER SON JACOB (14 YEARS OLD)

My biggest regret was having him think they were going to go away

When Jake was seven, he said to me, "My eyes are bothering me." Within a day or two he started blinking super-rapidly, non–stop. He said, "I don't know why I can't stop blinking." I took him to the pediatrician, who said, "Ignore it and they'll go away as mysteriously as they came." Well, within months Jake developed more tics. My biggest regret was having him think they were going to go away.

We went to a neurologist and he was awful. Jake had only been having tics for a little while, and the neurologist said, "This is what kids act like when they have Tourette's." I'd done research, and I'm thinking, "You can't diagnose Tourette's after only two months." And he specialized in Tourette's. I thought, "If this guy is a specialist, I'm in big trouble." We didn't see him again.

So we saw another neurologist, who we liked, and he said it's likely Tourette syndrome, but he wouldn't diagnose because it hadn't been a full year. It was perfect. We had a home base, a good supportive doctor. A couple of months later we got a letter saying he was going to pursue a new career. Well that's just our luck. What new career are you going to? You're a neurologist [*she laughs*].

I was getting way more sad than I needed to

Jacob had a bad overbite so an orthodontist gave him headgear to prepare

---

23   Cognitive Behavioral Intervention for Tics. See Chapter Ten and tourette. org.

him for braces. We told him right up front that Jacob has Tourette syndrome. I don't know what he thought Tourette's was, but he said it wouldn't interfere with the headgear.

Within a month Jacob developed a tic where he'd open his mouth really wide, and he broke the headgear brackets on his teeth. The orthodontist fixed it for free. Three weeks later the same thing happened. I brought him in and they said, "That'll be $55." I said, "He has Tourette's and that's why he broke it." They didn't care. So I paid the $55, I dropped him off at school, and I cried [*she laughs*].

A week or two later the same thing happened. We went back and they were rude. "I told you guys he has Tourette's," I said. "He can't help it." The orthodontist said to Jake, "You better knock this off. You're costing your mom a lot of money."

Every time the thing broke I brought him into that office and I was pulling out the credit card. I wouldn't let Jake see me cry, but I couldn't get it together. My son was in this situation where he can't help that he's breaking this thing. They're being mean and they're charging us. And he's up in the bathroom putting toothpaste on it, thinking he can repair it. Finally I said, "We're done." And we found a new orthodontist.

I was getting way more sad than I needed to. At first I was blaming myself. But I eventually realized TS was genetic, and that released me. His tics bothered *me* more than they bothered him. So a big step for me was coming to terms with TS and embracing it and saying, "You know what? There's a mom out there with a kid with epilepsy, who would switch places with me in a heartbeat. I need to put on a positive attitude and remember this isn't so bad. We'll be okay."

Everything I've worried about for Jake, he's shown me it's not a big deal. He thoroughly accepts Tourette's. When he was younger, he could say, "I don't like it, but I can accept it." He's continued to prove me wrong about my worries.

They're required to make these modifications

Every teacher Jake had was supportive. First grade, Jake needed to stand in class, so his teacher moved him to where he could do that without bothering anyone. That's where he's been lucky. He's hit the teacher Lotto. Teachers who didn't need to teach him how to conform.

I got him a 504 plan[24] and that's helped also. A 504 plan is different from an IEP. For a 504 you don't have to be behind in school, you just need some kind of disability that interferes with your learning. It can be stressful for someone with Tourette's if the class is taking a test, it's dead quiet, and they don't want to make noise. With a 504 plan you can get it written in that they're allowed to take their test in another room. For the ACT[25] they're allowed as much time as they need to finish it.

With Jacob I'm like, "Whatever works." He likes to chew gum, he almost *needs* to chew. It helps release energy, I think. So I buy him gum by the case at Costco [*she chuckles*]. And I asked that he be allowed to chew gum in class despite what the policy is. They're also putting in there that if he needs to leave class for a little bit, he'll be allowed to do that. The 504 plan gives a kid these protections by law. They're required to make these modifications. If you don't have that 504 in place, they don't have to do anything.

Jake's an eighth grader now and he's explained to the kids that he has Tourette syndrome and everybody accepts it.

My tics were cut in half

In 2011, we had a big snow storm here. My son was having fun playing in that snow, digging this giant tunnel. With the repetitive motion, he gave himself ulnaritis in his wrist. The orthopedic doctor said it was serious, and Jake needed to wear a brace and not take it off until the nerve was completely healed.

So a couple of days later I walk past his room and see he's taken the brace off and he's bending his wrist. It's not one of my proudest mom moments [*she chuckles*]—I yelled, "What are you doing! You're gonna end up with permanent nerve injury. Get that brace back on." He looked at me, he kind of had teary eyes, and said, "Mom, it's a tic." I felt about an inch tall. I'd never yelled at him about his tics and now I'm like the orthodontist [*she laughs*].

That really stinks, that he has a tic that could injure him permanently. So I did some research about controlling tics and I came across Dr. Douglas Woods and his CBIT treatment. I found out Jacob might qualify for one of their research studies and I said, "Sign us up." So Jacob came home from

---

24   See the 504 plan and IEP references at tourette.org.
25   A standardized test that measures college readiness.

school and I said "Guess what, buddy? I found this CBIT and I got you an appointment." He looked at me and said, "Nope. I don't want to." So I did what any good mother would do—I bribed him [*she laughs*]. He'd been wanting boxing lessons, so I gave him a little incentive. And he agreed to go.

They evaluated him and where I thought he had only three or four tics, it turned out he had eighteen. He was doing a lot of tics I couldn't see, like he would squeeze his hand, he would curl his toes.

The CBIT was fun. It was once a week, a two-hour drive. We'd pack a lunch or a dinner, and we had mother-son time. Jake was young enough to have a good attitude and old enough to understand what he was doing. 'Cause I look at my son now, at fourteen, and there's no way I could drag him to CBIT.

The folks who worked with him were graduate students, and one of them himself had Tourette's. Jake enjoyed meeting him. And when we were at the end of it he said, "Mom, my tics were cut in half." If you talk to him now he'd say, "I don't do CBIT. It's stupid." He's a fourteen-year-old boy. I know he may not be doing the exact procedure they taught him, but he's modified it and made it his own.

The face of hope

When you're first doing CBIT, they want to be sure you're aware of your tics. They let Jake choose which ones we worked on. We started with the most bothersome tic, and focused on one tic a week.

They had us do homework. During the week we had twenty minutes where we'd watch just that tic we were working on. We'd read a book or watch TV, you could choose your activity, and I would keep count and he would keep count. I think this was to make sure the child is aware of the tic. Because if Mom is marking down a hundred-and-twenty times and the kid is marking down two, he's not aware yet.

So we'd go in and the CBIT trainer would talk to Jake about what sensation he got *before* he had the tic. They'd have a conversation and every time he felt it coming on he'd raise his hand. So they talked, Jake would raise his hand, and then we'd see the tic.

The trainer would teach him a competing response. So like for a vocal tic, you have to breathe out your mouth. If you're breathing *in* your mouth and out your nose, you can't make that sound. So he'd do something opposite the tic.

For Jake's eye blinking tic, he would still blink but they'd have him do a slow blink. So they taught him, when he felt it coming on, to do this competing response until the urge went away. So you didn't *have* to do the tic to make the urge go away.

At the end of the program there was a real decrease in his tics. For me, as his mom, I felt like I gave him a tool for the toolbox. Something he could have for the rest of his life. After that, he was so much more confident. He felt more in control. And I learned a lot about what Jake was going through because I was with him for every session. CBIT helped him and me.

I think CBIT could help so many people. I figure everybody ought to *try* it. See if it works. There are no side effects to it. And for what it did for my son, I think of him as the face of hope. With Tourette's you can still be a very successful person. You can have a great life. Six years ago Tourette syndrome was a big part of who my son was. His tics were a big part of his daily life. Today, he's a good kid, he's a good student, he's got a good personality, athletic, and oh, by the way, he has Tourette's.

Michelle brings up the tough issue of how to discipline Tourette children, especially those with behavior issues. She and her husband work together rearing their family; teamwork brings double creativity to the task. She emphasizes the importance of parents making time to enjoy each other as a couple, so that each may return refreshed to the task of parenting. Her life as a Tourette's mom is a journey of personal growth into compassion and patience.

MICHELLE, ABOUT HER SON ANTHONY (6 YEARS OLD)
at Kenneth Michael Staebler Tourette Spectrum Camp

We videotaped Anthony ticcing on different days and different times

I have three boys and Anthony, my boy with Tourette's, is six. His tics became significant just after he turned three. Originally they told us he was having seizures. I wasn't comfortable with that diagnosis, so I started researching. I discovered these "little quirks" were actually tics. So somewhere between a year-and-a-half and two years is when he started ticcing. He got diagnosed just before he turned four.

You have to be persistent in your search for a doctor. When they see you know what you're talking about, and you're going to advocate for your child, they listen better. In the beginning we had doctors say, "That might be your theory, but my theory is this." I asked for second opinions. Finally you get the doctor who says, "Yes, I see this."

Doctors, a lot of them, are not as educated as they should be about Tourette's. I've had doctors tell me, "He's definitely not having tics." So we videotaped Anthony ticcing on different days and at different times. I went to the neurologist and she said, "He's young. I'm not going to diagnose Tourette syndrome yet, but I'm going to pass you to a psychiatrist." We got a good psychiatrist and started getting somewhere. So the video footage was helpful.

There definitely is a grieving process

It was challenging. We got a diagnosis for our oldest son of Asperger's at around the same time. So it was a big hit to find out two of our kids have special needs. But we're Christian and we felt God gave us these children for a reason and they're blessed with different gifts. You make the best of it. There definitely is a grieving process. I think that's normal, and we went through that. And then we said, "Okay, now it's time to move forward." There are still moments when you get sad, or you are overwhelmed or frustrated. But we did the best we could.

Anthony's in kindergarten now. He's a bright boy, but he has a learning disability. We have not been able to identify what it is. We know there's a discrepancy between what he knows and what he can produce, so he's in Special Ed. If we mainstream him, he would not be able to keep up.

We're starting to question whether we should home school. I was a teacher, so I have some knowledge. I think with a year or two of that, maybe we could mainstream him and he would do okay on his own. Which is ultimately what everyone wants. We want him to achieve his potential. Our feeling is, we can try it and if it doesn't work we can put him back into school. We're definitely learning as we go. And making mistakes. That's part of the growing process.

The behavior is bad and the child is good

Anthony has a lot of behavioral issues. And he does often say he can't control or he feels like someone else is controlling him. But sometimes it's hard to tell. Is he being a naughty little boy or is this something he can't control? That's where it gets wishy-washy, like how far do you let it go? And we've messed up sometimes. We've punished Anthony for things we probably shouldn't have. Our extended family tries hard to be supportive, but they don't understand fully. Sometimes they do things they think are helpful that aren't. If it's hard for *us* to determine what is behavioral and what's Tourette's, they have a really hard time when they come to visit.

Our parents are older, and back when they were younger it was black and white. You were good or you were bad. There wasn't this middle road where the behavior is bad and the child is good. We just say, "This is not a behavioral issue. This is part of his disorder." And they say, "Yes, but he can't do that, it's not appropriate." We can tell him it's not appropriate, but we have to understand he can't control it. It happens so quickly sometimes, and we discipline him and then realize we shouldn't be so hard on him.

It's too complicated to figure out by yourself

My husband and I are working together in this. There definitely was a learning curve, where we had to figure out how we're going to change our discipline styles and work together. It's easy to get angry, but with this kind of child that's the worst thing you can do. Anthony does get very aggressive, so we have to work together as a team. When one parent sees the other starting to lose it, they can take over. And that other parent takes a time out. Because it's inevitable. There are times we disagree, but we're at a good place. We see the same way how to handle things. And we've had a lot of help from our psychologist and psychiatrist. We go as a family and work together. It's too complicated to figure out by yourself.

We have to make ourselves take that time

I think through this, my husband and I, our relationship has gotten much stronger. We've learned to be not so heated when things come up, and to communicate in a nicer way. We have to be more patient with each other when we get stressed. There are many days he comes home tired or stressed from work, but I'm at the end of my rope from being with the kids all day. So we both have learned to be more understanding. I have needs and he does too, and we have to be patient with each other.

We are lucky that the military has a program they're trying out in certain cities. It's through the Armed Services YMCA. They have what's called an Exceptional Family Member Program[26] for family members with special needs. If you are a certain level of that, you can receive respite care, and it's forty hours a month. We just started getting that and it has allowed me to take a break. And as a couple, it's allowed us to go out. This has been invaluable because as soon as he comes home it's all about the kids, it's never about us anymore. So we've learned we have to make ourselves take that time.

It's hard to know people are thinking that of you

Going out in public is challenging. One of the parents here at TS camp said you try to make your child feel normal as he is, so you don't feel embarrassed, or embarrassed for them. I'm still learning how to accept that other people aren't going to understand. Learning when he does things, how to handle it. Recently there was a little girl, and she was in his space and did something he wasn't comfortable with, so he said, "Get away from me, you little freak." I was embarrassed and told him that wasn't appropriate. Then I said to the mom, "I'm sorry, he has impulse control issues, he has Tourette syndrome." And she was very understanding.

I've had that experience where people, understandably, get very defensive of their children. It can make for uncomfortable situations. In public, I try to ignore some behaviors. Not major ones, but on a smaller level. Other people don't always appreciate that, and you get looks, you hear comments. I know they're thinking, "That parent does not know how to handle her child." It's hard to know people are thinking that of you.

A challenging card

Society is uneducated about disabilities. When people understand, they are generally more accepting. I think the disadvantage to this disorder is

---

26   efmp.amedd.army.mil. Each branch of the services has its own program.

that the children look normal. You can't go, "Oh, he's in a wheelchair." It's a lot harder to tell.

I have a friend, her son is autistic, and she actually puts buttons and labels on everything that say, "I'm autistic." I don't agree with that approach. I don't think they should literally have a label. It should be something you choose to share with people. But it does make it harder, because people wonder why you're not saying anything to the child. You have to pick your battles.

Anthony has more anxiety and self-esteem issues than we're aware of. He's not as verbal about it, but he holds it in or expresses it through his tics. It's interesting that Tourette's takes place in years that are so formative to children. They're being dealt a challenging card at the same time they're forming their self-identity.

You just know

These Tourette camps, talking with other parents and the Tourette Syndrome Association, it's invaluable. It's a wealth of knowledge. We've had some great doctors, but when I asked, "Are there any other families I can meet?" they weren't interested. We have not been able to get involved in a support group. That's what we need.

Anthony doesn't have many close friends. He's very social with adults and has a hard time socializing with children. The place he's finding closer friends is with other kids who have needs. He identifies with them more. He's in a social skills group with two other boys the same age and they're becoming friends. The other two moms and I are arranging play dates. We're also tolerant of each others' children and we *know*, so if there is a squabble we know why that happens, and we're not going to get irritated at the other person. We can see beneath the surface.

It's about personal growth. I've definitely fallen flat on my face a couple of times, and will continue to. But I've learned from that and discovered how to handle things better. I'm definitely growing as a person. I'm much more patient than I ever thought I could be' cause you have to learn to be [*she laughs*]. I'm much more accepting of other people. Not that I wasn't compassionate, or didn't accept people before, but now it's easy to spot other parents with children that have special issues. I understand. I've even gone over to parents who were overwhelmed and asked if I could help. I've been there. You just know.

———————————— ✑ ————————————

How fortunate to have a loving family, true friends, and a supportive school system. But Tourette syndrome still can create an arduous journey, personal and familial, and Meg set a hopeful tone by advocating for her son and teaching him to advocate for himself. He was active in this way throughout his school career, and became a Youth Ambassador for the Tourette Association of America. Despite their worries about TS disrupting his last years of high school, Ben is now attending university.

MEG AND HER SON BEN (17 YEARS OLD)

Some days were bad, some weren't

Meg: When Ben was four, he started blinking his eyes a lot. We took him to the doctor, who said it was probably a habit and not to worry. Then that stopped and about a year and a half later he started twirling. Then, in second grade, he was head ticcing. So we took him to a neurologist. We weren't crazy about her because she was reluctant to diagnose. She called it Transient Tic Disorder. And then he started with the verbal sounds and noises. So we pretty much knew, because I had done my own research—Tourette's. So when he was nine we took him to UCLA, to the Tic Disorder Program, and that's where he was formally diagnosed. He went through the Habit Reversal program… now it's called CBIT[27].

Ben: They told me to sit on my hands if I felt like I had to flare them out. Just sit on my hands for sixty seconds, then I'll learn to control my tics a little better. It was *so* hard to do. I don't use it much anymore. I probably should, though.

Meg: It worked for a little while.

Ben: My tics are a lot more extreme now than they were in third grade.

Meg: They were mild. And then fourth grade, the verbal tics got really bad. But fifth, sixth, seventh, you know, he'd tic but you wouldn't know he had Tourette's. Some days were bad, some days weren't. And then, I think there were four months left to eighth grade, and he started with coprolalia. Really bad. I mean in school it was … yeah, a nightmare.

———————————————————————————

27   Cognitive Behavioral Intervention for Tics. See tourette.org.

Luckily our school was so supportive. The teachers were wonderful, the kids were wonderful.

Then they went crazy

Meg: Starting in third grade he would give presentations to all the classes.
Ben: I showed this video, *I Have Tourette's, But Tourette's Doesn't Have Me*[28], to all my classes. I didn't give as complicated a presentation as I give now.
Meg: Things were calm in the beginning of this year and then they went crazy.
Ben: I'm a junior in high school. I know I'm going to college, just not where. I want to be a math teacher, high school, at least that's what I'm thinking right now.
Meg: Eighth grade was fantastic. We were at a small school. In ninth and tenth grades, nobody would have known he had Tourette's, the tics were so minor. Then this November all hell broke loose. So it's been a disaster. But again we're so fortunate. From the principals to the counselors to the teachers to the kids—everybody has been supportive and accommodating.

What's happening now, though, is before this semester he had a 3.8 average. Now, if he gets straight Cs we're going to be happy. He just can't do *anything*, he's so stressed. As soon as I talk about homework he starts freaking out. You know, it's a college year. He's supposed to take the ACT[29] in June, but at this point we don't know if he'll be able to. We already got accommodation for the SAT. Extended time in a one-on-one setting. And then the ACT, we're asking for a reader and that it can be taken over five days. English, right now? He couldn't read an article.
Ben: I have this tic where I crumple up papers and that really gets in the way a lot [*he chuckles*]. It's frustrating, but I get used to it.

Everyone looks up to you for your courage

Meg: Yeah. But you know what? We've had many a day this year where he has called me in tears because it's so bad he can't stay at school. He's woken up on mornings where he can't go to school.

---

28   Available at tourette.org.
29   A standardized test that measures college readiness.

Ben: I tic so bad I can't get in the shower.

Meg: How many times have you had to leave class?

Ben: Oh, I've... countless. My teachers understand. At school I can suppress a *little* bit, but when you're holding in a tic it takes a lot of energy. You can't focus on anything else. So I have to choose between holding my tics and letting everyone else learn, or ticcing and letting myself learn, and other people have a harder time. Sometimes I'll suppress my tics for awhile, then go outside and let them all out.

Tourette's gets in the way of social life, but it doesn't ruin my relationships. All my friends know about my Tourette's. They don't know what it feels like, but they understand it's frustrating and I'm going through a hard time. I've had so many friends say, "Everyone looks up to you for your courage." That helps me a lot.

Never mind

Ben: Then there's daily things I can't do sometimes. Like we're going to have study sessions for the AP[30] U.S. History test. It's a marathon study session. I don't know if I'm going to be able to do it. And movie theaters? They're hard for me. Last time I went was four or five months ago with my parents and my brother. I started cussing and stuff and people turned around and looked at me and went, "Shhh!" I don't know if they were doing it a lot or if it's in my head, but I remember it being bad. So I sat in the lobby, put my earphones in, and listened to music.

It's hard because a lot of people don't know what Tourette's is, and it's hard for you to go into a full-on description in the middle of nowhere in public. It's awkward. Just the other day I was at Subway and I couldn't control myself at all. I was flinging my hands everywhere and cussing. And the guys were like, "Okay... here's your sandwich." I said, "I'm so sorry, I have Tourette's." And they're like, "Okay. But you were cussing, and that's kinda rude." And I was like, "Well, you know... never mind."

Meg: Oh, you didn't tell me that.

Ben: No, I didn't. If I feel I'm going to have a relationship with them at all, I'll tell them. A substitute teacher? That's one of the first things I tell them. Before class I say, "I have Tourette's, it's a neurological disorder."

Meg: The other day this sub turned around, and one of his friends went like that [*she gives the finger*] and he said to Ben, "That's not a tic, I'm

---

30   Advanced Placement.

flipping her off." You know, because the sub was giving him a hard time.

Ben: The teacher was like, "Watch your language, young man!" And I said, "I have Tourette's." And she turned around and one of the guys flipped her off, "Oh, I don't even have Tourette's. I'm just flipping her off."

[*They laugh.*]

Thank you for your support

Meg: Did you ever have teasing or bullying or anything?

Ben: Well, there's been jokes, but they've always been light-hearted.

Meg: He's always had friends, teachers always have liked him.

Ben: Except one.

Meg: Except one. And we got out of her class quick. But with any other teacher, I would send emails, "I'm so sorry. We're going through this. Thank you for your support." And teachers would respond to me, "Oh, we love Ben. Don't worry about it." There's been *so* much support. He had an IEP[31] all the way up through tenth grade. Then because everything was so fine we switched it to...

Ben: To a 504.

Meg: That's for *medical* conditions. And then, like two weeks ago, we went back to the IEP, which is, by law, better. They *have* to meet with you. You have to sign off on things. Whereas a 504 is a little bit more loosey-goosey.

Eighth grade, and especially this junior year, has been really, really hard for all of us. Luckily I've got a boss who's super-flexible, 'cause Ben will call me at ten-thirty, I'll have to pick him up and bring him home and go back to work. So for my husband, for me, for his brother, it's been very, very stressful. I think mostly for me, because Ben and I are together the most out of everybody. And what's freaking me out is that I know he's got so much potential, and so these *grades*—this is so not fair. It is *not* fair. You know, about getting into college. And I'm going between being the empathetic mother—'cause I know he can only do so much—to, "You've gotta do your homework. You gotta get your grades up." That actually makes it harder for us because we see him suffering so.

---

31   Individualized Education Program and 504 are Federal programs. See tourette.org for details.

Everyone has something like *Tourette's*

Ben: I think one of my best qualities is I'm a really nice person. I'm not a jerk at all. I've never been in a fight. Every time someone starts challenging me to a fight I just walk away. I don't care what they think about me. I'm not going to hurt anybody, you know?

And also, this sounds corny probably, but having Tourette's helped me not make fun of people with other disabilities. But even if someone's making fun of someone for being poor, or for not having nice clothes, I usually stick up for them. I know that everyone has their own demons they fight. Everyone has something *like* Tourette's. Nobody has it perfect.

Meg: My sense is generally he feels pretty good about himself, but boy, those times when he's down, it's *down*. He's really good about talking, at least to me and my husband, about his feelings. And if he is depressed, since we're both struggling with that now, there's this kind of 'code thing' that we talk to each other about depression.

Ben: We can tell when each other is depressed. Super powers.

[*They laugh.*]

Meg: We've been blessed and I think a lot of that is because we've been open and forthright with each other. We've been willing to share, of ourselves and our stories. He's a bright kid, so even at nine, when he was being diagnosed with it, he was part of the process in learning what it was.

I've learned that I have to advocate for my child. That it is better to be open about it and encourage him to be open about it. We try to be supportive. We've had our arguments because *I'm* so stressed about school this year. The way his teachers talk about him makes me feel really good. And also for me, I learned as a parent, my mindset has to change. Things may not go as I've always thought they would go for Benjamin. We may have to shift gears a little bit. Accepting that, and being okay with that, and supporting him in that.

I'm going to have to learn to deal with it

Ben: It's hard to say what I'd tell other kids. I think just, "Keep going. You'll learn how to deal with it better." My tics are worse now than they've ever been. But I'm more accepting of my Tourette's than I've ever been. I don't bring myself down as much because of it. I bring myself down for other reasons, but I'm like, "My Tourette's I'm going to have for the rest of my life. I'm going to have to learn to deal with it." It's nothing that will ever go away, so I have to accept that. That makes it easier.

I went to the Youth Ambassador Program[32] and they taught me a lot about Tourette's. Soon I'm going to middle schools and elementary schools around the area to talk about Tourette's. I'll go into classrooms and talk about how it feels to have Tourette's and what it is.

Meg: Yeah, the Youth Ambassador Program. We went to the TSA conference in Washington, D.C. They gave him a formal presentation he can use as a base, but adapt it to who he is. And then he took a trip to Capitol Hill and talked to a representative, staffers, and senators.

Ben: I put my story into it. Like when my tics started, when they got worse, how they are now, and when my coprolalia started. I can deal with it, but it still gets in the way of daily things. I've found ways, like instead of the F-word I'll say, "Fuh."

Meg: When we went to the TSA conference, it was the first time we were around people with Tourette's. He made some really great friends. He's going to Georgia to a summer camp, Twitch and Shout. But he definitely picked up some tics at the conference. It's like crazyville, 'cause they're all shouting things and doing things. One night at dinner he started knocking and the girl next to him started knocking, somebody at the other table said, "Who's there? [*she laughs*]"

More like a community now

Ben: It was weird. I was like, "Other kids with Tourette's!" For a while, whenever they'd tic I was like, "What are you doing?" And then... "Oh, yeah [*he laughs*]." I'm not used to it, seeing other people. Having Tourette's is more like a community now, rather than just by myself.

Meg: I felt that way too, meeting moms. And now we've got friends in Ohio and Arkansas that we're texting. You know, my friends try to be empathetic, but they don't get it. Whereas other moms that are dealing with it, or dads, do get it.

There was a lot of training for parents as well. Particular things I've learned, like when we're applying for college, make sure in his personal statement to address this semester, what was going on. That was helpful.

---

32   See tourette.org for program details and how to apply.

We've talked about different medications. And we were encouraged to go back on the IEP.

We're on Tourette groups on Facebook, so that's good, being able to give advice. We went to a couple of support groups, but his tics weren't that bad, so we didn't want to *make* them bad. We thought, "These people are way worse than we are." Now we're in a different ballgame. We met the group leader, they're doing social things, there's a lot more to get involved with. That's huge for us.

My husband and I now go on a date night every Friday night and have a couple of cocktails. That's kind of what gets us through... [*she laughs*] through the week. Looking forward to having alone time on a Friday night.

Don't just give us your disapproval

Meg: So anyway, Ben was bad before we went to the conference in D.C., but he was a lot more animated when we got back. And I said to him, "Was it wrong? Should we have not gone to D.C.?" And he kept saying, "Please don't regret it, mom. That was the best week." He said his tics weren't worse, he just picked up some new ones [*she laughs*].

Ben: Oh, and on Capitol Hill, when we went through security, I had the urge to say, "Bomb."

Meg: You know why? Because somebody told a story about one of the kids had gone to the airport and he kept saying, "Bomb, bomb, bomb."

Ben: I was going [*softly into his shirt*] "Bomb, bomb, bomb." Once I had gone through security, I went by myself in a corner and said, "Bomb! Bomb! [*he laughs quietly*]."

Meg: But it was hard in the airport because he was ticcing like crazy. And on the way back, the airplane, there was a woman sitting right there, she looked at him and... eye contact, and he said, "I'm sorry, I have Tourette's." And she said, "That's what I figured." But a guy in front of us just kept half-turning around. You know, turn *all* the way around so we can tell you. Don't just give us your disapproval. What's bothersome is when people are not giving him eye contact.

It's magic

Ben: To relax I play basketball. It's a big stress relief. I'll go to the park, I'll go to the gym, and play pick-up games. People there, I don't have to explain that I have Tourette's because I don't think I'll cuss a single time, or maybe a single twitch.

Men: Tell about the free-styling.

[*They chuckle.*]

Ben: It's kind of embarrassing [*he laughs*]. My friends and I, a couple of buddies, we do this thing called free-style rapping. It's like, think up rhymes off the top of your head. When I'm doing that, I usually don't tic at all.

Meg: His friends pointed that out.

Ben: It's pretty fun. It's so challenging. I don't know how it works. It's magic.

CHAPTER FOUR

DISABILITY AND SOCIETY

I spoke with a woman who, as a child, was ticcing on the school bus when kids tried lighting her hair on fire. Ridicule, shun, attack: by and large, and throughout history, this conduct has been society's response to the differences of others.

Intuitively we know better. All major religions teach the unity of human beings. Science proves the same. The great physicist Richard Feynman called humans "atoms with consciousness, matter with curiosity." It's not a metaphor that we are all one.

And yet, so often, we see nothing but differences.

In this chapter you'll hear from four individuals who feel that by creating "The Other," society loses contributions from some of its most creative members.

We are responsible for one another. Our language helps us understand this. If you break down the word *responsibility* it becomes *response-ability*. Our challenge, as individuals who form a society, is to respond to one another with open hearts and minds.

TS—Treat Society. That is Bill's interpretation of the acronym TS and his message to the medical community and the culture at large. Meds are right for some Touretters, but coping strategies, support at home, and other sociological and psychological approaches build self-esteem in a child. If the ambient response to disability is acceptance, then where is the disability?

BILL
48 years old

I had to be strong and do things on my own

In junior high, I was diagnosed with TS by a neurologist. He treated me with Haldol. I remember taking it for the first time and my tics were completely suppressed. I was in Toronto at the Hockey Hall of Fame, and I was able to stay focused and read the displays without ticcing. Then, for some reason, after two or three weeks, the tics came back. So for me it worked very short term, but I stayed on Haldol for *years*, probably unnecessarily.

I was embarrassed and humiliated by my symptoms and would constantly try to hide them at school and at home. Unfortunately, my brother and dad teased me, and this led to more anxiety. I used to hide out in my room a little bit, to escape that. But in terms of my self-esteem, I was a good student, I had a close network of friends. And, in general, my parents were supportive of me.

I had no school accommodations, no interventions to help with teasing. So I had to be strong and do things on my own. Nowadays the medical community might be doing some harm by over-accommodating parents. Both parents and kids need to learn coping skills, and to be assertive with issues that come up with school, for example.

I couldn't hold it in any longer

To be honest, I did get beaten up, too. There was a lot of stuff that happened. One of my favorite tics, in elementary school [*he chuckles*], I would go outside... you know, there's a window in the classroom looking out to the yard where we played. The window glass has putty around it, and my tic was I'd pick the putty off. I couldn't stop myself. And I would get into so much trouble. So I decided, "I won't go out to play for the entire year." When I was older, I remember working on a paper for weeks. But you know, you can't finish it. It has to be perfect. You erase and rewrite. I handed it in and it looked like a tornado hit it. I remember how frustrating it was because I worked so hard on it.

Yeah, this was in Kansas, early-80s. I remember my Bar Mitzvah, when I was thirteen, in a pretty religious temple. It was a service that lasted three hours. There were maybe 250 people watching me up on the stage. I had to suppress all my tics. For *three* hours. Basically I was just trying to get it over with. So finally, I couldn't hold it in any more and, [*he laughs*] you know, with tics you just have to release it. It was during a prayer, and I couldn't hold it in any longer, and I said, "F— God." [*He laughs again*]. I was completely in shock after I said it. It was a *big* release. And it was humiliating, of course. I never talked to anybody about it afterwards. I always wanted to ask the rabbi what he thought. My parents never mentioned it.

Some of the doctors I saw were role models

Academically I was a good student, and I had confidence because of that. I was also a competitive athlete. Some of the doctors I saw were role models. I eventually went to medical school in the Midwest and finished up in New York. When I finished my residency in psychiatry, I was recruited to do a Fellowship for a couple of years. It was learning how to design and implement clinical trials. Fortunately, they were running several medication trials focused on TS, ADHD, and OCD. They needed a psychiatrist, so I began the rotation. I worked with one of the largest Tourette syndrome clinic populations in the country. I would see patients clinically during the week and do research at the same time. One of the studies involved trying to locate the genes for Tourette's[33].

---

33   Almost all cases of Tourette syndrome probably result from a variety of
      genetic and environmental factors, not changes in a single gene. However,
      there are two uncommon mutations, SLITRKI and HDL (histamine), found
      in a small number of people with Tourette's.

PANDAS is a true entity

We also started investigating PANDAS. That's Pediatric Autoimmune Neuropsychiatric Disorders Associated with Strep. Some of the first cases were presented to Sue Swedo at NIH[34], where she treated children using plasmapheresis[35]. The idea is that an autoimmune reaction to strep affects the basal ganglia, which influences motor activity, learning, and emotions. This can cause acute onset of anxiety, OCD, tics, and other behavioral and emotional symptoms, about three to six weeks after the strep exposure. I believe I had a true PANDAS reaction when I was a child.

Initially this was controversial, but now I think most experts in the field would agree that PANDAS is a true entity, and merits future research to help diagnosis and treatment. The NIH is conducting a couple of trials, looking at immune-based therapy, as well as plasmapheresis.

I think some immune therapies seem promising. Plasmapheresis might be a little risky because of side effects. Antibiotics work, but I do not think kids need to be on antibiotics continuously. Right now the recommendation is to treat strep throat immediately, and hopefully this will decrease the chances of a PANDAS reaction.

We're watching all these people leave

I'm like many physicians with Tourette's, who go into the field to help others. Sue Levy Pearl[36], from the TSA, told me numerous M.D.'s have this condition. I feel the obsessive-compulsive characteristics are conducive to detail-oriented and perfectionistic types of work, like being a doctor.

It wasn't until medical school that I wanted to specialize in Tourette's. I did an elective in child psychiatry and became more focused. I went to a couple of TSA National Conventions, which piqued my curiosity. Here were leaders in the field giving presentations about the latest research and treatment. That was inspiring.

---

34   National Institutes of Health.
35   A process in which the liquid in the blood, called plasma, is separated from the cells. In sick people, plasma can contain antibodies that attack the immune system. A machine removes the affected plasma and replaces it with good plasma, or a plasma substitute.
36   One of the founding members of the Tourette Syndrome Association (now Tourette Association of America at tourette.org). She was the liaison for medical and scientific programs.

At one conference, I overheard a couple of experts in the field say that medications just don't work for TS. Both of these people were involved in the tic community for at least 20 years. Like them, I believe some medications do initially work, but there is limited data that they work long-term.

I definitely felt at home during the TSA conventions. It was cool to be among all these ticcers. And you know what? I realized I had a mild case. A friend of mine from Toronto, he's a doctor who specializes in Tourette's. His vocal tics are probably the worst I've ever heard. It was the saddest thing. We went to a restaurant in New York, and his tics were so loud, most of the people left. I felt so bad for him. It's terrible. We're watching all these people leave. On the other hand, despite his tics, he went on to get his Ph.D.

The other good news

I've been in private practice for fifteen years. I wasn't sure, even after the fellowship program, if I wanted to specialize in tics. But I was curious. I had TS, I could definitely help others who had it. I could empathize. I'm pleased to be a role model for some patients. They're interested to get to know me. We share stories. Right now I see adolescents and adults. I specialize in ADHD and tics, mood disorders like bipolar. I only have a handful of ticcers.

With Tourette's patients, it helps to remember how it was for me. I feel like I'm helping a friend, or my own child. I don't want anything to get in my way. I want that patient to have the best treatment. The kids coming through the research clinic, I'd say a large percentage knew I had Tourette's. So I'd talk with them about it. Hits to self-esteem, being embarrassed, humiliated, misunderstood, being punished for your symptoms, coping with symptoms, all this can be addressed by relating my own experience.

The other good news, of course, is that about seventy pecent of kids outgrow their tics as they get older, especially in their early twenties, due to brain maturation.

It's true that if the family and school are supportive, friends are supportive, a child's self-esteem can be pretty good, even with bad tics. I think self-image has a lot to do with the culture in the family. I see kids all the time whose self-esteem is low. They're embarrassed, humiliated, have difficulties functioning socially. It's interesting—in the clinic we looked at teasing as a target for meds. So it's, "Are you being teased? Okay, we'll give you medication." I do not think that's proper treatment. Obviously we cannot use medications to help with social issues. You have non-medication types of interventions. Coping strategies probably would be first-line treatment. You're also talking about getting accommodations for school, educating teachers, issues with family dynamics.

He did well mainly because of the culture around him

I had a 16-year-old female patient who had a simple eye-blink tic. She was on medications for mainly social reasons, where looks are very important. She definitely did not need medication, and I spent a lot of time trying to teach her that. But she did not want to tic, and was adamant about taking Clonidine.

Then I had a 35-year-old with severe Tourette's, who had painful tics affecting his neck and head. He was always breaking his glasses, and had a special deal with the local optical shop for getting replacements at a discount. He had no accommodations at school. I think academically, and at work, he did well mainly because of the culture around him. He lived in a small town in New York. He was able to endure without treatment because he was accepted as a family member and a friend. Pretty much everybody around him was socialized to be supportive.

As a doctor, my prescription has always been to treat Tourette's by treating society

I think for some patients medications are effective. But there are bad side effects, especially the risk of tardive dyskinesia[37], even with the newer meds. There are a few medications where the side effects aren't that bad, but from my standpoint, we have to be very cautious giving out meds. I think we, the medical community, probably have been overprescribing, especially the Big Guns, like Haldol and Risperdal. I think these should be used as a last resort, for painful, violent tics. I think we should focus more on effective social interventions.

As a doctor, my prescription has always been to treat Tourette's by treating society. That's my version of TS—Treat Society. It's a cultural

---

37   A difficult-to-treat and often incurable disorder resulting in involuntary, repetitive body movements.

change. This is huge. There needs to be a shift from meds to psycho-social interventions. Teaching communication and coping skills, dealing with kids in school, assertiveness training, networking, school accommodations. If kids come through with severe tics, definitely I recommend meds. But we should be very, very conscious of when we prescribe these medications.

I think the TSA does an amazing job educating everybody. I'd like to see them put even more money into education and less into basic research. Focus on what's going to help patients in the near future. As far as searching for a cure for TS, what if some of these symptoms are advantageous? I'm sure there are some adaptive features you don't want to manipulate. Many doctors have some obsessive-compulsive symptoms. It's part of our profession.

This whole idea of needing to 'fix' TS kids is off base

You have to learn to live with your tics for a while. They're either going to go away or lessen in your late teens, early twenties. You have to learn coping strategies. The thing I keep going back to is the meds work only mildly, and side effects can be incredibly bad. So my belief is the best way to treat Tourette's patients, or people with disabilities, is to treat society and not so much the people with disabilities. Again, for me, this is what TS stands for—Treat Society.

This whole idea of needing to 'fix' TS kids is off base. What's important is listening to their stories and giving support. Support as they grow up, in school, in relationships, at work. I want to educate everybody about disability studies. It's a new way of thinking about Tourette's, a move away from medication and research. The Tourette's business will take a hit, but we have to challenge the view of Tourette syndrome as a deficit that needs to be fixed by modern medicine. We also have to explore the social, political, cultural, and economic factors of every single kid who passes through a specialty clinic.

———————————— ❧ ————————————

Of all the ways out of self-hatred, the surest vehicle is another's love. Andrew's wife began his healing, and his own accomplishments completed his release. He is not the only one in this book to complete that journey of reanimation. His new perspective taught him an important lesson: Tourette's is a natural thing. Disability exists only in the eye of the beholder.

ANDREW
37 years old

I was good

I was eight when symptoms first appeared. I don't think I got a lot of attention because of my parents' divorce. I think this is typical. They understand the kid's not going through a good thing and try to compensate and make things nice. But they were so wrapped up in their own stuff, I don't think they had energy to figure out what was going on with me. My parents didn't reject me, but they didn't understand my tics and the doctors weren't giving them any information. I wasn't diagnosed until I was twenty-one.

I was 'very energetic' [*he laughs*]. I had a lot of nervous tics, although it's possible part of it was the divorce. Until I was twelve, I went through a barrage of experiments on my father's part where he would offer me different incentives not to tic. He was a psychotherapist, and part of me as an adult had a hard time resolving that. That he was stuck enough in his own baggage he didn't realize I had Tourette's. He now says he more or less knew, but was going through so much he couldn't come to terms with it.

So he offered me money. I remember being in a toy store and him saying, "If you can walk around for five minutes and not do that thing, I'll give you a couple of bucks for a toy." So I'd go around the aisle, where he couldn't see me, so I could do my tics. And I'd come back and say, "I was good,' and he'd give me the money.

Down in flames

When my tics came on, I was in a small grade school that was sort of run by the parents. I have images of my dad building the play structure with other dads. I was in that school from first to fourth grade. Everyone knew everyone else. If I'd stayed there I probably wouldn't have had so many problems with confidence and socializing. But in the fifth grade I moved to a magnet school. There were problems as soon as I moved in. My tics were severe. I was coming out of my desk with these big arm movements. I couldn't contain it at all. My friend Tim went down in flames with me. He would have been the nerdy kid anyway. I remember a kid in class giving a presentation, drawing concentric circles on the board. "The inner circle is all of us cool kids, and there's the outer circle with all the losers, and then outside all the circles are Tim and Andrew." And everyone laughed. Looking back on it I think, 'Poor Tim.' [*He laughs.*]

I could have done with somebody telling me to tell those kids to go fuck themselves. Those were some of the stories that made me cry when I became an adult and got diagnosed. Kids who had parents or mentors present enough to say, "Those kids are idiots." And then to *say* that to those kids? It's amazing. But I was swimming in ignorance. I knew I couldn't control it, and I knew it made me different. I felt like there was something wrong with me, but I didn't have a name for it. And when I got the name for it, it was a big emotional weight lifted.

I decided I was like a thing instead of a person

So my school experience was pretty ragged. I had *a* friend, who happened to live across the street. I didn't have people over, I didn't go over to anybody's house, I wasn't part of any groups or included in social circles. I've talked to people who didn't have Tourette's who had similar experiences, where you feel like an outcast, but there was a different quality to how the kids related to me. It was more like someone with a disability. At some point, there was an aversion to teasing me that left a kind of quietness. I think kids were weirded out by me. The same way you tend to treat Special Ed kids. They tease nerdy kids because they understand nerdy kids. But you don't go around giving wedgies to kids with Down syndrome. You sort of leave them alone. You might make jokes about them, but what's the point of teasing them? I think this gave me a pretty bad view of myself. Plainly spoken, it's self-hatred. I think I decided I was like a thing instead of a person. That went on until I was in my twenties, when I met my wife.

Because she loved me

I had a lot of anger issues. It wasn't usually the big life stuff that threw me. I would have rage fits based on small things, tiny accidents like mismeasuring for a recipe. I would go off on myself and tear the place apart. I punched holes in walls. And I hit myself. I had a lot of self-injurious behavior. These were not tics. This was rage, self-directed, maybe exacerbated by my active, Tourettic brain, which allows you to obsess in little loops of self-hatred. It just piles up on itself

My wife, Melissa, was helpful in dealing with this. I'm a typical Tourettic person—I'm always on the edge of my seat, always have a comment. She is the opposite end of the spectrum. When I'd get frantic, she'd try to bring me back around. And she wouldn't blame me. She'd get mad if I hurt myself, because she loved me. Her love helped. And patience, probably. I think my wife has the right kind of energy that allowed me not to keep spiraling in those self-hating ways.

I came from therapists, who were unaware I had Tourette's. Her family's more straight-up, hard-core Philadelphia people. She'd say, "I don't care if you have Tourette's. But you can't flip out like that." It wasn't about talking. It was, "How can we change that?" She is about fixing what's not working, not talking about why it's not working. It got me down to practical solutions.

I got down off my horse

Because I had such a bad experience with school, another big piece of my changing self-image was going back to school. I think part of my self-hatred was that I felt I was broken and wrecked and wasn't going to be able to achieve anything. The first couple of times I tried college were failures. I didn't learn study habits. I just went in and tried to do the English and Biology or whatever and would fail at them. It wasn't until I went to the Learning Disability Center at Santa Monica College that things improved. The first thing they do is test you to gauge your ability to handle standardized learning. And of course, I scored poorly. But they immediately say, "This isn't your fault. You need to learn habits." So they teach you study habits.

They teach you that you have the right to bring a recorder to class. A teacher can't object to that. If they do, you refer them to the Disability

Office. This became empowering. I didn't want to be known as somebody with a disability, somebody who couldn't do it on his own. But I got down off my horse enough to let them help me. I really turned the boat around. I went from getting Fs or Ds to straight As.

I transferred to Humbolt State University for my degree, then moved back to Philly so Melissa could be close to her family. That's where we had our daughter, Maya, who is three now. Melissa and I are both practicing artists, and now she makes mobiles and kids' toys she sells online.[38] But at the time we were making our living being graphic designers and webpage designers. It was hard to make a living like that so I got a software development job. That wasn't very appealing—it was in a cubicle. I learned a bunch of programming, which ended up being beneficial. But I decided to apply to graduate school because my skill set was moving me toward cubicle work.

I wanted to prove I could do it

One of the things I made that helped me get into grad school was a thing called the Tourette-A-Tron. It's a device that allows people to experience what tics feel like. It's got an accelerometer, like in a Wii remote, and you wear it on your arm or leg or head with a Velcro sweat-band. It picks up motion. When you move a certain amount, it considers that as normal. When you move outside normal, it considers that a tic. You also wear an ear-bud that generates a very obnoxious sound in your ear. Then, in a random way, it brings the volume up gradually, like a Tourettic urge. You can ignore the noise, until it gets louder and louder and gets to the point where you can't hear anyone talking. But if you move outside your normal range, that's a 'tic' and the noise stops. And people report this wonderful sense of relief. It sounds a lot like how we experience a tic. And after a while, people even stopped noticing the sound coming on or that they were ticcing to stop it.

So what helped my self-image was my wife, doing well in school, and getting into grad school at Ohio State. It's why I don't like being associated with having a disability. This is coming up as I work on my thesis—not being identified as a Tourette's person. It would be irritating to me because I'm trying to prove I'm not dumb. And that worked against me in the Learning Disability Education stuff. That's where I would shut down

---

38   sqrlbee.com

and not get help. I didn't want to be somebody with a disability, who gets through class because he has a free pass. I wanted to prove I could do it.

There are tropes about Tourette's and that's what I want to pry out

This is a hot topic for me right now. As I write my thesis, I am trying to outline what my work is about[39]. It's difficult, talking about each piece I made over the last two years. I'm noticing these patterns—that I shut myself down from making work about Tourette's. I did make pieces about Tourette's and then, as I was breaking down a student show, another grad student said to me, "Oh, all your pieces are about Tourette's." You know, in this mock voice, with a little flip of the hand. I know she was being goofy, and she doesn't know how it's affecting me, and that I'm too sensitive. But it really messed with me. I didn't like how it felt when she said it, but I didn't own up to how it affected me. That encouraged me to stop using Tourette's as a theme. These little comments that make me feel, "I don't want to be the Tourette's guy."

Now, for some of my work-in-progress I've been collecting instances of Tourette's in the media. I think I've got every movie or documentary and TV episode that's been made. I have *South Park,* I have *Ally McBeal, Touched By An Angel, Seventh Heaven, Niagra, Niagra, Deuce Bigelow.* I have *Matchstick Men,* which never mentions Tourette's but it sure seems like the guy has it. I've got ten documentaries, six or eight movies. There are tropes about Tourette's and that's what I want to pry out.

Tourette's is a disorder of other people's perceptions

My wife didn't seem scared of having a child, given my Tourette history. We'd been married ten years, so we had ten years of dealing with my stuff and making it better. And from her perspective, it wasn't just a disability. It was also energy and creativity and a bunch of other things. And for me, at that point I'd managed to get over my hatred of it and of myself. I saw Tourette's as part of a... a rich life experience. All the other people I've talked to, who had weird problems or whatever, have the most interesting stories, anyway. They seemed to have the best perspective on life.

---

39   See more of Andrew's work at andrewfrueh.com.

The thing that's stuck out most to me in learning about Tourette's is giving somebody confidence to say, "You can't make fun of me for that. It's a normal thing. It's a disorder." It *is* a disability, and you should have the leverage to talk about it. Anybody who hangs out with somebody with Tourette's doesn't have a problem with it. It's always the people who've never seen it before or who don't know what to do with it. And everybody with Tourette's has friends and family who say, "I don't even notice your twitches." So it's mainly a disorder of other people's perceptions. And mainly those perceptions are thrown off by ignorance. So who actually has the disorder? That's what I've come to—Tourette's is a disorder of other people's perceptions.

Who would have guessed Matthew and I have in common attending British private schools in the Caribbean? We both survived, and benefitted from, that paradoxical mixture of high-level education and 19ᵗʰ-century treatment of children. One of my teachers would take his seat, light a cigarette (yes!), and, as we readied to review homework, he'd glare at us and say, 'If you have tears, prepare to shed them.' Andrew and I share something else. Our conversation illuminated my hidden response to Tourette's—the fear of calling forth the demon by saying its name.

MATTHEW
45 years old

A cool nickname

I was born in the U.K. but grew up in Bermuda. Tourette's was brought to my attention in Cub Scouts. I wasn't really noticing the tics, but clearly others were. I remember asking my mother what the word 'mental' meant. In one evening I had distinguished myself as 'the mental kid.' I thought I'd been bestowed a cool nickname, and it was with great enthusiasm that I shared the news with my mother that same night. She broke it to me as gently as possible that the other boys were teasing me. There was a fierceness there, as any mother would feel in defense of her child. She made it clear that, despite what others said, I was not, under any circumstances, crazy.

As my symptoms increased, I became more conscious of my condition, as did everyone around me. I started tapping my forehead with my knuckles and succumbing to a compulsion to duck-walk. I was making noises, which created a disturbance in the classroom. I was around seven years old.

The Pink House on the Hill

The 'experts' at St. Brendan's, the local mental hospital, suggested I stay for a while, an invitation my parents patently declined. Bermuda is known for its pastel-colored buildings, and St. Brendan's was jokingly referred to as The Pink House on the Hill. "That's where Matthew lives," the boys at school would say.

I felt very much excluded by my peers. School officials followed suit, on the premise that my tics were too distracting for me to keep up with other students. I was homeschooled for a time, but in the end, I insisted my parents return me to a proper school environment.

My symptoms increased in severity and variety, and the prejudice of my classmates took on a weight I hadn't experienced before. The whole point of returning to regular classes was to be around normal kids and feel more normal myself, but this proved too great a hurdle. This was the '70s, an all-boys school in a British colony, where it was routine for a teacher to strike a student with the boy's own gym shoe, and caning was also a popular method of correcting bad behavior. I took my share of licks.

Reluctant heroes

My parents were desperate for a solution. They arranged for me to visit specialists in the U.S. for several weeks at a time, only to return to Bermuda no better than when I'd left. I did have the good fortune meeting Dr. Donald Cohen, at Yale Children's Hospital. After learning I was a fan of Superman, he presented me with two phonebook-thick anthologies from Marvel Comics. One showcased heroes, and the other villains. Dr. Cohen explained how these heroes were social outcasts. Spiderman, the Hulk, and the X-Men had powers that were more like amplified medical conditions.

These people were all struggling to overcome the social displacement that comes from being too different. They hadn't chosen to be this way. They were reluctant heroes making the most of the special gifts they'd been given. Dr. Cohen let me draw parallels on my own between the plight of these characters and living with Tourette's. It was under his tutelage that I realized I had superpowers of my own, in my writing and drawing abilities.

This body of mine

By the time I was fourteen, I'd interviewed with several boarding schools on the East coast of the U.S. catering to kids with learning disabilities. My parents settled on a school in upstate New York. Classes were small, which allowed for significantly more individual attention. Gone were the tyrannical teachers and their corporal punishment, the school uniform, and the social stacking of an all-boys school.

My symptoms had also begun to dissipate. By senior year, I was as close to normal as a seventeen-year old can hope to be. I stood five-eleven, was physically fit, I even had a girlfriend. So this body of mine, the bane of my existence for so long, had become something I was proud of. But once I felt the freedom of being 'normal,' I put too much emphasis on it. I was always afraid of being found out because, even on my best day, I would still tic, even though it went largely unnoticed.

During my senior year, I returned to my old school on holiday break. There were a handful of teachers who had taken the time to relate to me and work with me, and I wanted to shake some hands. As I glanced out the second floor window, I clocked one of the old mob in the courtyard, a kid who'd coined some of the more stinging nicknames that had so fixed my identity. We locked eyes. He pointed at me, grinning, then bolted towards the other kids milling about on their lunch break.

The dude who descended the steps

I emerged from the building to find a small crowd waiting for me. News had spread that an old punching bag had foolishly returned, and there was fun to be had. They weren't prepared for the dude who descended the steps toward them. I was a head taller than most of them, stronger, and ready to tangle. I watched their grins drop. They just looked me up and down in silence, then someone shook my hand, and the questions started about boarding school, about the snow, and about all those girls. Nobody mentioned my Tourette's or made any reference to the old me. For the first time, these guys were showing me respect. I didn't even have to fight for it.

That was a profound moment, but not the turning point it should have been. Rather, it was all the more reason to hide, and fear, my Tourette's. Tourette's remained my dark secret. I never talked about it. My family never talked about it. You don't want it to come back, you don't want to jinx anything, so you don't talk about it. Because if you whisper the name it might… you know, knock on your door again. I was in my twenties before my family and I started talking about it. We were able to have conversations about that whole time, and the fallout from it, and why I might still be carrying apprehension.

There's so much more to a person than the immediacy of tics

I'd been trying all my life to adhere to a convention of normalcy that didn't suit my personality. I'd been trying to force a square peg into a round hole based on something that overshadowed the rest of me. Conditions like Tourette's can dictate what others think and how they behave toward you. What gets lost are the individual's nuances. There's so much more to a person than the immediacy of tics.

The tics have never fully gone away. As you get older, you get more responsibility and accompanying stress. There's been a resurgence of my tics over the last fifteen or twenty years. As a parent, as a divorcee, and the list goes on [*he laughs*].

When I was very young, I'd lock myself in my room and write and draw, write and draw, write and draw. In a fever. That was my out. But in high school, with the changes in me, I didn't feel compelled to run to that as much. Then I stopped creating altogether for a couple of years. It was only in college, after I committed to majoring in theater, that I picked up pencil and pen and tapped into that facet of myself again. And I ultimately went to art school and got my graphic design degree.

One glorious teardrop after another

I was invited to attend a Tourette's-based performance by a group called

Band of Artists[40]. I thought to myself, "Who'd want to see that?" I was still harboring my dark secret. But I decided to attend. The show started with a neurologist giving a short presentation on the history of Tourette's, followed by a split-screen video demonstrating how the dance troupe took tics and translated them into performance. One half of the screen showed a patient ticcing, and on the other half the dancers performed the same motion in unison, making it something beautiful. And that's when I started crying.

The performance hadn't even begun. That was me watching video of people experiencing different levels of tics, some quite severe, and many I'd forgotten I suffered as a child. So many things came back to me. A rush of childhood remorse. I was thinking about my parents, what they were dealing with, what parents now are dealing with. I had buried so much and for so long. And then I was watching the dancers unfold this tremendous performance—torment transformed into art. I shed one glorious teardrop after another. That night was the pivotal moment that had eluded me as a teenager on the steps of my Bermuda high school.

Something so beautiful

It was incredible. It lifted this whole veil I'd been looking at myself through. That performance completely changed the way I view myself—my Tourette's and Tourette's in general. Because they made something so beautiful out of it. Today I feel like I have a tribe. I have pride in the boy I used to be, and what he was comprised of, including Tourette's.

I've since had the honor of contributing to Band Of Artists on a creative level, producing animation and artwork for various shows. And another artist, who subsequently joined the troupe, told me it was one of my animated pieces that gave him the resolve to open up about his Tourette's with confidence, and draw from it much the way I had. Paying it forward feels good.

You learn your way

I have two daughters, eight and ten, and they both exhibit tics. My eldest asked me about ADHD, because her mother had arranged for her to be tested. And she said, "I know that you have it too, and that we're kind of

40   See Sutie's interview in Chapter Eight.

alike that way." And I said, "Here's the deal. A lot of people do things one way, and there are people who do it another way. Sometimes it takes the rest of the people a while to catch up to you, if you're doing something differently. You learn your way. Just because the rest of the world hasn't caught up with you doesn't mean it's the wrong way. As you get older, and develop your skills, as you develop as a person, you're going to find people like the way you do stuff. It's hard because it might not be a popular way now. But there are a lot of people, who started off being unpopular, who changed the world. So try your best to only worry about what you want to do. Don't fuss about what other people think you should be doing with your life. You should be too busy living it."

She didn't say anything, but my daughter's smile let me know she got the message. I hope everyone reading this gets it too.

Jaesy is blessed with a group of friends who have stayed loyal to her since childhood. When her Tourette's blossomed, this loving circle was her safe haven in times of stress. Her intimate, accepting society of pals shows us how the idea of 'normal' is simply what people make it out to be. I admire Jaesy for following her creative needs and feel confident that she will someday forge a career from her talents. I also admire her because she has courage enough to look at herself with clarity and honesty and say, "This is who I am."

JAESY
28 years old

That was jarring

I am South Korean but I'm adopted. Culturally speaking I was raised in an Italian-American home, but I do look Korean [*she chuckles*]. I grew up in suburbs, middle to upper-middle class, pretty much white and Jewish neighborhoods. My family is Catholic.

I didn't notice my tics as much as other people did. I don't know why. I guess the thing about tics is if you're not conscious of them they go by without you noticing. But it got really bad really fast. In first grade I made squeaking noises before going to bed and within a year it got terrible. We moved and I changed schools and started shaking my head very violently. That was pretty much my only tic at that point.

I moved from a neighborhood school where it was a lot more diverse in my class, with Indians, Asians, Blacks. We moved to a town where there were only four kids who were not white, including me, and that was *it*. That was jarring. This was in second grade.

About Tourette's, my story is similar to a lot of other people's—we didn't know what it was. We had no clue. It was sometime during second grade that I was diagnosed. I did go on medicine, but it made me sleepy and didn't do anything about the tics. I didn't want to take it anymore, so it was a joint decision with my parents for me to go off that.

Between second and fifth grade, my tics were mostly the head shaking, but it did become violent blinking also. Towards middle school, the head shaking went down and now I don't do it anymore. But as that became calmer, new tics came in to replace it, like facial grimacing. It got better in middle school/high school, maybe half as severe. Then in college it halved again. I still tic now, but since I was twenty-three or so it's been a pretty mild case.

For me, Tourette's helped me read people better

When you have Tourette's, you understand when people notice. It's very apparent. For me, Tourette's helped me read people better, what they were thinking about me. It's not what people say, it's also how they act around me. I truly do believe that a lot of people don't notice. But then I tell them and they notice. I can feel it. It doesn't change their behavior much.

Social life for me in school was smooth, kind of/sort of. I always had a good core group of friends. I'm very happy about that. The friends I made between second grade and into high school, they're still my best friends today. It was a group of maybe ten to fourteen kids. So they always accepted it. They never brought it up; it never seemed they were uncomfortable with it. The thing was, my other peers in school gave me a bad time.

A lot of it was in my head. I was way too sensitive. What I've realized is kids weren't necessarily making fun of me—eventually they did—but for the most part it was curiosity. So a lot of it was how *I* responded. I handled it poorly and it became worse. I should have done what I do now, which is explain it to people. That works well for me, makes me feel more comfortable. I know the result we're looking for is honest and open communication. That's generally the key to not being so much an outcast and to fitting in a little more. Getting in front of it.

I think one of the best ways a kid with Tourette's could succeed is to see other kids with Tourette's succeeding. To see that they can be good people, and can have good friends, and could love themselves.

If I could use my creativity to make a living, that would be tops

My worldview opened up a lot in the past five years, but I still don't know what I want to do with my life. In college, first I wanted to be in creative writing, then I went for film, then I went for English, and then science. Then I was on this kick where I wanted to do languages and translate. But you need to commit to something, and instead I would switch. Every time I got closer to any one thing, I saw a future I didn't want to be in. I didn't want to be stuck.

I'm always interested in doing a lot of things. I always have projects. I like to create. So I know that's the direction I want to go down. But it's tough to use your mind in a creative way and make money. That would be the dream. I don't even care if it doesn't pay well, but if I could use my creativity to make a living, that would be tops [*she chuckles*]. Ya know?

It's a labor of love

Right now my friend Josh and I are writing radio shows, parody scripts. It's a labor of love. Back in the days of radio, there were dramas. There was a show *The New Adventures of Sherlock Holmes*. We find that so funny. It's just such a backward time and it's ripe for parody. So we're writing our own Sherlock Holmes adventures and it's so bad, just like the radio show [*she laughs*].

Mostly I do music. I play a lot of instruments poorly [*she chuckles*], but my best is guitar. I play piano and I also play accordion. One of my dreams is one day to play accordion in some orchestra pit for a musical. But I'm more about lyrics. I record my music, play the instruments, make my own songs.

I was living in another town but gave up the apartment. I live with my mom currently, in the basement, which is nice because it's far away, so I can be kinda loud [*she chuckles*]. I have a nice little set-up to do music in my room.

It was a weird, lucky night

I think electrolysis would be a good job for me. It's laser hair removal. It's really good because I'm trans and that's a huge thing in the trans community—for any male to female—you gotta get rid of the body hair. And since I'm very much in the community, I have a clientele base already.

I didn't realize I was trans. I blocked it out for the longest time. I never humored it fully. But I know that every single day of my life I did tell myself, "Oh, I wish I was a girl." It was about the same as, "I wish I had a billion dollars. I wish I was an astronaut." It felt that impossible. I know now that it's a lot more achievable, but back then it did feel equally as impossible.

The day I realized I was trans, I was on vacation with my girlfriend. This is when I was twenty-three or so. My life was not in the best shape or place. I quit college and was starting to give up on stuff. I was in kind of a low place. I was drinking a lot more. But that night there was nothing bad going on. We were having a good time and suddenly I just started crying. Then I got really angry and mad. I didn't know why I was feeling all these emotions so intimately. And then I said out loud, "I wanna be a girl. I'm not a boy." I said it without thinking. Not like Tourette's. I said it but didn't know where it came from. In that one moment, everything made so much sense. It was a weird, lucky night. Then I could honestly start thinking about it. It wasn't blocked out anymore. I said it out loud and that was the most important thing. That was the first important thing I needed to do to become me.

You should love the person you are

My girlfriend was very supportive. She was one of my childhood friends. We eventually did break up. At the end of the day, it came down to she's not gay. By that logic alone, we couldn't be together. It didn't match. She wanted to be with a boy and I couldn't be that anymore. As far as my friends go, it's kind of a mixed bag. Some of them support me and really get it. In fact, all of them support me. None of them left me. I'm extremely lucky and fortunate for that to happen. In transitions, statistically speaking, you *will* lose family and friends. That's just the bottom line. I haven't heard of anyone I know in real life who hasn't lost a friend or family member.

As far as my friends go, some of them understand—it's like intuition. You say, "I'm a girl inside and that's just how it is," and they go, "Okay," and they feel it too. They *feel* it, you know? Then others are supportive but I don't think they *understand* it. We're good friends and always have been, so that does pull a lot of weight. But I think they feel it's a choice I made.

You should love the person you are. To think that maybe I could still be a boy and express my femininity, like be gay, that's not it. So they miss a little bit of the situation. It kinda makes sense because transition is extremely complicated and it *is* full of contradictions. So I'm a little more distant from some of my friends because they don't totally understand it. I do think some of it could be peer pressure. In this world I grew up in, it's not cool to be bigoted. Very liberal area. So if they feel something, it's not something they could say out loud without people thinking less of them.

For me, with my differences, Tourette's is the easy one

Tourette's gets better every year because knowledge about it becomes more available. That makes a huge difference. People are more open to listening to me and trying to understand Tourette's. But for me, with my differences, Tourette's is the easy one [*she laughs*].

I'm *in* transition now, so I didn't make the whole change. I did in terms of me presenting female. But as far as the way I look, I'm not completely there yet. You know, it takes a little time. I take estrogen and I also take testosterone blockers. So my hormonal levels are the same as a biological woman. I don't think it's affected my tics much. What I'm going through right now is literally puberty again, so it is a bit of an awkward time. Not like pimples, not like that [*she chuckles*], but awkward in terms of my looks. I'm slowly gaining female features and losing male features. Not ugly or off-putting, but just a little awkward, like not clearly a guy or a girl. Physically I actually do feel better with the hormones in me. They really do help align my body with my mind. I don't miss testosterone at all. It kinda feels awful to me—no offense [*she laughs*]. It's like what I *should* feel—estrogen really helps me feel the way I should.

I've wished society were more inclusive.
I guess that's our goal, to change it

Any time I've become confident in one area, it doesn't necessarily make it better in other areas. It took me a while to feel comfortable with the fact that I *do* have Tourette's. But that didn't help when it came to how I was different being Asian. You know? It took me a while to be proud of my race. But those two aren't helping in my strength with transition now. There must be some other thing I need to work out before confidence comes naturally. It's about trusting yourself. That's the goal.

I have pretty low self-esteem, but I hide it well. People tend to like me, people tend to want to be around me, and they compliment my confidence. But it's not like that inside. I'm hypersensitive to what people might be thinking of me. I get down on myself and compare myself to others, which isn't smart, but I can't help it. The word 'normal' comes to mind. One of the biggest questions I've asked myself all through my life is, "Why can't I be normal?" But what is normal? I don't know. Not having Tourette's, not looking different or being trans. Even with a career, I wish I could be like everyone else who knows what they want to do. But I've read about late bloomers and that makes me feel good. It's a first-hand example of how it's not a wrong path.

But I've wished society were more inclusive. I guess that's our goal, to change it. Through talking. I'm a big advocate in my everyday life. Not like marching in parades or writing blogs. I talk. I'm good at explaining things and getting people to understand things. If I can say something that rings true to someone, that could help for a more positive worldview, and if *they* say it to someone else, then I did my job. Just by talking.

CHAPTER FIVE

TOURETTE SYNDROME CAMP

I lived fifty-nine years before I met another person with Tourette syndrome. That encounter took place at the Kenneth Michael Staebler Tourette Spectrum Camp in California, as I began work on this book. As a child, I had never met another person like me, nor could I imagine one existed. I felt alone with my tics in the world. Even a correct diagnosis wouldn't have assuaged the loneliness of never hearing another person say, "I know how you feel."

Belonging is what Tourette syndrome camp offers. It's a chance for children to forget their tics (finally!) in the freedom and safety of an accepting community. With the ground cleared in this way, children find other, self-affirming qualities that distinguish them. They have an opportunity to believe themselves to be more than their tics.

This is why I feel Tourette syndrome camp can be more effective than medication to relieve a child's suffering from TS. Camp can form a foundation that allows a child to gain confidence and to build a happier life.

So next you'll hear from TS campers. They're happy because they delighted in the outdoor experience and camaraderie. And they're joyous because their lives changed for the better at camp.

For a list of Tourette syndrome camps in the United States, see Appendix A.

"We are a tribe." With these words, Shayna evokes a child's great relief at finding kindred spirits at a Tourette camp. For many kids it's the first time in their lives they've met someone else with TS. The doors of isolation burst open. They experience friendship, they experience sunburn and bug bites, blue skies and laughter. Tourette kids are liberated from fear, from suffering, and this freedom returns home with them. I believe, like Shayna, that Tourette camps are a wonder, indeed a necessity.

SHAYNA
24 years old

Being at camp normalizes the child's condition and their sense of the world

At the Tourette camp where I volunteer, we were told to say it's not a 'therapeutic' camp. If you use that word people think there are therapy groups, or that it's about making the tics better. Ours is a regular summer camp that fits the needs of a Tourette syndrome child.

Being at camp normalizes the child's condition and their sense of the world. We are human beings, we can have friends, we can enjoy ourselves, we can experience social interactions without bullying. This is the one week out of the year where someone with a difference can feel normal, like any other regular person.

Some kids have never been to camp before. Some have never been away from their parents before, or stayed with anyone other than family. Some kids are looking forward to it and when they get there, they realize the shock of their parents leaving them at the cabin.

It's the teenagers who make the decision to come. They'll fundraise to come, because maybe their parents don't support it, or are still in denial about Tourette syndrome. Teenagers will do that work to get to camp. Not only that—they stick around. They eventually become counselors and they'll do great things in the Tourette community or special-advocacy communities.

We put assumptions on other people

What's really cool about Tourette camp is we become like our own nation. It's a place where we're free to be ourselves, where it's weird to *not* have Tourette's, where we have our own social system. There are so many unwritten rules about tics. Most people on the outside would think it's a free-for-all, as if you laugh at any tics you want. But we have an innate understanding of when someone's having a tic and when someone is suffering.

There's a unique social structure, because most everyone is the 'freak.' We do have some kids who are popular and they're jocks and stuff. But at camp that hierarchy is taken away—the bully, the popular kids, the kids who socially isolate others. At camp you have no one to isolate yourself *from*.

However, the thing with isolation is that some of us cause our own. I'm not saying bullies don't bear responsibility—of course they do. But we have responsibility too. We put assumptions on other people that they're going to hurt us, and we push them away. So we can isolate *ourselves* just out of habit. The way to break out of that is by being proved wrong. Camp is a thoroughly good way to do that.

They leave with friends

What I find most striking is these kids have never spent an entire week of their lives without video games and Facebook. They're going to bed at night truly exhausted, in a good way. They're seeing in person that trees are green and the sky is blue.

A lot of the kids have OCD and never let their hands get dirty. But at camp they do. It doesn't mean they'll always do it, but at camp they did it at least once. And each of them is contributing to a community, the kind they don't have outside of camp. What kids leave with, besides bug bites and being sun-kissed [*she chuckles*], is they leave with friends.

The age range of the kids is seven to seventeen, which is extremely interesting because it falls into the Piaget criteria for theories of child development. At camp, an eight-year-old kid can have someone to play with. That's all they see—"I can play with whoever I want."

They take from camp, "I was able to do this." That opens the door for them to do those things again, because they experienced it.

They experienced friendship once, they can experience friendship again. And some of these kids truly have never experienced friendship before.

It's so beautiful

Friendship for adolescents is different. It involves sharing, and our kids share *a lot*. They share experiences of oppression, of being bullied, they know what it's like to suffer. And they share Tourette syndrome. That's a huge thing they can't share with many other people in the world.

So we see this camaraderie form among teenagers that's quite beautiful. They are very supportive of each other. We have some teenagers who experience mental challenges and the kids don't treat them any differently. They'll even be a little more patient and understanding. It's so beautiful, these teenagers. They're so incredible with each other.

What I call the 'side effects' of camp are things like feeling normal, friends, happiness, confidence, the ability to be yourself, acceptance of tics by other people *and* by yourself. There are positive role models in the form of counselors. These kids have a sense of community and teamwork, they experience their own courage and strength and gain new hobbies. And smelly laundry. That's what parents get at the end [*she laughs*].

We are a tribe

At a Tourette conference, a parent asked if they should send their recently diagnosed child to a TS camp or to a regular camp. A professional answered, "Regular camp." I was horrified. This is a child whose entire identity is changing because they have to include tics in their life. At a regular camp, they'd be in contact with people who do *not* have an understanding of Tourette syndrome. And be forced to live with them for a week? Can you imagine that? Without being able to go home and cry to mom if something bad happens?

It's my belief that if children are reinforced that they are okay, that tics are okay, and if they are in a place where they can be themselves, without fear of judgment, they will be better off. It's my opinion that being put with normal children sometimes is not the best solution. Sure there are wonderful children out there. But I don't believe it's best for TS children to *not* have the experience of being with their own people. We are a tribe. We need to connect with our tribe. We need to understand and know that it's okay.

Notice how often Sydney says, "Camp taught me..." She doesn't mean canoeing and bonfires. She's referring to a Tourette syndrome camp, where she experienced deep, personal insights. TS camp changed Sydney's life. This is why I believe that, in substantive ways, Tourette syndrome camps are more effective than medication at relieving the emotional stresses of tics. Kids and adults, all Touretters, living for a time in freedom and safety, discovering who they are and what they might become. Think of that. What would such a camp teach you?

SYDNEY
21 years old

You're one of the smart ones

My parents didn't know how to handle Tourette's. I was diagnosed around six and they said, "We don't think she has Tourette's." My mom dragged me from doctor to doctor [*she chuckles*] trying to get *any* other diagnosis, and it was always Tourette's.

My father grew up with epilepsy and could not get over that he had it. So he didn't accept that I couldn't control my tics. It was, "If you can't get rid of the tics, you can't do anything with your life."

It didn't matter how high my GPA was, it didn't matter how many friends I had or how many clubs I was in, how many hours I was working—it was, "You have Tourette's and you don't work hard enough at getting rid of it."

Going into sixth grade, my parents were told by a neurologist—a well-known guy around here—he said, "Based on the tics she's having, there's no way she's going to make it in school."

No one thought I would get good grades. But that gave me the determination to say, "No. Fuck you. I'm going to do this. Just to piss you off [*she laughs*]."

Tourette's taught me to set my mind on something and get it done. At the end of high school I was taking AP classes and I graduated with honors. A kid came up to me and said, "Emily, you're one of the smart ones. Can you help me with this?"

I need to meet another person with Tourette's

I went to Argentina for a year abroad and my parents said, "This will be your year to get rid of your problems." I was terrified I'd get sent home because my parents told me, "If you tic in front of your host family, you're gonna get kicked out of the program." That fear made me suppress until that was all my brain would do. I shut down emotionally, my sensory system shut down. I would blank out all the time. My mom told me to sit on my hands and all my weirdness would go away. But Tourette's doesn't work that way, and that's when I started to question my family's view, and accept my TS.

I realized this wasn't a choice. I didn't choose to have Tourette's. Then I heard about Camp Twitch and Shout and thought, "I need to meet another person with Tourette's." So I applied to be a counselor and was accepted. I ended up doing that for three years.

Tourette camp was a life changing experience for me

One of my co-counselors said, "Why aren't you ticcing?" He could tell I was suppressed. I told him I'd never ticced because my parents had decided it was a choice. I believed everything they said. They said, "Parents who don't love their kids let them tic."

It was this huge concept—you're just ticcing? I didn't understand why people were letting themselves tic. You're *supposed* to hold back. Tourette camp was a life changing experience for me.

My turning point was seeing the kids at camp. I saw how people were able to live having Tourette's. I wanted a healthier attitude, and that's what I saw people doing. I saw that if I could be out, I would have a chance at a better future. Then you'll have a husband, you'll have a boyfriend, you'll have friends—you're fine. It's not a big deal.

I definitely had trouble learning how to let my tics out. Definitely. Even alone. I was uncomfortable letting anyone see my tics. I was uncomfortable not suppressing. I had to learn it's okay to let people see. That took at least a year and a half of hard work. I looked up to people who were out and spoke about it. I wanted to be like them.

Camp was my only Tourette support system for awhile. Then I slowly came out to my friends, and they are amazing.

CBIT is not a cure

When I was a kid I always wanted to go home. I couldn't understand, because I was at my house. I was home with my parents but felt there was an emotional home for me somewhere else. It didn't make sense. When I went to camp, a lot of those emotions became valid and things in my life made sense. I saw that people were ticcing and knew I wanted to live my life that way. So my emotions became valid, which was huge.

I had always felt rejected. At school I was the weird kid, the different one. My dad used to say, "If you tic, it's so weird that no one will be your friend." So in fourth grade my parents had a therapist teach me how to not tic using CBIT[41]. In a way, that was my saving grace because I learned how to make it look like I wasn't ticcing. Learning those techniques is how I was able to make it through school.

But my parents decided CBIT was a cure for Tourette's. It's just a coping strategy to deal with what life has given you. CBIT is not a cure. If you think it's a cure, that's detrimental and harming. When you redirect a tic, it doesn't look like you're having one but your *body* is still having a tic.

Suppressing is like tearing your muscles apart. You still feel like you have Tourette's, even though your physical symptoms don't look as bad. If you're suppressing all day, you're going to have that bad tic attack. People didn't see it, but I could have a tic-attack that lasted from half an hour to, high end, six hours of relentless ticcing until I fell asleep.

So I would recommend CBIT, understanding its limitations. But at the end of the day, the best thing is the people around you accepting your tics.

If you tell someone, you give them the opportunity to be compassionate

You see some of these kids at camp, the transformations in them, it's beautiful.

---

41   Cognitive Behavioral Intervention for Tics. See tourette.org for details.

It's stunning to see them *finally* not be the only one who has to deal with it. They bring home this new-found confidence. Camp teaches you you're not the only one. You have a friend, maybe he lives in Iowa, but he's a friend you can text or call and say, "I had a really bad day." You can tell him things other people wouldn't understand. That's why community is so important.

Camp teaches you how to tell people you have Tourette's. I learned that if you can't tell anyone, no one knows what Tourette's is. If you tell someone, you give them the opportunity to be compassionate. That was a turning point for me, also.

Camp taught me to not be ashamed. It taught me I could be proud of it. And it taught me there was a lot of good that came out of it in my life. In a way it made me a better person.

At camp I learned how to accept my Tourette's and be okay with it. I saw there was a possibility to *not* be ashamed of my Tourette's. It's not a bad thing, it's who I am. Camp taught me how to embrace that.

I have, and a lot of people with Tourette's have, a very high patience level. People ask, "How are you so patient? How do you never raise your voice?" And I say, "It's Tourette's."

Tourette's taught me that you have control over your mind and over your decisions. It taught me to look at the bigger picture and to look deeper. It's insightful. Coping mechanisms I learned for Tourette's transferred easily into adult life. How to be determined. How to do things people didn't think were possible.

—⁂—

Add Molly to the long list of artists—among them Willie Nelson, Ry Coder, and Carole King—who have recorded an album of original music in Austin, Texas. Intelligent, dedicated to learning, she's a role model for kids in the TS camp where she volunteers. She urges every child to attend Tourette syndrome camp, where they will meet their peers. Tics fade to the background and children are free to recognize other qualities in themselves. Molly acknowledges the strength Tourette's has forced upon her, noting that her tics often cause people to underestimate her, and this serves as motivation for her to excel.

MOLLY
24 years old

Trade-off

I was four when a lot of my tics started. My parents said it was after I had strep throat.[42] They used to joke, "I hope she doesn't have Tourette's." I started doing a lot of vocal tics and my parents diagnosed me themselves. They're both clinical psychologists, and it was, "Uh oh, I guess she does have Tourette's." My parents told me recently they had decided they'd never put me on medication because of what they'd seen kids go through. They said they'd homeschool me if they had to.

I loved school so much, and it became so important to me, I insisted on taking medication in order to go. I was desperate. I had a lot of bad experiences with meds and my parents never wanted that for me. But I stayed in school. Trade-off. I loved it, probably because I felt it wasn't a given for me. A lot of kids hate going, but they take it for granted. For me, sometimes I couldn't go because I'd be having such a bad day. I loved it when I could go.

Tics and ticks

When I turned nineteen, my tics got much more severe. I was on the ground flailing. I was non-functional. I couldn't walk or talk or feed myself

---

42   PANDAS is Pediatric Autoimmune Neuropsychiatric Disorders Associated
     with Streptococcal Infections. See Bill's interview, Chapter Four.

or bathe myself. It seemed to come out of nowhere. That time is kind of a blur now. It really affected my parents. My mom felt a particular brand of helplessness. She tried lying on top of me to make me stop seizing. That didn't work. Just really scary. The only thing my doctors could think of was brain surgery, and I did *not* want that.

I went to a top Lyme disease doctor. What we found is I had worked at a summer camp when I was nineteen, and that's when my severe symptoms started. He tested me and I had Lyme disease. Mosquitoes and ticks, some people they don't bother, but they always go after me. I get tick bites all the time living in Missouri [*she chuckles*], which is kind of funny—tics and ticks. But yeah, a lot of the weird movements I thought were tics were actually pseudo-seizures. We think Lyme could've exacerbated my tics. I've been on antibiotics since I got diagnosed and I'm a lot better. I went to college at University of Missouri and transferred to Stephens College. I had one year left, but because of the Lyme disease, I've been taking time off, trying to get my health back on track.

I don't understand how that's okay

I've realized I don't like feeling weak. I like to be independent and do everything myself. So having mobility taken away was frustrating. Now, every time I can do something, even if it takes longer, or I don't know how to do it, I prefer to do it myself.

I feel people underestimate me a lot. Or they assume I'm incompetent. I always have to prove I'm not weak, for some reason. I'm kind of paranoid that people will think I'm incompetent because of my disability, and I have to prove them wrong. Maybe it's having to prove to *myself*, because I've been limited.

My tics are subtle right now. But when they're not, people stare, they say rude things. I usually take the higher road and ignore them. I used to have a thin skin and I'd get upset. When I was in high school, every time someone made a Tourette's joke—which was, for some reason, really often—I would get a panic attack and have to leave. If you don't have Tourette's, you don't realize how often people make jokes about it. So every week I'd miss a day of school because someone made a Tourette's joke.

I found it necessary to get a thick skin. I wouldn't be able to leave the house if I wasn't tough enough to handle people staring at me, people yelling, "Retard!" I don't understand how that's okay, but it happens. I try to not acknowledge them, but it makes me mad.

Do I dare finish?

I'm a singer-songwriter, play acoustic guitar. The past few years since I had to take this hiatus, I recorded a CD in Austin, Texas. Just finished this last month. One of my dad's best friends is a songwriter and he mentored me. His friend owns the studio I recorded at, and they helped me. We sat down and did arrangements for the songs. It was really fun. And we called in musicians they know in Austin. Yeah, it was really cool. The last step is artwork. And for some reason, I'm taking so long with it. I don't know if I have problems finishing things, or if I am holding on to it, like do I dare finish? It's not even a hard step. I'm just freaking out about finishing my CD. The title of the album... it's either "Nothing Is Enough" or it's going to be self-titled.[43]

He's going to talk about Tourette's

In eighth grade, I was at a Youth Group convention. I never told anyone I had Tourette's, even my closet friends, until recently. So I was with some friends from Youth Group, and the organizers said, "We're going to have this speaker today." And I don't know why, I had this feeling, "He's going to talk about Tourette's." I just *knew* it. I knew it before it happened. It was Marc Elliot, who is a motivational speaker. He talked about Tourette's and people thought he was so cool. That's the first time I thought maybe Tourette's is an acceptable thing. He told us about his Tourette's and some of his experiences, and how we should accept people with differences. After, I went up to him and said, "I have Tourette's too. Can I have a hug?" I was nervous, but it felt so nice. Throughout the weekend he'd come up and ask, "How're you doing?"

That's the first time I met someone with TS. And then, I was maybe twenty, I went to the National Tourette Syndrome Association conference in D.C. and Marc was speaking. I wrote him on Facebook before I went, thanking him for that talk and how it helped me as a kid. And in D.C., we hung out with him, me and my mom, the whole weekend. I gave him a demo CD of my album [*she laughs*].

---

43   Available at http://mollytrull.bandcamp.com.

That's what I'd recommend to any kid with Tourette's—go to a camp

This will be my fourth summer counseling at a Tourette's camp. Camp was when I met people with it and learned so much about myself. Not just having Tourette's and who that made me. I started to find out who I was in *spite* of Tourette's. I found parts of me that had nothing to do with Tourette's. In camp, when everyone has Tourette's, you realize, "This is what makes me uniquely me." It's interesting. If everyone has Tourette's, then what differentiates us?

The camp I work at is Camp Twitch and Shout, in Georgia. We had this guy from Dateline Australia who made a documentary about us[44]. It's beautiful. I cry every time I see it. It does a good job of showing the joys and also the dark parts of Tourette's.

A lot of my camp kids are Youth Ambassadors for Tourette's. I would've loved to be a Youth Ambassador, but I'm too old. When I was in school, I always wanted to get involved. I wished I could go to a Tourette's camp and meet other people. That's what helped a lot of kids I know, meeting other people with Tourette syndrome. It helped their confidence so much. That's what I'd recommend to any kid with Tourette's—go to a camp. Try to meet someone else with it. That helps you feel so much better, and not so alone. Just being able to bitch about how you hate your tics and have someone understand, 'Oh, I had that one too."

Back to the real world

Being a counselor at a camp for kids with Tourette syndrome, I notice compassion. It's crazy how much these kids feel, and how much they've been through. I love these kids so much, I can't put it into words. At camp I usually have thirteen- to fifteen-year-old girls, and a lot of people would get really scared when they hear that, I think [*she laughs*]. Oh my God, there's going to be so much trouble and drama. But no. These kids, it's amazing the things I witness.

I've worked at other camps that were sleep-away. At one of these, there was a girl who was developmentally challenged. She was in a group with thirteen-year-olds and they shied away from her and left her with the

---

44   See the documentary at missionmanmedia.com.

counselor, and never included her. That same girl at a Tourette camp, you wouldn't even have to talk about it with the others. She'd be part of the cabin, she'd be included in everything. All the girls, there's so much love outpouring from them.

Going to Tourette's camp helped me develop a sense of humor about it [*she chuckles*]. I think I have a dark sense of humor. It helped me become more okay with having Tourette's myself. And also, getting used to people acting like jerks, I guess. As I got older, too, I feel like I just didn't care as much.

The Tourette campers feel so at home and accepted, they're always sad to leave. I remember, I was on airport duty and some of the kids were ticcing [*she chuckles*]. A few people in the airport were staring at them and one of the boys said, "Well, back to the real world, I guess." It's not like camp anymore, where everyone's making noises and no one's noticing or looking at you funny. Now people will stare at them.

You are such a strong person

My tics have been mild lately, thanks to a biofeedback machine I've been using called the Ondamed[45]. That's a huge relief. I've also found meditation helps with tics. Breathing exercises. I think they're originally for anxiety attacks, but I use those. Playing music helps me calm down. Laying in bed, sometimes [*she laughs*]. Changing my diet. We've been looking into that. Certain foods might set me off. Finding triggers like that. Also, as a woman with Tourette's, I think tics are more tied to your hormones. Tics flare up around our period, and that's what we talk about at camp in the cabin. We talk about when we have our periods our tics get so much worse.

It's hard to keep going sometimes. There are going to be hard days, but there are always going to be good days too. I never take a good day for granted. The fact that you are still alive and here, that you have Tourette's syndrome and are living with it, means you're so strong. That's something I've come to realize. People don't understand how it makes you such a strong person. You can handle so much.

We don't often realize how much we can handle, how much is thrown at us on a daily basis. We have to deal with so much, on top of having tics. We're multi-tasking all the time. Pouring a cup of coffee, with tics, that's

---

45   A naturopathic treatment using low-frequency pulsed electromagnetic fields.

a huge challenge, if you think about it. So you are, with Tourette's, just the fact that you *have* it, you are such a strong person. That's something to always remember. That's an accomplishment.

I admire individuals who see a need and find a way to satisfy it. Maybe it's the same impulse and energy Scott uses to run marathons. Whatever its source, he harnessed that power to create Tourette Syndrome Camp USA, and he's been changing children's and parents' lives every summer since 1994. He has seen firsthand how TS camp brings confidence and hope to entire families. I also was struck by his daring sense of humor. After the first date with the woman who would become his wife, Scott found what must be the world's most inventive idea for a second date. I'm sure it sealed the deal.

SCOTT
51 years old

I turned to him and said

I worked at a YMCA camp when I was in college, Camp Lakewood, Missouri, on the north end of the Ozarks. I did a lot of growing up there. I remember talking to people about how I would love to do something with Tourette syndrome and camp. This is like 1984, '85, '86.

In February of 1990, I come home, it's a cold evening, Chicago, I get a message from a program director I'd worked with. He was now director at a camp in Virginia and he'd signed a contract to do a Tourette camp. He said, "You always talked about doing a Tourette's camp. Now you've got the opportunity."

So the next five summers I volunteered for a week. This camp was not as much fun as the one in Missouri. I got some staff from Camp Lakewood, and they agreed it was not the same. Then, on my way to a resort area in Lake Geneva—I went there after camp to recover—I passed a YMCA camp. I was with one of the volunteers, I turned to him and said, "I gotta stop talking about a Tourette camp. I gotta start doing it."

They thought I was nuts

By this time, I was President of the Tourette Syndrome Association of Illinois. My board said, "If you want to start a camp, go for it." They thought I was nuts [*he chuckles*]. About five weeks later I presented to the board, "I got a contract for a camp." Then they *really* thought I was out of my mind.

The camp has become Tourette Syndrome Camp USA[46]. That first summer, it was myself and a volunteer, who was there part of the week. We had thirteen kids. The following week, I did the Virginia camp, and realized I cannot do two Tourette camps anymore.

We did it differently from Virginia. There they had kids, their least amount of problems was Tourette's. They had bipolar, all the associated disorders, and then some. So we screened kids more closely. And it took a while to bring on staff. We don't take volunteers without experience, like Virginia did. They had staff walk out in the middle of the night. Plus, the one in Virginia was run at a fundamentalist Christian camp, which is all right, but you can't ask twenty kids with ADHD to sit and do Bible study for an hour and a half.

The camp I found, Camp Duncan, was more interactive. They just want the kids to be kids. That's what I liked about it. Sixty percent of their programs are 'special-needs camps,' so that made us a good match. I don't think they knew what they were getting into. Me either. But here we are, twenty-one years later, and it's almost like clockwork with them. I mean, forty to forty-five kids with Tourette's is never smooth, but yeah, the structure works real well.

The inspirational, emotional reason I started a TS camp here in Illinois is I got damn tired of driving a day and a half to Virginia [*he chuckles*]. I can't give you a heart-warming reason why. I thought there was a better way. And I was tired of driving.

One week at camp and kids get fifty-one-weeks' worth of confidence

The advantage of Tourette's camps is that kids learn they're not alone, and they meet other kids like themselves. They develop camaraderie and

---

46   tourettecamp.com. For a list of Tourette syndrome camps in the United States, please see Appendix A.

friendships. They also find some coping mechanisms. One week at camp and kids get fifty-one-weeks' worth of confidence.

We keep our kids very structured during the day. We might do a rap group, but one thing we do not do is workshops. We do not bring in speakers. The kids learn from being at camp and having fun. And from our staff being role models.

Most of our staff have come up through the program. That's one of the most unique features of our camp, compared to other Tourette camps. Not only have we been around the longest, but a lot of our staff comes from within. We get a lot of campers or adults who want to be staff members. But if they can't deal with their own Tourette's, they can't help a child deal with it. It is the role model. I want kids to see that getting older, you can succeed, you can enjoy what you're doing. And for younger kids to understand that it does get better.

Sometimes it's hard for parents to figure out what's a tic and what's not. In camp we deal with this too. We're sometimes not sure, but we try and muddle through. Some kids with Tourette's [*he chuckles*], they use it to get out of trouble. Hearing some of these stories is humorous, even though they shouldn't be doing that.

For parents, it's important to see that their child isn't going to be in the basement until he's fifty years old. They can have a satisfying life, a productive life, and not be isolated. Yes, I know it's tough, but just keep chugging away, hang in there. You'll find something to do in life, something of meaning.

Camp helps children accept Tourette's

The way parents and kids respond once they get a TS diagnosis, it varies. I've got families, the kid accepts the diagnosis, the parents can't. Or the parents accept the diagnosis, the child can't. But I think parents do eventually come to some acceptance of it. Not often, but I've had parents who drop the kid off and the wheels are squealing to get out of there as quickly as possible for a week's respite. I get other parents who, I can't get them to *leave* camp.

Camp helps children accept Tourette's. That's the feedback we usually get—the child is much more confident. They're not as scared to make friends. And again, the end result is seeing these kids grow up. I've got one alumnus who's a doctor, a couple are teachers, one's an engineer. That's what tells me we've made a positive impact.

A lot of these kids suffer from isolation. I had that myself. I didn't have time to get a relationship. Though I was helping hundreds of other people, the camp was actually a negative. So even though I was a successful adult, doing all this great stuff for kids with Tourette's, I had my own isolation issue.

How about going to an opera?

I was in therapy for relationships for almost ten years. If I hadn't spent all those years in therapy, I don't think I'd be as open as I am today. I just got married, in September of 2012. It was nice, after getting married, to be able to fire my therapist [*he chuckles*]. My wife and I met on eHarmony. I was looking through all my choices and I saw this person, her name was simply the letter A. That intrigued me.

Yeah, I was nervous. I broached Tourette's on the first date. My profile picture, I had the Tourette camp shirt on, so that was a give-away. Aimee likes the theater, the arts, and I don't. On our second date she said, jokingly, "How about going to an opera?" I sent her a link, "How about this?" I'm a big fan of Star Trek—it was a Klingon opera [*he laughs*]. They do *A Christmas Carol*, that Christmas story with the ghosts, but they use Klingon characters and they speak Klingon, and they've got subtitles on the screen.

Seven families

My symptoms started when I was seven, and I was diagnosed with TS before my thirteenth birthday. When I was diagnosed, no one had ever heard of Tourette syndrome.

I grew up in the All-American, state-of-the-art dysfunctional family [*he laughs*]. The Tourette's caused a lot of friction between my mother and father. Why was I doing this? After I was diagnosed, the big argument was whose fault it was. It doesn't matter! Growing up, it wasn't solid, but we muddled through.

Then there was an article in the paper that my parents, and five other families, saw about another family dealing with Tourette's. Once they read the article, my parents never worked more cooperatively, trying to get in touch with the other families. My mother kept bugging the reporter for names. My father worked in purchasing at a major hospital in Chicago, so he went to the medical director, who said, "I've never heard of this. Let me see what I can do." It took him a month and a half to find the Tourette Syndrome Association in New York, and two doctors here in Chicago who knew anything about it. And those seven families founded the Tourette Syndrome Association of Illinois. That was way back in 1976.

I'm doing it through the camp

If I were to write an autobiography, I would call it, "Excuse me, sir, do you need a tissue?" Because of my tics I get, "Do you have allergies? Do you have a cold?" I used to say, "Yes, my allergies are bad." I was in an urgent care office last week, someone asked if I needed a tissue because I was sniffing, and I said, "No, that won't help."

It's not the denial method, but I'm not here to educate the world *all* the time. I'd go insane having to do that. That may be counter to a lot of things you hear, but that's just the way I found to deal with it. I spend so much of my life dealing with Tourette's in this camp. I've got other things in life than to educate the world about it. There are enough other people doing that. I'm doing it through the camp.

What to do when the child is good and the behavior is bad? These are the opaque situations that arise for parents of kids with Tourette syndrome, OCD, and other comorbids. Interestingly, the extreme stresses Jonathan underwent as a parent taught him patience and tolerance. I also find that, if Jonathan, a surgeon, and his wife have difficulty deciding about medication, it highlights the conundrums faced by non-physician parents. Frequent visits, monitoring, and good communication with physicians and psychiatrists are keys to success.

JONATHAN, ABOUT HIS SON SAM (13 YEARS OLD)
at Kenneth Michael Staebler Tourette Spectrum Camp

I went out and read five books

My son, Sam, was diagnosed at ten. He developed tics but they were relatively mild. The way we got the diagnosis was that both my wife and I figured out what it probably was. We went to a neurologist who said, "This meets the definition and here's some medicine to take." We were looking for something more substantial. But getting the diagnosis was a sigh of relief. I went out and read five books and that helped. Now I had a name for it. We felt empowered to get the right kinds of help. And I think we did, although it didn't forestall a big crisis.

I think Sam gets his OCD from me. It's actually an advantage for a surgeon, where calling someone compulsive is a compliment. But gradually Sam's OCD has gotten to be more of a problem. When he would make a new friend he would then feel compelled to threaten that friend. He would obsess about the new friend and then have this compulsion to disrupt the friendship. Also, it got him expelled from school, which further exacerbated the problem because all the friends were now barred to him.

And then it gradually got better

He was home, just rattling around being miserable—he had a right to. He would wake up crying and go to bed crying. He would talk incessantly about school and friends he was barred from. My wife and I were talking about homeschooling, putting her career on hold, that kind of thing. We didn't end up needing to do that. But it was certainly very dark and stayed dark for a good several weeks. And then it gradually got better. Gradually. Having seen Sam come through the dark period, we can face other dark times, if they occur, with much more confidence.

He's made a lot of progress since then. He's got counseling, we're getting him behavior therapy, and we're getting him medication. A while ago I would have given some years of my life to picture Sam fifteen years in the future, self-confident. Didn't seem like it could happen because he was such a wreck. But now I can kind of picture the future. And seeing people at this TS camp, with some of these high-functioning, successful adult Touretters—that's inspiring.

A high level of self-esteem

It seems a lot of successful Touretters you meet are people who have found their way to a higher level of self-esteem. I think from the parents' point of view, that just requires showing love and support, even when applying discipline, and even when applying pressure. It's critical for a kid's self-esteem. I heard a girl here at camp say that her dad told her, "I want you to know that you can do anything." And I use those words with Sam. We think of things he might be better at and things he might be worse at, but we do say, "You can do anything and you do not have an overwhelming disability."

This isn't the first time he's met other kids with Tourette's. We've been to a local TSA support group and to this camp twice. He was looking forward to coming back. The way he looks forward to things is to say, "This is stupid, I don't want to do it because it's a disruption in my schedule." Anything that's a disruption is automatically a problem. But then, when he remembers what he actually did here, he enjoys the prospects.

We went through crises of confidence about the medications

It's very hard to tell what works with medications or behavioral therapy. None of it forestalled the crisis. When this business of threatening other kids started, we thought we were on top of it. It escalated despite our efforts and despite the efforts of the professionals. And it ran its course in a very destructive and unpleasant way. So I don't know what's working and what just seems to help. It's hard. You have to decide what seems to make sense and then deal with it.

Someday I would love to have Sam off medication. Some of the stuff he's been on has been pretty worthless. He's now on Fluoxetine—Prozac—for the OCD. He's on Abilify for tics. And he's on Concerta for attention deficit. And he's doing better in school with those medications. It's often hard to know with the passage of time if it's maturation you're looking at or if it's the meds.

We go through crises of confidence about the medications. We went to some pediatric-medicine-type folks, who said, "It doesn't make sense to be on three meds at high doses." We got the impression that it's the custom of child psychiatrists to use medications on an individual-case basis. Like Abilify for tics is widely prescribed, but it's not FDA approved for tics. Child psychiatrists tend to be more comfortable with polypharmacy[47] than pediatricians. And they tend to use medications *they* think work regardless of whether the literature says it works. So we're reconciled to that.

Psychiatrists who go to TSA meetings are comparing notes, things that haven't been published, coming to conclusions about what seems to work, and trying it on patients. So sticking with your psychiatrist is key. And frequent visits are key. I made a resolution I was going to work a little harder to pay for Sam's care. We've been paying cash for his psychiatry and behavioral therapy, and it's hard if you can't do that because you don't get the frequent visits. It seems medical treatment for TS is labor intensive.

Having faith and taking the long view is key

We have four children. We noticed we were obsessing over Sam, and the fact is we wanted to treat all our kids equally. It's hard to when one child has special needs that seem to override the needs of the others. But you really shouldn't. That's part of mainstreaming all your children, if you can use that term within your own family. You don't want to view them, unless they're critically disabled, as the ones who require more attention than everyone else.

We're trying to adapt our family customs to what Sam needs and what we need to maintain peace. Sam's got the room at the end of the

---

47   Taking multiple medications at the same time to manage coexisting health problems.

hall where he can be when he wants to go to a private place. We used to be upset that he'd go behind a closed door and disappear. Now we think it's okay.

Also, we don't get nearly as excited as we used to. I'm more tolerant since Sam has come along. I'm more mature. I'm better with my patients. These experiences have been good for me. I've gotten a little more spiritual. I attend religious services more regularly than I used to. I've gotten some refuge and support there. Whatever faith you have, it's good to have it. And to try to strengthen it.

I think having faith and taking the long view is key, especially when you're angry. Sam has these rage attacks and what it elicits in the normal person is more rage. I try to take a deep breath. That probably helps *him* because when he sees the person he's talking to doesn't escalate the confrontation, it tends to de-escalate.

We, as a family, are feeling more successful

When Sam gets teased for his tics, he can pretty much hold his own. I don't know how he got there. He's got some basis of self-esteem. And I'm hoping that he will get to the point that he will be a spokesman for himself. He's gotten a little older and wiser, and maybe more mature.

So we, as a family, are feeling more successful these days. And I think that reflects in Sam being able to tell someone who's teasing him—he still uses bad words—but he can also tell them, "I have Tourette's. I can't help this. Don't bother me." I don't think he's developing a thicker skin, I think he's getting more articulate.

Sam had his bar mitzvah. We're trying to mainstream him in that sense as well. And so you read this long thing in Hebrew and learn the cantillations and he used his OCD abilities to study that material. He learned it cold. When it came time to read it in public, he was in a black mood and decided to sabotage it. It was sort of embarrassing and also heartbreaking. But the way the community viewed it was as a kid with a disability doing his darned best. Everybody clapped him on the back with tears in their eyes and said, "That was an inspiring experience for us."

Do a little bit of work on it every day

I think you can find happiness and fulfillment in many places. Our general approach to Sam's interests is to encourage them and also not be too critical when he drops something. We found that to be counterproductive. We cannot help placing familial expectations on Sam and we're trying to equip him for success. And we are trying to modify our ideas of what constitutes success for Sam. We hope that he will get married, we hope that he will be able to love and be loved, that he will be able to be satisfied. For him our hopes are more general, more fundamental. We want him to be able to love and be loved and feel fulfilled on a daily basis. We want him to be independent. There are a lot of good things to do in the world.

I would remind parents of the success that people with TS have. I would remind them to look around and notice that sub-clinical psychiatric and neurological stuff is everywhere. Their kid is not disastrously different. And I would remind them, as I have to remind myself, to take the long view. Do a little bit of work on it every day is a good idea. We like to say that we're not compelled to finish the job, but we are also not free to desist from it.

CHAPTER SIX

EDUCATION, ADVOCACY, AND ACTIVISM

TS—Treat Society, advocates Bill, a psychiatrist with Tourette's (see Chapter Three). He believes teaching society to accept people's differences should become a first-line treatment for Tourette's.

We must educate people about Tourette syndrome. We must advocate for tolerance of differences. We've got to stand up to work for changes in the law and public policy, alterations in workplace attitude, accommodations in school, funding for research. No child should be backed up against a wall and bullied. No adult should suffer indignity or prejudice at the hands of others. There are legal rights we need. There are human rights we deserve.

My dear friend Jack Healey[48] writes about rallying people to work for human rights: "To those with nowhere to turn, I say rise up. Believe in your own talent when you feel weak. Believe in your dreams and make them a reality. I know you will produce plays and poems and art and music and be able to step into the breach when needed. Take your place. Demand your rights and protect others that need help."

It begins with education, advocacy, and activism. It's on us to help each other. We are the ones who must Treat Society—TS.

Here are stories from those who are rising up.

---

48 *Create Your Future: A Memoir.* Jack Healey is Director of the Human Rights Action Center. Find him at humanrightsactioncenter.org. He is also the former Executive Director of Amnesty International USA.

Kevin responded to Tourette's by writing his story and encouraging others to do the same. Helping others, that's his spirit. Kevin's story illustrates how maddening, and sometimes crippling, tics and co-morbid conditions can be. He now grapples with the frustrating balancing act between having tics and working with side effects of medications. People so misunderstand Tourette's, many say they would choose tics over side effects. Little do they know. So what a role model Kevin is, living in hope as he does, and working to get the word out about TS.

KEVIN
44 years old

I wanted to raise awareness

My mom suggested I do research to find if any books had been done to show the spectrum of Tourette's. I wanted to raise awareness and thought an anthology was the best way to do it. There were a lot of books about Tourette's, but hardly any of them were written by people *with* Tourette's. Writing about their own experiences, most people I got for my anthology said it was like therapy for them.

For my own story, a lot of things happened to me that have happened to no other person. My mom went into the hospital for a cancer treatment when I was six years old. When I was finally diagnosed at age twenty, they said the stress of seeing her in the hospital, not knowing if she was going to live, brought out the tics, probably. She was weak from the treatments, so my dad tried to raise us, but he wasn't used to it. He was working a full-time job, but at least he tried. Then my mom got better and she was able to take care of my brother and me, and my sister. But the treatments killed her at sixty-four.

333

I had never been a good student, but was able to get along. When I was seventeen, I started making lists of things. I would make a list of cars, or NBA basketball teams. I was obsessed with making those lists. I couldn't study. Many times I'd be up all night. I didn't want to do it, but my brain made me. I didn't tell anyone about the lists. I thought because I didn't know why it happened, they wouldn't either. They'd think I was crazy because I had thoughts in my head.

When I graduated from high school—I barely did that—I started having trouble. It was almost like dyslexia, but it wasn't. I would read sentences backwards and forwards until it seemed right in my head. I tried to go to junior college but had to drop out because I was making lists constantly. I started being obsessed with numbers. If I was obsessed with the number 333, I would do every single thing, my daily activities, like brushing my teeth or combing my hair, it would be 333 strokes. Or I had to write down 333 things on the list. If I couldn't, I'd be up all night. Eventually the thoughts subsumed every activity. The biggest number I thought of was 555. It was always a multiple of the same number, an odd number. Luckily, big numbers didn't happen that often. Usually the numbers were like 111.

Kinda useless

My mom heard a radio program talking about Tourette's. So they took me to a neurologist and I was diagnosed right away. I was glad there was a name for what I had. They tried all the treatments, like Haldol, Klonopin, and none of them worked. And my Tourette's, the tics were still really bad. Orap was the only one left. I tried it and it works, but it gives me bad side effects. I don't have a clear mind, like cognitive dulling. I'm really tired all the time. But the tics are gone and the OCD disappeared a couple of years after I started medication.

Right now I'm a high school swim coach. It's a small team, a private school. None of the kids know I have TS. I don't have tics, so they don't know. Only my folks and friends really know. And people who read my book. I'm gonna coach soccer with my best friend in the fall. I've been coaching for many years and we always get a couple of teams every season, ages nine to twelve. We always get girls, for some reason. That's who needs coaches the most.

I'm on disability, so I can only work a certain amount. Many jobs I can't have because of the side effects of the medication. All these years, before I knew I had Tourette's, I would get fired or had to quit because of it. Same thing, once I was taking pills. So all these jobs were bound to fail from the minute I got them. It made me feel, I don't know, kinda useless.

He'd crumple it up

My mom was the only one in my family who stood up for me with Tourette's. My dad just says, "I don't want to talk about it." I'd print out stuff I wanted him to know, he'd crumple it up and throw it on the floor. My brother and sister are the same. They say if they had Tourette's, they would handle it a lot better than me. That's my family for ya.

They said I used Tourette's as a crutch. I don't think I ever did. I admit, I've been bad to the family. There were underlying causes. That's what I always tell 'em. My neurologist says I have Oppositional Defiant Disorder. I have learning disabilities and mental illnesses that are undiagnosed.

They think I don't go out of the house or get a job because I'm lazy. Even though my dad sat there with me in the disability hearing. He was shaking his head like he didn't believe what the guy was telling him.

Everybody should do their part raising awareness

I do a lot of things to keep myself busy. I like writing, playing soccer, I like to sing, and I write songs. I took a songwriting class and whenever I feel like doing it, I sit down and write whatever comes to mind. I'm taking vocal lessons now.

I live in one of those residential hotels in Oakland. It's not the best area, but it's all I can afford, so… I'm doing the best I can. Hopefully the books—I didn't write them to make money, I wrote them to raise awareness for Tourette's and OCD. But making money from them would be nice.

I wish I had been more open about my Tourette's when I was younger. I hid in a cocoon for a long time when I was first diagnosed. If I had started telling people about it twenty years ago, when it was very misunderstood—I mean, it still is—I would have been getting the word out all this time. I think everybody should do their part raising awareness.

They don't know what it's like

Sometimes I isolate myself. The medication makes me so tired, there are a lot of times I just can't go out. But I'm a happy person, and if I was able to, if I didn't have side effects, I would be out all the time. Sometimes my doctor takes me off the meds to see if the tics are better or worse. It only takes a couple of days before my tics are back full force. I would never want to go back to how I was before I took meds. I don't think I would be here today if I was back like that. I would have killed myself. There's no way I could have… I mean day after day, multiple tics every two or three seconds.

There are many things I can't do now, but before meds I could barely even eat. I couldn't have a job, I couldn't have friends, I couldn't have a conversation. There are so many things I couldn't do then, that I can do now. Whenever I tell people how it was before medication, and how it is since I've been on, they say they would rather not have been on medication. They don't know what it's like.

Everybody's given talents

But I'm a happy guy. Yeah, pretty happy. I think I am, yeah. I mean, there are my books. I can't write every day because sometimes I'm just too tired. But usually I write a little every day. I play soccer three or four times a week. The swim team's gonna end pretty soon, but that's fun. So I consider myself to be happy.

As far as kids with Tourette's, I just say that everybody's given talents. Try different things because you never know what you're going to be good at. I've learned about having hope. If you don't have hope for a better future, or hope of improving, then there's way less chance it'll happen. There's a better chance it'll happen if you believe it'll happen. A positive outlook. I used to be kinda negative, but that doesn't help anybody, especially yourself. But if you have hope, are positive about things, there's a good chance things'll work out.

Chris characterizes the spirit of accepting, even welcoming, challenges. He's got a muscular spirit and an inspiring message. I imagine his rich baritone voice ringing out in classrooms, lecture halls, and on stage. Becoming a stand-up comedian is his unique contribution to advocacy and education about Tourette syndrome. (A personal note: In describing the difficult life of a standup comedian to my mother, I mentioned how exposed they are on stage, the loneliness of travel, hostile audiences and hecklers, the cold-sweat of having a joke bomb. As innocent and self-conscious as she was, mom intuitively understood the risks of stand-up comedy and she added sympathetically, "And all that standing.")

CHRIS
38 years old

I'm on this Earth for a reason

I battled Tourette's and OCD all my life. I battled addictions. I couldn't get out. So I had a decision to make—was I going to walk alone or was I going to walk with God? And I surrendered my life to God. Within a short time I was substance free. When I got delivered from substance abuse, I realized I'm born with a disability. No one's gonna owe me anything in life, no one's gonna give me nothin'. I gotta accept I have Tourette's.

I said to my wife, "I want to be a role model out in society." I have a gift to make people laugh, so I decided I was gonna take a comedy class. I had to face my fears. And God revealed to me, "Put Me first in your life and I'll show you that you can do anything." So I went up in front of the class.

I'm on this Earth for a reason. I have Tourette's and I have the gift to make people laugh. I intertwined the two together. I could talk about Tourette's *and* educate people. I never wanted to be a regular comedian. I wanted to be an inspirational comedian. I wanted to be a Tourette comedian. If we can get the world to know what Tourette's really is, things would be so much easier. A person with no arm, people know what it is. With Tourette's, you're not different, you're not an alien.

How are you going to be good at something unless you do it?

In that class I finally honed a five-minute set, and in the comedy world five minutes is like eternity. At comedy clubs, someone famous will show up and they'll put them on, even if they weren't scheduled. So, it was like my third show ever, and Darrell Hammond from *Saturday Night Live* showed up, and they put him on. Then Judah Friedlander from *30 Rock* showed up and they put *him* on. He does a lot of crowd work and they were really into him. Then I was up. I was scared. It's like going on after Celine Dion. But you never want to say 'no' in the business. The crowd was still high on Judah and I went up and I bombed. But I *did* it. I learned from it. How are you going to be good at something unless you do it?

I don't use Tourette's as an excuse

When I got off stage, I knew it had nothing to do with my Tourette's. People weren't staring at me because of my disability. It was because I didn't do what I set forth to do. I wasn't prepared. It takes practice. You learn on the fly. I don't use Tourette's as an excuse any more. I don't. I look at every situation as a learning experience.

I made it to the top, to Caroline's on Broadway. People came up to me after and said, "Chris, I didn't know that about Tourette syndrome." I was educating them. Wow. I'm entertaining and I'm inspiring. What better thing to do in life?

Then I produced my own show. I got in contact with Craig Carton and his Tic Toc Stop Foundation.[49] He sends kids to a Tourette camp once a year, Camp Carton. He also raises money for awareness and research. I gave all the money from my show to him.

They gave me a hockey stick instead

I was very, very blessed as a child with a supportive family. My dad had OCD, but he'd say, "Chris, it's all in your head. Don't think about it." But people don't realize the more you mention Tourette's, the more we tic. It's better not saying nothing at all.

Growing up with Tourette syndrome, my jobs were very limited.

49   tictocstop.com

Coming out of high school, I wanted to be a cop, but who'd ever give me a gun? They gave me a hockey stick instead [*he laughs*].

I was very active in sports because when I was part of a team, I felt I didn't have Tourette's. It's the camaraderie. You're a *team*. I got very involved in roller hockey. At first, no one wanted to let me play because I was small. But as soon as they let me play, and I started scoring, people started believing in me. And you know what? It was just like Tourette's. When I got accepted, I could excel. A year later, I was captain of the team. That goes to show that practice makes perfect. I finally joined the U.S. Dek Hockey National team.

Light a light in a dark place

When I speak in schools, I deliver a strong message of what Tourette's is. I make it fun. I give kids a story of hope. Everyone battles something. But look at me now. I'm not rich and famous, but I'm successful. I tell people, "I'm only a minority because the world makes me a minority." I'm videotaping my presentations 'cause I can't be in every state. So schools can purchase it, and—you know what?—it's gonna save lives.

I'm making a website, it's called TICS—Tourette's Inspirational Champion Speaker. That's me. Schools, churches, anyone can contact me to speak. Businesses can hire me to motivate their employees. What separates me from the rest is I do a comedy show for the first ten minutes. I get the crowd loose, and then I motivate them.

I play a game when I go into schools. I say to the class, "Whenever I say the word 'Tourette,' stamp your right foot." Because unless you do it, you don't have an idea. And I'll say, "Tourette. Tourette Tourette Tourette." Some people laugh, but you know what? They're getting an idea of what it's like.

Light a light in a dark place. That's one of my favorite scriptures. I got troubles, I got Tourette's, I battled addictions. I know that. But if I focus on that, I'm gonna kill myself doing it. The first half of my life I battled disability, and now I accept what I have. I'm substance free. And I'm taking everything I was blessed with and using it to my advantage.

Find what makes us happy in life

I used to get beat down a lot, and bullied as a child. Kids in my school, they scared the teachers. When a teacher turned their back, kids would mock me. I'd make a joke, because what was I to do? You fight the demon in your mind and you can't win.

I see what kids go through. When I look at the world, there are no positive role models. I had so much to offer kids, but I didn't have a voice. So I set forth to become that person. When I wrote my book,[50] I didn't realize what transpired for these kids. I recently posted on my Facebook page and my website[51] that 4,400 kids a year take their own lives because of bullying. People see disabilities, they don't know what pain it causes. I tell people, yeah, I have Tourette's, but we all have something.

I tell kids, "We're born with good and bad. The bad is we're born with disabilities—we're all born with something. The good is we have gifts and talents. We all gotta find what makes us happy in life."

Are you cooking naked for me?

I met my wife in an online dating site. It got pretty serious, and we started calling each other. I had a joke that I was going to cook naked for her. So she called my house one day, thought it was my cell phone. My dad answered, she thought it was me, and said, "Are you cooking naked for me?" My dad said, "Excuse me?"

My mom's dream was to swim with dolphins, so I took my parents and my wife to the Dominican Republic. And mom fulfilled that dream with me next to her. She was laughing, she was like a little kid. My dad's like, "Okay, let's get this over with." Then we went to swim with sharks and stingrays, and my dad, he just jumped right in the water. There are sharks in there and he's like, 'Okay, whatever." Very tough, old Irish-German.

I have a story that could save lives. In my book, I wrote things my wife didn't know about, my parents didn't know. When my dad read it, he broke down in tears. My *dad*. It's about how I battled Tourette's, how I battled substance abuse, and inspiration at the end. I wrote it to give people hope.

---

50   *How God Saved Me: My Inspirational Story* by Christopher Fox on amazon. com and barnesandnoble.com.

51   chrisfoxcomedy.com.

❧

Daniel is irrepressible. He speaks rapidly, plunging into topics, he digresses, he returns, he chuckles, he consults his mother on details. His speech is emotional and his message is gratitude—for life, for his family, for his creativity, and for the opportunity to spread the news about Tourette syndrome.

DANIEL
43 years old

Why is it so quiet?

I grew up most of my life in New Jersey and we were close enough to where we could see the New York skyline. On 9/11 we could see the buildings burning. The smoldering for weeks after. I lived right near Newark airport, which was for the first time ever shut down. The silence was deafening. Why is it so quiet?

If you went over to Hoboken, the view of Manhattan was breathtaking. It's where they'd film a lot of movies. It was picture perfect. You could almost reach out and touch the skyline. Somebody said as the wind blew, weeks and months later, you got the scent of death. It made me cringe. I had never needed an anti-depressant, but after that I did.

My mother is my guardian angel, my rock

My mother said I was born smiling and never stopped. My personality shined past my Tourette's. My older sister said, "There was nothing that came Danny's way that he didn't conquer." I didn't think of it like that. You know the deal; it's just survival.

My sisters and I went to a Catholic school and the principal, a nun, became good friends with our family. She did what people should be doing today—she educated every class about Tourette syndrome. She said, "If you cough or sneeze you can't control it, correct? Think of Tourette's like that for Danny."

Growing up it was love, it was support, my family. Any broken home disturbs me, but for someone with Tourette's, I can't imagine. My mother is my guardian angel, my rock. Not everybody has that. She didn't have the internet back then so she did things on foot. She went to the Board of Education to get me into a special school, where I was among peers. I didn't have to explain myself. I never felt so comfortable, and I graduated from there.

Not that life is easy, but it's easier

I was a guinea pig on medications from five to twelve, then we stopped all the medications and I went through a remission for about ten years. Symbolically it felt like I came out of a coma. By the time the tics came back, they were mild. It was like, "Okay, I can deal with it [*he laughs*]. This is nothing." I have none of the emotional scars others have. I'm blessed, I have to say.

The only thing I hated was on one medication I blew up like a balloon. That's common. But I'd rather have that than emotional damage. I got a lot better and moved on. To be able to button my shirt, tie my shoes—things that were difficult as a kid—I'm good. I can drive a car, get a job. Not that life is easy, but it's *easier*.

I consider my story nothing less than a miracle, which is why I'm doing a documentary.[52] For inspiration. It was time.

This is what I was born for

I've always been an artist, I've always done creative things, and it's therapeutic. A lot of Touretters get into the arts. There's definitely a pattern there.

I had done a lot of background work on films. I did *The Basketball Diaries* with Leonardo DiCaprio and Mark Wahlberg, I did *City Hall* with Al Pacino, I did *Copland* with De Niro and Stallone, *Law & Order*, *West Wing*. But I didn't want to keep doing extra work. I didn't need to be another Tom Cruise, but I wanted to make a living at it. This is what I was born for.

Mom always said, "Don't use Tourette's to take advantage of things in life." So with the documentary I thought, "I'm *gonna* use it to my advantage, but in a positive way." Not only for exposure for myself, but for others as an inspiration. That has taken off so strongly. My newest saying

52   Daniel continues working on his documentary called *My Life, My Story, My Tourette's*. More information at mytourettemovie.com.

is, "Every time a door opens, ten others blow open." God is steering the ship, opening those doors.

All of a sudden there was this epiphany

The idea for the documentary was floating around in my head a long time. Five years ago, I worked with a young man who was graduating from film school, and he agreed to do the documentary. He took a stab at it but never completed the project, and I got discouraged. So I put it on the back burner. I have a lot of things on the back burner. It's a little crowded back there.

In the meantime, I met my friend Peter Giunta, who shoots video. Then my middle sister reconnected with an old school friend, who now had three kids, and two of them had Tourette's. Oh, my God. I called her, we became friends, and she told me about Brad Cohen,[53] who was having a conference in Georgia.

I told her about the documentary I'd been planning and all of a sudden there was this epiphany. I said to myself, "I need to take a road trip and make this Brad Cohen conference part of the documentary." And that's exactly what we did.

Pete and I kinda went in blind, but we worked out the kinks and interviewed lots of people. When we were going in I said, "I'm giving you fair warning, it may be loud in there with people ticcing."

It was quiet. You wouldn't know anybody had Tourette's. The way everybody spoke and their body language, it seemed they felt like a million dollars. To witness it, you know—wow.

Everybody has some thing in their life they struggle with

It went smoothly and we got our footage. Brad's message, it seems to me, is that with Tourette's you have to be your own voice. You have to educate people. Everybody has some thing in their life they struggle with. I don't care who you are. Here's what I say to myself, "A problem is not a problem until you make it a problem." Your house is on fire—that's a problem. I broke a nail—that's not a problem [*he laughs*].

53   A motivational speaker, teacher, and school administrator. Brad also wrote, with Lisa Wysocky, *Front of the Class: How Tourette Syndrome Made Me the Teacher I Never Had*, which was made into the Hallmark Hall of Fame TV movie *Front of the Class*. Find him at bradcohentourettefoundation.com

It's therapeutic to meet other people with Tourette's. It's therapeutic to talk about it. We interviewed a young man for the documentary, and after that interview he decided to start doing a blog about Tourette's and his life. I think we're all taking advantage of networking to get the word out. We all advocate for ourselves. We have to. If we don't do it, who will? Nobody else gets it but us.

Working on the documentary I felt not just comfortable but, "Wow, I've arrived." It was a sense of calm and inner peace for the first time. I was on the road to something that was going to make an impact.

I embrace it

I've always been confident, even with the tics. I never got discouraged because of Tourette's. Embarrassment? Been there, done that. Discouragement is half the battle. If you can get over that, you're gonna get somewhere. My mother would, sympathetically, say when I was a kid, "There's always somebody worse off than you. Don't feel sorry for yourself." And I'll take that to the grave. Keep plugging away in life. Everything's a challenge and I love it.

I tend to just work through situations. So if you struggle with Tourette's, and go through that personal hell as a kid, everything after that is cake. I would get frustrated because it took me ten minutes to put on a T-shirt. Mom would say, "Take your time. Where are you going?"

I never forget what it used to be like. I embrace it. If you've made it through childhood, you've already got the strength. But to let Tourette's define me? No. I'm good. I enjoy the reminder because it keeps me fresh, it keeps me humble and reminds me how blessed I am.

———————————— ❧ ————————————

For a high school student, Leslie has a sophisticated point of view about the world. She already understands a deep lesson: you can always find someone whose suffering is greater than your own. This perspective diminished her own anguish and motivated her to ease the pain of others. She's one of several in this book who draw parallels between the difficulties of Tourette syndrome and social complexities experienced by the LGBT community.

LESLIE
17 years old

I kept saying, "I'm trying. It's not working."

I'm a junior in high school and plan to go to college.[54] I'll probably study education or social work, I'm trying to figure that out. If I teach, I'm thinking about elementary school.

My first tic I remember, I was twelve years old. I flapped my arms like a chicken. I thought I had just formed a bad habit. I have a habit of cracking my knuckles, so I thought it was like that. But no, it wasn't. My parents didn't understand, so they kept telling me to, "Stop," and, "Stop and don't do that." I kept saying, "I'm trying. It's not working." I didn't like it. I'm one of those people who likes to know what they're doing when they're doing it [*she laughs*].

At the time, I went to a school for kids with learning disabilities, because they labeled me with ADHD, bi-polar, Asperger's, dysgraphia, anything that was popular at the time. So things weren't as bad as they would have been at a normal school.

Then, in seventh grade, we moved to South Carolina and I went to a public middle school. I stopped the arm flapping tic, but had head twitching and a sniffing tic. The tics were getting really bad.

I like to stand up for people who aren't considered the norm.

It was difficult, but not because I had Tourette's. I went to school with a

---

54   Leslie graduated high school and is attending university, studying elementary education.

thousand kids and there were only three Jewish people. Two of them were me and my sister. With my religion, in South Carolina, I would explain Judaism to them, what we do, how it's different, but they didn't really understand. Like, one time I was asked if I had horns. Yeah. They weren't very knowledgeable. I think it was more ignorance than cruelty.

But my tics didn't help things. I couldn't relate to people because of my Tourette's. They just kept asking me, "Why do you shake your head? Why do you sniff so much?" I tried to explain as best I could, "I can't help it. I don't know why." There was a lot of hostility and teasing. I don't really care when people make fun of me because I can stand up for myself. But I do care when other people are made fun of. If someone who doesn't stand up for themselves is made fun of, I will stand up for them.

It does anger me sometimes, the lack of teaching that people do. Parents are supposed to teach kids that other people are different, and you shouldn't make fun of them for that. People should be *taught* when they're young. I don't get angry in situations, for the most part. I try to think out my argument. It's one reason I wanted to be a Youth Ambassador for TSA. I like to stand up for people who aren't considered the norm.

I finally knew why

I wasn't diagnosed until eighth grade, when I was fourteen and we moved to Ohio. I was more relieved than anything, that I finally knew why I was doing those things. At the time, I had a bending-over-sideways tic, and I broke four ribs doing that. Getting the diagnosis was good for my parents because they didn't understand I couldn't control it, so they were always saying, "Yes, you can control it. You have to stop." I guess they finally realized the extent of why I did what I did.

When I got diagnosed, my mom and dad joined the local TSA chapter. They got an email that the Youth Ambassador Program was going to happen, so I filled out the whole application, and a few weeks later I got in. I was fifteen at the time. I was really happy because it sounded like a great program and a way I could help people.

Everyone has struggled

I went with my dad to the TSA Conference in Washington, D.C. The first two days were training on how to present the Youth Ambassador message and how to say the correct information. Then we were given a presentation similar to the one we would give, and we could add our own personal information. That was really interesting to me because I got tolerance and acceptance out of it. Not for myself, but to teach others. It's a great thing to inform others about people who are slightly different, so they can learn to deal with their reactions. They can know the facts before they judge.

Tolerance, to me, is being able to say, "Okay, she might be different than he is. But they both are people, they both are human. They're not the same, but they are alike in many other ways. We shouldn't treat her differently than him or vice versa."

We didn't have time for sightseeing, but we sat around and talked about our experiences and got to know each other. I learned that everybody has something unique about them. Everyone has struggled. *Everyone* has. So we need to learn from each other.

On the last day, we went into Capitol Hill and spoke to our Senators and Congressmen to pass a bill that funds the TSA through the CDC.[55] That was interesting, because I liked seeing how political people think. It was interesting how the whole system works.

There's a similarity with disabilities and the LGBT community because you can be marginalized

They had a banquet at the end of the conference, where you could say what most struck you. I stood up and talked about my experience, and what I thought, and a little bit about myself, and I found it thrilling to speak to a large group.

I made friends there and still talk to some. One is Carlos Guevara, who was on *X-Factor*.[56] He finished thirteenth out of everybody. He's a singer, a really sweet guy. His Tourette's was so bad he had to leave school and was homeschooled. Another is Justin Bachman[57], and he does a lot of tolerance speaking to school groups. He has a whole line of YouTube videos and he does the Tolerance Festival[58] in Cleveland, in the spring. It's interesting because it's not just Tourette syndrome, it's all disabilities and all aspects of the community, like LGBT. All different groups that are <u>misunderstood in</u> some way.

55   Centers for Disease Control and Prevention.
56   Search youtube.com for Carlos' performance on *X-Factor*.
57   Find Justin on youtube.
58   honorgooddeeds.com.

There's a similarity with disabilities and the LGBT community because you can be marginalized. But, in some ways, being gay you have it harder. There are always going to be people who don't like you. For us, our symptoms might go away, and a lot of people will accept Tourette's, if they know what's going on. If you're gay, you may not have as much acceptance.

If you feel awful and you hear someone else's story, you might not give up

One of the things I like to say, when I am giving speeches about tolerance, is you may not get along with everybody, but you should try to understand where they're coming from, and who they are, and why they do what they do. If we see through the eyes of someone else, there are infinite possibilities we can learn. Things I couldn't learn from being just me, in my little world. If we learn from other people, are tolerant of other people, the world would be so much better. The world wouldn't be perfect, it wouldn't be the prettiest or the nicest, but it might be just a little bit better than it is now.

I posted a thing on Facebook that said, "Fight like a girl against Tourette's." I meant that because so few girls have Tourette's—I think it's three guys to one girl—I wanted to post a little girlpower. You can get through this. One of my goals is to inspire someone to reach their dreams. You could succeed. If you feel awful and you hear someone else's story, you might not give up. You'd be inspired to overcome. It's important not to give up, even though it's hard sometimes.

My main goal in life is to be happy and help other people accomplish something or improve their lives in some way. I go to temple and I say the prayers, but I don't believe someone is going to help me through this, without me doing something for myself. I have to help myself before someone else will help me. I don't know if all people believe that, but I definitely do.

--- ❧ ---

The cruelty of children is breathtaking. What links me most to Lynda is the dehumanization she was subjected to by schoolmates. How is it possible to move past such disgraceful treatment? She has done it, through creativity, humor, and the simple act of helping others. And what a treat to know that her father wrote songs that kept me hoppin' and stompin' when I was young in Mexico: "The kids in Bristol are sharp as a pistol..."

LYNDA
45 years old and holding

I tic less when I'm painting

I first started doing drawings when I was little. My parents gave me three books; they were all nature books, one on reptiles, one on mammals, one on birds. I first started copying the photographs and that interest grew. Eventually I got an Associate's Degree in Liberal Arts and I took courses at Tyler Art School, at Temple University. I wound up working in commercial arts for advertising agencies.

I've exhibited paintings several times in the Philadelphia area, in New York City, Boston, and other cities. I have a permanent painting in the C.A.R.P. Art Gallery in Washington, D.C., and I've exhibited my paintings in shows for disabled artists, including with Chuck Close.[59] He's a disabled artist, very established.

I tic less when I'm painting. It's because I'm concentrating on something. I've read that when you sing, you tic less but that's not one of my options. I'm a pretty bad singer, even my relatives will tell you that [*she laughs*]. My father can sing.

I'm still shy

I write for my blog, I'm a co-writer. It's called Society For Dainty Damsels.[60] It started off basically as a take-off on an etiquette manual.

59   Chuck Close's work has been the subject of more than 150 solo national and international exhibitions, including a number of major museum retrospectives. In 2000 he received the National Medal of Arts from President Clinton.
60   societyfordaintydamsels.com.

These two middle-aged women, they're very dowdy, very old-fashioned, and they are self-proclaimed etiquette experts. The tagline is "'50s style etiquette in the 21st century." Their names are Auntie Carol, who's really friendly, and Lady Lynda, 'cause no matter what she does, she's always a lady. Her husband is Seymour Toes, because he works in a shoe store [*she giggles*]. I also get a lot of pleasure being on Twitter. And I'm on Facebook. And I also write my own blog,[61] and that's a personal blog concerning my experiences with Tourette and Waardenburg syndromes, and whatever I feel like writing about in my life.

I also write poetry. There are places you can read your poetry. I don't like to go unless I go with a friend. If it's an open reading, I do read. It wasn't difficult to get up and do that. Put it this way—one place I go, there's a woman who has a hand puppet and she plays it back and forth to a song. If the audience can be polite to her [*she laughs*], then they're gonna be polite to me, okay?

I'm still shy. I find some people are more approachable than others. And I do have close friends. So for the art openings, I usually go with somebody I know, or if somebody I know will be there.

Someone who yelled out profanities and ethnic slurs

My disabilities are mood disorder, depression, OCD and ADHD. I was first diagnosed with a mood disorder in my early twenties, and the rest came a bit later. At the time, I wasn't diagnosed with Tourette's. I was diagnosed with Tourette's just last year. My image of Tourette's was some-one who yelled out profanities and ethnic slurs. Since I didn't do this, I thought TS could never be a part of my life.

I remember my mother, around the house, having tics. Over ten years ago, I found out about Tourette's because my male cousin on my mother's side has it, the full package. So I called up the Pennsylvania Tourette's Association and, I didn't realize I was doing this, I was repeating the last couple of words that the person said. And the woman said, "You have echolalia. There's a possibility you might have Tourette's." That was the first time I heard that. Hearing 'Tourette syndrome' kind of freaked me out because I'd heard so many bad, negative things about it, especially the cursing, the coprolalia.

61   mayappells.wordpress.com.

I remember not having a very good image of myself

During my growing up years, my mother took diet pills. Amphetamines. I think it made her tics worse. She yelled and screamed at me and called me terrible names and said some really terrible things to me. I suspect it was a combination of the drugs and being frustrated, not knowing how to deal with a kid like yours truly. My mother got on my case because she thought I was being disrespectful. It was rough. At any rate, when she finally got off the drugs, she recognized how she had treated me and apologized. I accepted her apology and she became a loving mother to me. She more than made up for her past mistreatment. I forgave her.

I remember not having a very good image of myself, at least partially because of the way my mother treated me. She could be either very loving or very critical. One extreme or the other. My father was very laid back. My father noticed about me what he called idiosyncrasies. He didn't call them tics, he called them my 'schticks.'

The kids sure noticed in high school, and I was teased unmercifully. I was called "It." And this was a school for kids with learning disabilities. It was a school for kids with 'minimal brain damage.' But they got on my case. They were really cruel to me.

I met a boy there, in high school, who, years later, became my husband. So we met there, then went our separate ways, separate boyfriends, separate girlfriends, then we re-met in 1982. And we were together since that time. Jerry passed away from acute leukemia on the eve of Obama's election. We have a child, we produced a girl. She was never diagnosed with Tourette's, but there might be a chance of Asperger syndrome. I'm not sure.

When you've got it, you've got it!

My father was born with a syndrome called Waardenburg. I got that from him. Waardenburg is a leading cause of deafness. My dad is hard of hearing but I suspect that is because of his age. He's ninety-two. In fact, he is a retired musician.[62] He did arrangements for Earl "Fatha" Hines and Benny Carter.

---

62   Dave Appell also co-wrote: "Let's Twist Again" and "Limbo Rock" for Chubby Checker; "Mashed Potato Time" for Dee Dee Sharp; "Don't Hang Up," "South Street," and "Wah Watusi" for The Orlons; "Wild One" and "Swinging School" for Bobby Rydell; "The Bristol Stomp" for The Dovells; he co-produced "Tie A Yellow Ribbon Round the Old Oak Tree" and "Knock Three Times" for Tony Orlando and Dawn. He died five months after this

I don't play any musical instruments. My talent is listening to music on YouTube [*she laughs*]. My father plays keyboard these days at his home. One of his favorite sayings is, "When you got it, you got it!" as he looks at himself in the mirror.

I felt like I accomplished something; I helped people

The last twenty-five years of my working life, I did advocacy for people with disabilities, especially psychiatric, in rehab centers in Philadelphia, Upper Darby, and Media, Pennsylvania. I advocated politically in 2008 when Bush, with his budget cuts, tried to cut off intensive-case managers. Those cuts didn't go through.

The other big thing for me was the issue of photo ID for voting. This affects people with disabilities, physical or developmental, because they don't drive. The only acceptable forms of photo ID are passport and driver's license. It's also low-income people. How many low-income people can get a passport? They are disenfranchising people. The incidence of voter fraud is as common as... a person with three eyes [*she chuckles*]. The reason I'm not there anymore is the place lost its funding.

I felt good about being an advocate. Being helpful. I believe in disability rights and especially invisible disabilities, those you can't see, like ADD, or deafness, for that matter. The history of disability on both sides of my family, that's what helped me get into it. And I felt like I accomplished something; I helped people.

I believe people should look at the whole person, not just the disability

I believe that people should look at the whole person, not just the disability. Everyone with disabilities has rights. I'm all for the Americans with Disabilities Act. I'm also for fairness, like with accommodations, let's say a restaurant. That goes for employment and higher education too.

In public I don't have to explain much because when I clear my throat and cough, most people don't think of that as Tourette's. So I don't think I need to explain myself. It's a socially acceptable tic. I also have palilalia, where I repeat words of my own. Now, some people think I'm being a

interview.

smart aleck when I repeat things. I've been teased about that, pretty much throughout my life.

Tourette's is not your fault. It is not your parents' fault. It's not faulty parenting. You're just as good a person as anybody else and you shouldn't be ashamed of yourself. I've found that it's very helpful to get into a support group, either Facebook or out in the world. I'm on Facebook pages for Tourette's and Waardenburg. You're with other people who understand you. I can talk to people with the same thing and I don't feel different or out of place. I don't feel like people are going to criticize me. We're in the same situation. We're similar to each other.

I try not to let people get to me. At least people who are not import-ant to me. I think that's a good attitude. My mother had this expression, if she didn't think somebody was significant in her life, she would say, "He means less than nothing to me."

The other night I went to the corner drug store to pick up a prescrip-tion. I was in line and I was ticcing, you know, grimacing, nose snorting, clearing my throat, tensing my stomach. And this woman, she was very indignant, and I wasn't doing anything to her. At first, I thought I was in her way, so I moved. She very curtly said, "I'm not going that way." I said to her, "I was only trying to be nice," and I started ticcing more. And she said, "Get away from me."

At first, I was very upset and I started to cry. Then I thought about what happened. I came to the conclusion that, why am I letting an igno-rant bitch get the better of me? It's not like that woman is a big part of my life. I didn't think of that right away, but later on I did. I'm not sure why that came to me, but I'm glad it did.

The chameleon blends and disappears. This has been Guy's life for years, hiding his Tourette's and his true self behind brilliantly constructed disguises. The toxic homelife of his childhood motivates Guy and his wife to create a loving environment for their delightful son. Encouraged by new, young friends with Tourette's, Guy found the courage to break camouflage, go public, and talk about his own Tourette's. For the greater good, as he says. His compassion also brings him closer to who he really is.

GUY
age not stated

What I did in my life is build a façade

I used to fly for a living, and my whole life I've geared toward that. I wanted to fly, I wanted to be a pilot. So I studied people. People were like aliens to me, so I learned how to *be* like them. I've done that all my life. The problem is, it's not me. You can only keep up the lie so long.

What I did in my life is build a façade, a layer over top of me that I would present to other people. So I was a mechanic, language and all. Firefighter, the same. When I'm a pilot, depending on whether freight or airline, I act like the pilot. I practiced accents, studied cultures. So not only was I doing the accent, but I got all the rest right. And I hate to say, the airline pilot is the most *not* like me. That was the hardest.

With each new career, after a few years, the facade would fall apart. There was nothing I could do to prevent the collapse. I would cry many hours watching this play out, knowing there was no one I could turn to. I would watch others in amazement, how easy things appeared to come to them. Yet I would fight for almost everything. Frustrating is too light of a word to describe my feelings.

I'm always like this

I was a commercial airline pilot, though I never made the major airlines. The regionals are horrible. The only thing that saves passengers are the flight crew and the cabin crew. The company is not there for you in any way, shape, or form. I made it to Captain, but never got off the bottom, so I got all the worst runs, broken airplanes, for years. You're pushed sixteen hours a day, you get minimal rest. You don't get paid retirement, you make a quarter to a fifth of what major pilots do. And it was getting to me.

Airlines are very strict with how they want you to present yourself. I've had severe nail biting, and sniffing, and a myriad other things I dealt with. When I was getting older, these separate things were getting worse. The people I worked with, for them the biggest thing was the sniffing. "If you're sick, go home!" And I'd say, "I'm not sick. I'm always like this." In an airliner, in that closed environment, you don't want to be with someone who is sick.

Critical approaches

The hardest one to deal with, and this has been my whole life, is an eye twitch. It's so little you don't see it. It's when I'm doing detailed work, about every two or three seconds, I twitch. Just enough to where you lose your place reading, and it's made that mind bogglingly difficult. The hardest part flying is doing critical approaches, where you're on the gauges. The jet was a little nicer because it had CRT screens. But I was constantly having to reacquire my vision. It was exhausting. I couldn't tell anybody because I would be out on the street. We have aviation medicals—you have one every six months—to fly as a Captain. Well finally, what was happening every six months, I'd see my blood pressure rise.

I flew for a regional and the company was going downhill because of a merger with a major carrier. Those of us who worked with the regional, we got kicked down the road.

What money we had left

So my wife and I, we lost our house, we lost everything. We left with two cars and the stuff in them. We took what money we had, and with half of it we bought a boat in Rhode Island. It was on Craigslist known as The Floating Whorehouse. It was dirt cheap. The owner's nephew lived on it in the summertime, and it's right in the middle of the city. What would *you* do [*he laughs*]?

We were going to get local jobs, fix the boat up, and head to Europe.

But the economy tanked again. I found a job for a little bit, flying a twin-engine airplane going into Canada, the arm of Nova Scotia. During the winter, I fell getting into the boat and got hurt. I was down for the count in an enclosed boat, and I got very depressed. On the NPR I heard a program about Asperger's and I thought, "Boy, those people are a lot like me, but they aren't like me." I wanted to find out deeper what ailed me and someone recommended a neuropsychologist. So we took what money we had left—we had no insurance—and I went to see this doctor.

Spying on the Soviets

This guy saw me for one hour and said, "Have you ever been tested for a tic disorder?" And I thought the insect. I said, "Well, I've been bitten by them." He says, "No, I mean a tic. Tourette's." I said, "You must be crazy." He said, "Let me ask you about your father."

My parents had an extremely adversarial relationship. Not physical, but intellectually abusive. Every single night, *forever*. They were academics, highly educated, all kinds of degrees. I was expected to be the same. They looked upon me to carry the name, and I was failing. My parents would tell me what I had to achieve, but never give me the tools to achieve it. They gave up on me about fourth grade.

My mom was a painter, an artist, and a sculptor. There was so much hatred in the marriage her art was hidden away. I finally found it, rummaging around, and I have pieces of her art in the boat. My dad worked for the Eisenhower administration on top-secret military space payloads for spying on the Soviets. He worked hand-in-hand with the CIA and the Air Force. I got to know a lot of scientific people. I got to see their world, people who make history, and the politics behind all that. My dad made noises, made faces, all kinds of things that weren't diagnosed because he was extremely successful.

A horse out of the barn

So this doctor says, "You have a family line of Tourette's." I thought he was crazy. And he diagnosed me with Autism Spectrum Disorder. I said, "If this is true, I'm going to let a horse out of the barn that I don't know what to do with."

Under Part 121 air carrier rules, if there's *any* change to your medical, you have to disclose. It's a federal offense not to. So I lost my career and went into the deepest depression that one can do. I lost what I'd worked for all my life. My house was gone, the money was gone, I had a five-year old son I had to provide for, and I couldn't. We would run out of money for food. I was an airline Captain one year before. So the depression got worse and I started having more accelerated tics at night. I would be violently shaking. My wife would say, "You're just afraid." I wasn't afraid. I couldn't control what was going on.

My Tourette's likes her

My wife is salt-of-the-earth, from a farm family in Minnesota. She's the Rock of Gibraltar. I value our relationship. She's the best thing that's ever happened to me. It took me thirty-eight years to get a gal to marry me. She's there every day. Her warm body's there every night in bed.

Because nights for me are hell. That's when the tics are the worst. When they were really bad a few months ago, I was just *horrible*. My Tourette's likes her. How does it show it? By cursing all the time, and twitching, and saying bad things to her. It's absolutely horrible. So it worries me. It usually makes her cry, which none of us like to do to our wives. It's like cutting into your heart.

And what really hurts is I took a lot of pride in providing for my family. And now I'm the liability. I told her a long time ago, if I ever become a liability I'm getting a gun, and I'm gonna stand on the end of the dock.

It's refreshing to talk to young people because they're so open for ways to work with Tourette's

I always hoped finding out what was wrong with me would fix the problem. Now knowing, I am quite let down that there is nothing I can do. It is nice to know there are others like myself out there. Yet I feel sad for them, as I do not want *anyone* to go through this frustration.
That is why, when I see others going through difficult times, I cannot stand back and watch while nobody seems to care. Especially young people, with such potential. I will be the one that cares. I will try my best to help.

These last two years have been rather amazing, when I decided to go public with my YouTube videos. I've got about thirty of them. It all started about two weeks after I was diagnosed. I saw a gal on YouTube talking about Tourette's. We were commenting back and forth and she said, "You should do a video." I thought people would use it against me, ridicule me. And she talked to me about the greater good. I talked with young people on YouTube and they encouraged me, as an older person, to get out there. It's refreshing to talk to young people because they're so open for ways to work with Tourette's.

So about a week later I started making the videos about Tourette's. You know, "Here's my life today," sitting in front of the computer. I did a few of them while driving. I even did 'Tourette's on a bike,' riding to school. One time I almost ran into a guardrail [*he chuckles*].

One of the neatest things a parent can get

My son is six years old. Evan's physically my wife's family, Scandinavian and German. But inside, he's me, and that worries me. He already shows autistic stuff socially. I think I see tics, but it's hard to tell.

I view my job as critical. Once you have a kid, your life changes for the better. As parents, we give our children a full toolbox and the knowledge of when and how to use it. I tell him, "You need to take educated risks and see opportunity." I would like to take pride that Evan knows he's done his best. And when he reaches his goal, to turn back and help those having difficulty.

This weekend I got one of the neatest things a parent can get. We're at a McDonald's—that's our level of eating [*he laughs*]—it has a playground in it. Evan was climbing around, there were a lot of kids. Some older boys were bullying a group of girls, especially this little one with thick glasses. My wife and I are eating, and the little girl with the thick glasses, she comes up and points to my boy and says, "Are you Evan's father?" And I think, "Oh, my God, what's he done?" And you know what she said? She said, "Your son is standing up for us."

She said Evan gathered the girls together, took them to the mother of the boy teasing them. And he told her what happened, but in a positive fashion, so good could come out of it. I was blown away. Because I've been teaching him that. All the things I've learned. And it was so cute—the little girl wanted his phone number [*he laughs*].

CHAPTER SIX

MISCONCEPTIONS

I spoke with a young man who, as a high school sophomore, had searched for answers to his strange, sometimes incapacitating symptoms. Intelligent and motivated, he read the Diagnostic and Statistical Manual for Mental Disorders, all eight hundred eighty-six pages of it, to find a diagnosis for his inexplicable behaviors. He read the entire manual except two diagnoses—anorexia and Tourette's. Why? Because he believed that Tourette's is coprolalia and he figured, "I'm not cursing, so I can't have Tourette's." This widespread misconception often was detrimental to people in this book.

There are abundant misconceptions in the medical community too. I spoke with one woman whose psychiatrist told her, when she was a young girl, that her tics would disappear once she started menstruating.

Misconceptions impede Touretters and society from finding the common ground of understanding and acceptance. People with Tourette syndrome are often seen as flawed and weak, or drug-addicted, possibly schizophrenic, and often threatening. Sometimes a family, out of fear or pride, resists getting a diagnosis. The general population has difficulty believing we can't suppress tics. They don't understand how much tics can hurt, even endanger, us. And I'd like to acknowledge, for everyone in this book and beyond, how tiresome it is for us to hear Tourette's used as a punch line.

Our responsibility is advocacy and education; find creative ways to eradicate the simplistic, one-dimensional, and downright erroneous ideas about Tourette syndrome.

———————————— ⚙ ————————————

Rose's bright voice embodies her focus on positive attitude. She coined a beautiful phrase to describe the effort it takes for most Touretters, and folks with other disabilities, to make it through the day: "It takes strength to have this strength." This deep, constant effort is what the general population does not see. If they could, she says, those with disabilities might get the respect and admiration they deserve.

ROSE
19 years old

My first bully

My parents first noticed my tics when I was two. Whenever I would get really excited or upset, I would do weird arm movements, noises, shaking my head. My mom's cousin has Tourette's, so I think that's how my mom and dad thought of getting extra help from my pediatric doctors.

My Tourette's didn't impact the family much. They're very protective of me. My great grandmother would have us stand in front of the mirror and say, "My name is so-and-so and there is no one better than me." It was goofy, but she did it to bring up our spirits. As if to say to a bully, "Hey, that's not okay. I am who I am. And I love *me*."

In elementary school there was this boy who was bullied, and I felt bad for him. I would sit next to him and talk with him. But when he saw I had this new thing he would look at me with disgust and go, "You're so gross." So he was probably my first bully.

Imagine myself in a calm place

Out in public I was very aware of people watching me, so I would do something that is not good—I would suppress my tics. And this is really hard because it burns. It hurts so much to hold them in. If I *had* to tic, I would rush off to the bathroom and tic in there. When I got home (*she chuckles*), it was like a bomb would go off. I call them my 'Tic Attacks'.

Now my tics have gotten better. My therapist has helped me with relaxation. I went to hypnotherapy and habit-reversal therapy. My habit-reversal therapist had me twiddle my thumbs. I would transfer the tic into a non-noticeable part of my body—my fingers, my feet. That works great. If I wasn't noticing how bad my tics were, my mom would snap her fingers and that would trigger me to think, "Oh, the tics are bad. I'll twiddle my thumbs." That worked really well.

Once I got older and became more aware of how bad I was getting, I would take deep breaths and imagine myself in a calm place. At my high school, I was an advocate for Tourette's. I did seminars, 'cause there was an outbreak of kids with Tourette's. One of my brother's friends was diagnosed with it. And there were a few more who came to me with questions about what they should do.

I was in that confusion state

I have Tourette's, but I also have OCD, severe anxiety, and depression. I went through a hard part my sophomore year of high school. I started getting really depressed, but I wasn't diagnosed with depression yet. My best friend for the last seven years is Olivia, and she's the only reason I'm alive today.

I was at the peak of my tics, so they were horrible. I was applying for college, there was all this stress. I said, "I can't do this anymore." I was going for a walk and I was walking toward Calvin Coolidge Bridge. I started walking towards it. I was prepared to throw myself off the bridge.

Olivia called and said, "Hey, we need to go for a walk." And I thought, "I'm not going to leave and not go for a walk with her." Well, she took one look at me and said, "What's wrong?" And we went and got a pint of Ben and Jerry's and sat down and she said, "You need to go get help *now*."

It was scary walking to the bridge, because at that point I was so upset and I was crying and I was like, "I don't know what's going on." I was in that confused state. Now I look back and think of my family and the look on my mom's face…

I do feel other people's suffering

Ever since then, I look for positivity in everything. Even if it's the crappiest moment, I look for the positive in it. I've become a better person that way. We got a support group together at school. It's a group of people who are supportive of *you*. We kick the negativity out and keep in the positivity.

I do feel other people's suffering. Myself, I would emanate that I was the happiest person in the world, even though my smile was painted on my face. So I can tell a real smile from a fake one.

I am very good at helping other people. And through that, I became more calm. The peaks started to go down, and my tics started getting a lot better. I accepted it. "I have this weird thing, that's part of me, that I'm going to have for the rest of my life. Okay, I gotta deal with it." I think I became more accepting of TS when I had to stick up for myself around people who were giving me weird looks.

A love-hate relationship

College is going well for me. I'm a visual-arts major and I'm figuring out what I want to concentrate in. I'm thinking photography, but I also love drawing and painting. When I paint, I like to paint scenery. I'll take a picture from up on Mount Aston and you can see the whole landscape and the way the river curves right through there. Especially in late summer, early fall, when you can see the fields of different colors and patterns. I did a painting of that, and I just love it.

I wrote a poem about my Tourette's that I call *The Demon Inside Me*. I always thought of it like that. In my poetry I refer to Tourette's as a demon. As a monster. And I also refer to it as my friend. I know that no matter where anybody else goes, I'll always have that. It's a love-hate relationship. So all of that meshes together, my life experiences and the beauty of nature, in my art.

It takes strength to have this strength

My parents raised me to be accepting of *everyone*, no matter race, color, gender, we accept them. So I think there's a similarity between the gay community and people with Tourette's. Everyone is beautiful in their own way. Whether it's inside or outside, it doesn't matter. Because even the most beautiful people in society could be ugly on the inside. It's not fair to marginalize people.

I don't understand why people discriminate, because you shouldn't judge before you've stepped inside someone's shoes. I said to somebody who bullied me, "I want you, for one day, to see if you can live in my shoes and see how far you make it."

Everyone tells me, "You're such a strong person." I said, "Yeah, I am strong. But it takes strength to have this strength. Sometimes it can feel like you have a fifty-thousand-ton lead plate on your back. So let me see *you* do that. You might be big and macho, but can you do that every single day of your life?" But also, I can't judge that bully's life. I don't know what goes on in his home.

Dark chocolate

I posted a quote from Kurt Vonnegut.[63] I like it because whenever I was upset, I'd draw. It's a freeing thing. It takes your mind off the tics, and off the stress, and the emotion. And especially music. I'm horrible at singing, but I sing and play piano. Anything in the arts, I like to do. It takes my mind off the stresses and I feel like the bubble has been popped. I feel more free in that moment. I'll realize I'm not ticcing, and "Oh, gosh, I *am* free." And there's that moment.

I quit medications cold turkey. I was on Risperidal. I was on five or six medications for Tourette's my whole life. They had the worst side effects and I've been coping better without them. I'd rather have my tics and deal with them in my own, natural way than being doped up, confused, and not myself.

For women, tics get worse with hormones. I'd be agitated, like, "Leave me alone. Give me chocolate and I'll be fine." Dark chocolate is a very good thing to calm you down when you're stressed. Just a little calms your nerves. But just a little bit. Don't go overboard 'cause then you're gonna feel like, "I shouldn't have done that (*she laughs*)."

When I was younger, I was very thin and athletic and now I struggle with my weight. I've come to say, "You don't like the way I look, I don't care. I like the way I look. I'm good enough for myself." I look at myself and I see a healthy person. I don't have a six-pack and I don't have a thigh gap, but who wants that? I'm happy with myself, I'm strong and confident, and that's all I need. I just need to be good enough for myself.

---

63   Vonnegut's quote is about the enormous reward of going into the arts, not necessarily as a career, but as a way to make life more bearable. Do it well, do it badly, but *do* it. You will have created something.

I spoke with Arthur in the spring, after the hard winter of 2014, when Niagara Falls froze, and his voice had the lightness and relief of easier times ahead. He's overcome the habit of self-medication, the grip of deep depression, the pain of injuries and tics, and comes at life with enthusiasm. He's lucky to have a good wife, who helped him see the world with softer eyes. It's his daughter, Alice, who's caught in a tug-of-war of denial about Tourette's.

ARTHUR
30 years old

Oh, man, I ran with it

I'm a freelance sports and news writer for the local TV station. I grew up doing sports, almost went to college to play basketball. I just wasn't ready for college so I went into professional wrestling instead.

When I wrestled I didn't use my real name or act like my real self. I was Charlie Mudd. That was my character. I went out there real arrogant and tough. Oh, man, I ran with it and had so much fun. And believe it or not, I never ticced when I was in the ring. I would just go out there and do my thing. It was like I was in my own little world. It really took my mind off of things.

Entertainment is what I love to do and it's always been my outlet for Tourette's. I've been a radio DJ and I play drums, bass, guitar. Like everybody else, I get a little nervous before I perform, but I enjoy it so much it just disappears. I can go to the store and here I am ticcing and trying to hide it and I'm embarrassed. But get out in front of a thousand people, doing something I could mess up on, and it doesn't bother me at all [*he laughs*].

A superflex from the top ropes

What took me out of wrestling is I broke the lower section of my back. I took a superflex from the top ropes and my partner and I, our arms slipped and I landed wrong. What most people don't realize is the rings are extremely hard. They're plywood and metal. The big bang you hear is you're hitting plywood. It really hurts.

We had a doctor come in talking to us about the dangers of wrestling, what it could do to our bodies. He told us that every time we hit that ring it's the equivalent of being in a twenty-five or thirty-mile-an-hour fender bender, every single time. I did that for seven years. Yep.

Quit shaking your head!

I was six or seven when the Tourette's started. My mom said the biggest tic was me biting my shirts. I think the biggest one I started noticing was I shook my head constantly. I have a video of me playing baseball and you can hear my parents yelling, "Quit shaking your head!" And I can't do it [*he laughs*]. I didn't know why it was happening. But I knew it was something that was a part of me.

My parents saw a documentary on TV about Tourette's and mom looked at dad and said, "Maybe that's what is wrong with Arthur." I was thirteen. So she took me to a neurologist, who took one look at me and said, "Oh, yeah, he definitely has Tourette's." TS didn't affect my family life. My brothers never teased me about it. That could be because both of them are undiagnosed with mild Tourette's. They know they have it, they just never went to a neurologist.

School was a whole different ball game. When you're trying to focus on not ticcing, it's hard to focus on class. And with Tourette's, most of the time it comes with ADD and ADHD. It really hindered my school. Before I was diagnosed I had problems with teachers. They thought I was lazy, or making sounds to disrupt class. And I'm thinking, "I can't stop." I've always been good at suppressing and letting it out when I get home. But then it was a hellstorm, yelping and barking like a dog.

She died in my hands

At the end of my freshman year, I was fifteen, my dad and I found my mom having a massive heart attack. She died in my hands, quite literally. So I went through bouts of depression, real bad, suicidal. I was angry at God, I was angry at the world. My Tourette's acted up. I was ticcing to where they had to double my doses of medication.

I was on Tenex, Luvox, Adderall, and I definitely, honestly think they put me in a deeper depression. I've always been a happy, happy person. I never thought I would be suicidal. But I was [*he sighs*].

Dad got remarried. He was really lonely and just... you know. He met someone he thought was the right person. She was... she was not very nice. I'll just put it that way. So my senior year I developed bleeding ulcers on top of my Tourette's. I was out of school so much, going to counseling for the PTSD of mom dying in my hands, they said I'd have to come back next year. I said, "You mean I don't get to graduate?" Well here's the kicker. I was only a month and a half away from graduating early.

I had already put down money on the wresting academy. Three thousand, four thousand dollars. I'd put down another thousand on a rental house that my soon-to-be-wife and I would live in. I told the school, "I guess I'm going to not graduate." That put a kicker on me too. My mom would have been real disappointed, I'll tell you that much.

I'm accused of being on meth

For a while, my early- to mid-twenties, my Tourette's was so much better. I don't know why. It started up again about three years ago, real severe, how it was when I was a kid. It surprised and shocked me.

I'm on a lot of Facebook groups and educational pages about Tourette's. I've watched a lot of documentaries, trying to learn as much as I could possible. That way I could educate people. It's best to be straightforward. I almost always tell new friends I have Tourette's. That way, if I do something weird or off-color, they know what's going on. Any time I hear someone make a Tourette's joke, I'll say something. I don't jump down their throat, obviously, but I educate the crap out of them [*he laughs*].

I have coprolalia, but I've learned to slur words. It comes off as if I'm yawning or about to cough. People look at me, but usually I can keep it from coming out full force.

One thing that ticks me off is I've been accused of being on meth. Somebody started a rumor I might be a drug dealer because I'm always twitching and talking to myself [*he laughs*]. I never thought coprolalia seemed like you were talking to yourself. "He must be psychotic," or "He's probably schizophrenic." I've heard both of those.

People don't realize that Tourette's isn't just hootin' and hollerin' and moving around. It's very painful.

I haven't been on meds since I was eighteen. Doctors have recommended it to me but it seemed on the medicines felt like I was walking on clouds or I was sluggish.

For a long time I was an alcoholic. I started because of my Tourette's. Alcohol calmed me down, so that was the only way I could sleep. Otherwise I would just lay there and tic, tic, tic, tic, tic. I'm like that to this day. But now we go for walks. We also watch movies at home. We'll have movie nights with friends. I tic through them but nobody cares. I tic so much during the movie I can usually go to sleep 'cause I'm so exhausted.

People don't realize that Tourette's isn't just hootin' and hollerin' and moving around. It's very painful. I don't think people get that. We're sore most of the time.

Hold my new baby

I'm remarried, and my wife, she prepares my plates for me because I've broken plates and glasses. Obviously I don't want to go to somebody's house and start breaking their expensive china [*he laughs*]. And I've noticed whenever she's making me a plate, people are staring at me like, "Are you lazy? Or is she a slave? [*he chuckles*]." It's kind of embarrassing, but that's the way it is. She knows it helps me and I appreciate that greatly.

It's rare for me to cook 'cause I've burned myself so many times. And not on accident from a tic, but like an inhibition thing where I touch the burner. And oh—holding babies! It sounds funny but I don't like it when somebody's, "Here, hold my new baby." My arms start twitching. I'm thinking, "Oh, no, this isn't good."

Used to be, I was one of those people that couldn't relax. I was always stressed out. Oh, my gosh—what if, what if? I used to be the worst pessimistic person I knew. I've totally turned myself around. My wife kept saying, "When you're like that, bad things *are* going to happen." It just took a lot of her coaching, because she's real optimistic. It took the right person for me to be around. I don't think I realized how bad I was until I stopped and looked at myself. And now things are so much easier.

Here's the problem

My daughter will be eleven. My ex-wife and I did not know Tourette's is hereditary. Alice has displayed symptoms. She sniffs a lot and she wiggles her face. I've seen her do the shoulder shrugging, the eye blinking. And she does like she's clearing her throat.

Here's the problem. Her mom absolutely denies this. It turned into a battle, because she's having problems in school, right? She's having the same problems I had. I had to get a court order for an evaluation and I have an appointment set at a neurologist. But her mother's like, "There's nothing wrong with her." Her stepdad has told her to quit making those noises.

Alice, she talks to me. She said, "I have to hide it, dad." Whenever I talk to her mother about it, I say, "She's learned to suppress it." She took Alice to the school counselor, who actually said, "Oh, no, there's no such thing as people with Tourette's suppressing. They can't hold it back."

It's okay to let it out

So Alice is showing signs of depression, which happened to me whenever I suppressed hard. I told her, "It's okay to let it out. Yeah, you're not like everybody else, but it doesn't make you stupid. You can do anything that anybody else can do. As a matter of fact, you have higher grades than anybody in your class. So it doesn't have to stop you unless you let it."

My wife and I were counselors at our first Tourette summer camp, the Joshua Center[64] for kids with neurological disorders. Yep. We stayed in the cabins with the kids. It was an amazing experience to help kids with the same diagnosis. When we get that diagnosis for my daughter, she'll definitely be on board for next summer.

My hope, where we stand now, is keep living day by day and relax. I've thought about getting a high school equivalency. I've contemplated getting into college. If I could be anything, I'd be either a disability lawyer or a police officer. So who knows? Maybe one of these days I'll wake up and say, "I'm gonna go for it." That's the kind of person I am. I'm very, very spontaneous. You never know what I might do next [*he laughs*]. But it'll be fun, I can guarantee you that.

---

64   joshuacenter.com

On the one hand, media attention has been a valuable service to our TS community, answering urgent personal questions and educating the general public. On the other hand, the media have an uncontrollable urge to highlight extreme cases. It is shocking to see and, these days, what makes better entertainment than shock value? To combat this shock effect, Britney's parents kept her away from distressing images of TS and in this way helped her understand her milder Tourette's as something manageable, understandable, and quite natural.

BRITNEY
24 years old

It wouldn't make sense if I told her I couldn't help it

The first time I noticed tics I was on my way home from my grandma's house one night. It started registering, I guess, the urges to move my body. I didn't understand what was happening because I was only seven. I thought if I just did it, it would go away, this feeling I had. So I did it, and realized I had the urge again and again. My mom kept asking what I was doing. I told her I wasn't doing anything. It wouldn't make sense if I told her I couldn't help it. Shortly after that is when I started seeing the neurologist and got a diagnosis of Tourette syndrome.

My dad didn't want to accept the diagnosis at first because he didn't want anything to be wrong with me. But my grandma kind of knew because she babysat me. I have a big family and I'm close to all of them. They didn't get worked up about it. I don't know what I would do without each and every one of them.

My mom always taught me to stick up for myself and don't let anybody make fun of me

I had a decent time in school with my Tourette's, but I think it's because I let so many people know I have it. So they knew the noises I was making weren't something weird, it was something I had no control over. We didn't tell all my teachers. We told the ones I'd be in the classroom with most because the longer I sat there, the more it would come out. They let me take a walk if I needed to. I had problems with one teacher, who didn't believe me. So I kept my mouth shut when he told me to sit still.

I wasn't teased from what I can remember. My mom always taught me to stick up for myself and don't let anybody make fun of me. I wasn't mean, but if somebody said something, or I noticed them looking, I would say, "I have Tourette's syndrome. It's something I can't help." And it would turn into a conversation and them wanting to know more about it.

So many big life changes

Tics were getting worse toward high school. My junior year was the first time I went on medication. I have a milder case, but it can get bad. My senior year I had so many things going on—I was graduating, I was going to college. I'd been dancing forever and thought it was going to be my last year. I had so many big life changes, and my body wasn't dealing with all the exciting moments the way I wanted it to.

The Topamax definitely dialed down the tics. I did have a few problems, like stomach ache, and I didn't want to eat. So throughout my junior year I was on it, and my senior year I decreased it and got off it again. But I'm noticing the tics are making their way back into my life, and I'm on medication again, Topamax and Trihexyphenidyl. I started it a year before my wedding. I had a lot of excitement going on then.

I was stronger than what Tourette's made it seem I could be

My blog[65] has always been about Tourette's, but when I started it was mainly about my experience with it and explaining what the disorder is. I wanted people to realize it's not just what *I* have, because I have a mild case, but what others go through. I thought it was important to have their story told.

I've learned I really enjoy writing about Tourette's because it's so personal. I'm learning a lot more about it. I'm meeting all these new people and hearing their stories. Every time I write one of their stories, it's a new inspiration to my life. I find the people I'm talking to are inspirational because I learn what they go through. And for the most part, they have a positive outlook on life. It's an amazing thing.

---

65   writingmyemotions.wordpress.com.

Tourette's is not just what television portrays it to be. It really hits home when I watch the bad cases they show. When I was first diagnosed, my mom didn't let me watch anything like that. She didn't want me to get it in my head that there was something wrong with me. She wanted me to know I was stronger than what Tourette's made it seem I could be. She waited until I was older and could understand it a little more. Then we watched those shows together. I have my parents to thank for my self-image.

You have to look past the tics

I posted a quote on Facebook by Frieda Kahlo, how she imagined there had to be at least one other person as bizarre as she was, somewhere in the world. And she imagined that person might be thinking about her too. The first time I read that I related to it in an instant. I know I'm a very different person from most people, not just from my Tourette's, but in general. I will describe myself as a unique person. But growing up with Tourette's, I didn't know a lot of people with it. I've never really known *anybody* with it. My dad's friend has it, but I only saw him on occasion and I didn't really know him. So I never got to meet anybody who had what I had. And nobody understood what it was I went through. But I knew there were other people out there. I knew I wasn't the first case of Tourette's ever diagnosed [*she chuckles*]. And because I've gotten older, I've gotten more awareness and education about it. I think that's one of the most important things for people who are suffering with it—to know they're not alone, and there's somebody else out there going through this, and they can help or support you in some way.

I don't know what it would be like to meet somebody else with Tourette's. I feel like I might start doing their tics. I think we both would be able to learn from each other. It'd be like talking to anybody else because what they are doing is what I do every day. I wouldn't see it as a distraction. You have to look past the tics. If I'm sitting there trying to talk to somebody and I keep ticcing, I don't want them to stop talking and stare at me, and wonder if I'm okay. Or think what I'm doing is something off the wall and not normal. If you know I have Tourette's, you know that for me it's normal. For my body, it's normal.

It's against my will

I tic with my eyes and my mouth. Those are probably my most dominant tics. Sometimes somebody will ask if there's something in my eye. Or they'll straight out ask me, "What are you doing?" or "Why are you doing that?" I explain to them my Tourette's and what it makes me do. And you usually get into a conversation of, "So you really can't control that?" And I have to explain that no, I really can't. It's against my will. I would say that's one of the most frustrating things about it.

Usually when I walk, I kick with my feet. Like I start to scuff them across the floor. It happens if I have to walk for a long time. And so a lot of times in the grocery store, or if my husband and I are out on a walk, I have to stop because I have to do what my body needs me to do. Sometimes I'm stuck for a few minutes. That's what I don't like. My husband doesn't care. He's the most supportive person, and patient person in the world. But it's in my head that it's a bother, even though I know it's not.

When I move my arms and legs it's because I want to

I like to read a lot. Or I do crossword puzzles because they get my mind concentrated on something. Sometimes I'll go for a walk, even though I still tic. I've always liked to go on walks and exercise. When I have my bad days I get upset about it, and when I get upset, I get angry that I can't stop doing it. So sometimes I'll get on the treadmill and run it out.

Right now this is my eighteenth year dancing. I don't like ballet that much. I take jazz, tap, and hip-hop twice a week. I take classes mainly for the skill level they give me. My tics are pretty much gone when I'm dancing. Not only because I'm so passionate about it, but because I'm feeling free in my own body. When I move my arms and legs it's because I want to, and I'm telling my body to do it. Not because I can't help it.

I love dance so much. I love being on stage and dancing in front of a crowd. Knowing my body and knowing what it's doing. Under my control. It's just… amazing. After I have a bad day, of anything, really, but mainly if I have a bad day ticcing, if I dance that night, I come home and it's like I'm a completely different person again.

———————— ✿ ————————

As a former college disc jockey myself, right away I clicked with Jonathan's radio experience. I understand the satisfaction of the perfect segue, and I know his relationship with the deep beat of music. Jonathan's poetry also is a source of pleasure for him, and another example of the relief that comes from self-expression and creativity. He demonstrates that the compassion we give each other, and extend to ourselves, is what gives life richness and meaning.

JONATHAN
61 years old

You would cross the street to avoid walking next to me

I'm disabled, not because of Tourette's, but because I'm bipolar. When I try to work, I fall apart. Usually I last about six to seven months, then I fall to pieces. I'm on meds, but they only temper it. Like today, I'm feeling a great deal of anxiety.

I've more or less come to terms with my Tourette's, so I don't need a support group. I primarily go on Facebook groups in case somebody else needs support. Helping others helped me come to terms with my Tourette's and my bipolar. The bipolar is a bit of a bear. But with my Tourette's, the medicine I'm on, Clonazepam, has controlled a great deal of my bad tics. My tics used to be to such a degree that, if you saw me coming down the sidewalk, you would cross the street to avoid walking next to me.

Maybe I can help others

I really don't know how I came to terms with my Tourette's. It just occurred over time. I realized instead of looking at my disability as a, "Woe is me," I looked at it as, "I have this, and maybe I can help others who have it."

What also helped was having been a Philadelphia boy—I still am a Philly boy at heart—and we had a ball player named Jim Eisenreich. Whenever they had home games on Friday nights, he would hold a question and answer period for people, or parents of children, with Tourette's. That was him giving back to the community. I was talking to him and it turned out we were on the same medicines. And I felt a connection with him. I think what made me come to terms with Tourette's was seeing how *he* had come to terms with it, and had succeeded despite it.

I did the same thing being a disc jockey. I spent twelve years in radio. And I came to terms with the fact that I made noises for some reason. Before that, I was the first student to do a show in the radio station at my university. That was a fishbowl setup, so everybody walked by and saw me doing the show. I was told I had tics, but I wasn't aware of them. In 1997, the advisor to that station, who I maintained as a friend, asked me to come up and do a 25th anniversary show.

The perfect segue

What I loved most about radio… I tried to take five songs that were totally diverse and fit them all together. Avant-garde, classical, jazz, punk, electronic—the whole nine yards. And you're trying to fit these songs together so it sounds like one piece. The segue, moving from one piece to another, was crucial. One of the best segues I heard—it was absolutely perfect—I heard a disc jockey at a state college radio station do this segue—he went from Neil Young's *Cinnamon Girl*, which has that [*imitates the guitar riff*] at the end and went right into *Layla*, Derek and the Dominoes. The best segue I ever did was I went from Phillip Glass *Einstein on the Beach*, which had the rapid organ [*imitates the organ*] that suddenly stopped, and I went right into the long version of *In-A-Gadda-Da-Vida* by Iron Butterfly. It was the perfect segue.

The man I was began to emerge

I wasn't diagnosed until I was forty-one years old. But I've been able to determine I had Tourette's from the age of nine, when they misdiagnosed me. "Oh, he's got bad allergies, he has anxiety, and he has Saint Vitus Dance."

I was blessed with close friends, who either did not notice my tics or didn't care. I was not bullied because of my tics. I was bullied because I was smarter than everyone else and they resented it. Also, with the manic aspect of bipolar, I would lose my temper easily. So I was teased because I was giving them what they wanted.

My childhood was traumatic. I had two rotten parents. They were terrible. We left my father when I was nine. I've had no contact with him since. My mother was abusive physically. Any time I portrayed behavior that reminded her of my father, she would beat me. Unfortunately that included acting masculine, which a nine-, ten-year-old boy, you're beginning to act like the young man you are becoming. Any time I acted like a young man, she beat me. So I learned, as a matter of self-defense, to act effeminate around her. And finally, acting effeminate became who I was through my teen years, which of course got me in trouble in high school. In college, I was attracted to glam rock because of its androgyny. Then, living apart from my mother, the feminine aspects began to fade, and the man I was began to emerge.

Throughout this, I was unaware of my tics. The psychiatrist I was seeing, he asked me, "Are you aware you're doing this?" And I said, "No." The only thing I was aware of was the noises. And the only reason for that was I taped myself at the college radio station and heard the noises. I tried different positions of the microphone and eventually found one where the noises could not be heard.

I couldn't live with the shame

In my thirties I developed a horrible vocal tic, a chronic cough that was so bad I could not hold conversations. It was very difficult to maintain work with this disability. My bipolar was more obvious and more debilitating, until the Tourette's became more debilitating because of the cough.

When I got diagnosed in '94, they put me on Haldol and within a week the coughing was about seventy-five percent under control. It was like a miracle. When I would start a job I would tell them I had Tourette's, so there were no surprises. People accepted me. They knew I was a quirky, and I had movements, and they accepted that.

I did eventually come down with tardive dyskinesia from the Haldol, and went off it. But my feeling is, those twelve years, where I did not have coughing, the tardive dyskinesia was a worthwhile trade-off.

My first wife was very non-supportive. She made comments like, "Don't tell my family, I couldn't live with the shame. I'm embarrassed to be seen with you in public." When we divorced, she said, "I can't live with your Tourette's." In the midst of our bitter divorce, she swore out a protection-from-abuse order against me. She claimed that my Tourette's made me dangerous, and that she feared for her life. She knew it was a tic disorder, but she was betting on the judge not knowing. And she was right.

The most beautiful woman I'd ever seen

I met my current wife, Maureen, at a Parents Without Partners party. She was the most beautiful woman I'd ever seen. She was dancing with every Tom, Dick, and Harry in the place. Finally, she noticed I was glued to a pole and unable to take my eyes off her. And she came up to me and asked me to dance. We've been together ever since.

I must've been ticcing at that time, but it didn't bother her. She suffers from borderline personality disorder, so she has her own luggage of disabilities, and she simply accepted me for mine. I knew I was going to marry her, but it took me a month to work up the courage. And when I did ask, she was so excited, she was like, "Oh, God, yes." I wrote a wedding poem for when we got married fifteen years ago.

Because I am disabled, and my wife is disabled as well, we were able for the first year to get Obamacare at a very, very reasonable price. It ended up being the best thing that ever happened to us. Right now our finances are a total disaster. We can't pay our utilities. If my friends had not stepped up to the plate, we would not have electricity or cable right now, or internet, or phone.

Empathy is much better than sympathy

I believe God answers and God takes care of us. There is a great deal of similarity between Christianity and the teachings of the Buddha. The Dalai Lama is one of the most wonderful men on the planet. I think he is a breath of fresh air. Peace, love, and understanding, as us old hippies would say. The Buddha taught that, Jesus taught that. As Touretters we need understanding and empathy, from others and for each other. And empathy is much better than sympathy.

CHAPTER EIGHT

CREATIVITY

People in these pages often spoke of creativity's healing qualities. Writing about one's life, painting, performing, playing a sport, working with your hands and your imagination, these activities bring relief from tics and a transformative view of oneself.

Being creative, being expressive—"making something out of nothing" as one person put it—is a shining road to fulfillment and happiness. It's a way to nurture a healthy self-image. Innovative people are educating the public about TS; they're showing how it feels being captive to non-volitional action; they're transfiguring tics into beautiful actions; they're demonstrating with their own lives how to renew oneself by turning suffering into wisdom; they're using creativity to find a clearer view of oneself and the world.

The following is only a selection of creative individuals. Dip into almost any interview in this book and you will find someone involved in a creative endeavor.

Jamie was born in a trunk. Medically unadvisable? If your parents are in the theater, that phrase describes growing up familiar with the mysteries of back-stage life. Jamie was surrounded with people as creative as they were peculiar. This provided him two great benefits that help with his Tourette's to this day. Being unusual himself, he doesn't feel out of place. And he's tapped deeply into his creativity, bringing it forth in his worldview and his artistic responses to life. As you'll see, a second event—for Jamie and the nation—shaped his worldview as well.

JAMIE
20 years old

This new worldview

I have an unconventional brain. It's the only brain I've ever had [*he laughs*]. When I was in second grade, my mom read to me at night, and I started making noises. I went to school a few blocks from the Twin Towers when 9/11 happened, and there was already PTSD. We had special counsel-ors to work with us, who sent us to Dr. Barbara Coffey at NYU. She's a preeminent Tourette's doctor and she talked to me for ten minutes and said, "Yep, he has Tourette's." So then it was me working with occupation-al therapists, and figuring out how to deal with my Tourette's.

Being mature when I was younger was important in controlling my Tourette's. It forced me to grow up fast, and I was able to spend more time focusing on why I was doing these weird things, and why people were making fun of me. It allowed me to isolate that feeling and either stifle it or channel it into less overt expression. So if I wanted to fling my arm, I learned to twist my wrist and that gave me the same feeling.

Loud, crumbly noise

For whatever reason, I was good at letting stress roll off my back. I hate to thank 9/11 for *anything*, but I think my experience there forced maturity on me that made it easier to work through my impulses at a young age. I had seen people crying, I had seen people dying, it was... I think I was young enough that it's less a trauma and more a sad memory. But it gave me this new worldview.

September 11 was the second day of second grade. I was between four and six blocks away. I was out playing in the front area and we see the first plane go overhead and a few seconds later a huge explosion. We were shielded from seeing anything by a building. So we hear the first explosion and teachers are like, "Get inside, get inside." So we go inside and then we started… I remember we were outside again either when the second plane hit, or the first Tower collapsed. I remember we were walking down the street and there was this big explosion and loud, crumbly noise. And we ran to the side to get out of the way before all the bricks came flying by.

I found the bad dream

In school there was teasing, but I had pre-existing friendships. I had to learn to deal with it, when I realized it wasn't going to stop. My parents were on my side. It helps being from a liberal family. My dad's father was in the Peace Corps, my parents are actors, so they're used to peculiar people. They're good at accepting those differences.

My mom won a Tony Award in 1987 for Best Actress in a Musical for *Me And My Girl*. I wasn't born then. My dad is a familiar face to many people. He's had a TV and movie career, but his real passion is in the theater. He is an incredible Shakespearean actor. My mom is also a talented classical actress. Watching them in the theater is a privilege and I've learned so much from them about self-control.

When I was little, when I had a bad dream, my mom would rub my head and say, "I found the bad dream." She'd make an octopus-thing with her hands, a head massage, and pull her hand away and say, "I've got the bad dream. I'm going to throw it away." Now I do that with tics. I see it in my head. I feel the tension being pulled out wherever it is in my body. And if I let go too early, I feel it going back in and I have to grab it again and throw it down. It's weird, but it works for settling the stresses I have.

Less flourishy things

In public I was always stressed that I would say something and it would upset some other kid. I suppressed and used visualization techniques. Lots of lying on a beach and relaxing. Breathing exercises. Stress release, where you squeeze something really hard, until you can't anymore, then you let go. That's how I learned about isolating tics and how to push them to the side.

At this point, if I need to tic, and it isn't a particularly stressful situation, or if I'm not exhausted, I can sharply exhale once and that'll be my vocal tic. For physical tics, I'll move my ankle or kick my leg out and it looks like I'm shaking out a charley horse. Or I'll twist my arm, but it'll be into my body so nobody can see. So I've learned how to channel impulses into less flourishy things. Definitely it takes more of the motions to get it right. One big head snap to the side and my leg going up to my back would scratch the itch immediately. I can do six rotations of my wrist and one jaw clench and it does the same thing. Or I'll want to tic my elbow, so I'll move my pinkie finger off to the side, and twist my wrist, and that feels like I've done the elbow thing, even though I haven't. I call it 'isolation.'

Managing my tics improved over time. I've been doing it for more than half my life. Sometimes I'll catch a big one and think, "Okay, I need to deal with this one manually." But otherwise my control is on autopilot.

People don't look at it as defining me

Pretty much my entire life I've felt like I start as the outsider and learn how to engage myself. I'm aware of my difference, but I've learned to move past that. It's not like I've turned away from my Tourette's. It's that people don't look at it as defining me, and making me not worthy of being part of their group.

I'd gone to summer camps and been bullied a lot. But then I went to Super Camp and ID Tech Camp.[66] It was all about learning how to interact with people. And ID Tech was a nerd camp, so there were a lot of awkward kids, who loved playing video games. You could find common ground with them almost immediately. Plus you got to play video games and build video games. It was definitely very helpful. Super Camp was an academic camp, but also it was about learning how to have faith in yourself and be comfortable with yourself. I went to those camps every year until I graduated high school. Once I got to college, the teasing stopped.

---

66   Super Camp is an academic, life, and career skills camp. ID Tech Camp is a computer skills camp.

I realized I can do this

The first time I met another person with Tourette's was meeting Dash Mihok, who is an actor with Tourette syndrome. My dad was in *The Day After Tomorrow* and Dash played his best friend. So Dash and I got to hang out. I've always wanted to be an actor, and here is this cool, good-looking guy with lots of friends, very comfortable with himself, having a great time, doing a huge, blockbuster film, and he has Tourette's. So he was everything I wanted in my life, and he was right there in front of me proving it was possible. It gave me the drive. I realized I can do this if I'm smart about it.

The next time I met somebody with Tourette's was at La Guardia High School, a performing arts school that was the basis for the movie *Fame*. I was a drama major there. There were three people with Tourette's in my high school besides me. There was Julia. She was sweet. Loved her. There was Michael, a vocal major with Tourette's. It was cool to watch how he worked his tics around as he was singing. Then there was Anton, who was a visual artist with Tourette's. Anton is incredible. He's the son of... I'm not sure how the family dynamic works, but he's a child of people in the sideshow at Coney Island. For his sixteenth birthday, we got on a party bus and went to Coney Island and hung out with the Snake Lady and stuff. She was like, "Oh, Anton, I'm so proud of you! [*he laughs*]" And he's a great magician and animator.

It was cool to see these artists with Tourette's, each one doing a different type of thing, learning how to deal with their Tourette's. And apparently there's an instrumental major there now, who has Tourette's. And he's making his music too.

Shut up, brain

I'm a bad boy, except I'm really not. I'm about as much of a bad boy as someone with strict morals [*he laughs*]. I feel a lot of people with Tourette's are well aware of what they're capable of. "Oh, wow, right now I could yell fire in this theater." And part of you is—even if it's a small part—part of you is pushing to do that. That always scared me, but I've learned I am in control of it. I've learned I can tell it, "No," even when the urge is very much there. I'll be watching a play and part of me wants to stand up and yell. I'll feel the muscles in my legs getting tense, like I'm going to stand up. And I'll be like, "Really? You're not actually going to do that." And my brain is, "Well, I'm not, but I *could*." And I'm like, "Well, yeah, but shut up, brain. We're watching a play now [*he chuckles*]." I have a very interesting and dynamic internal dialogue.

Fear, and then amusement

My YouTube exposure,[67] it's nice [*he laughs*]. That's about the only word I can say. It's cool to get recognition for my poem. 'Cause there are so many things you can get famous for on the internet. It's good to know I'm getting attention for something I'm proud of as a performer and a writer, and has brought respect to me. Rather than, "Wow, this guy will eat *anything!*" Sure that might make you a crap-ton of money, but your grandchildren are going to watch that and say, "You shamed our family for generations."

I wrote about people's responses to me in sixth grade in my poem *This Time.* I say, "I see fear and then amusement, two reactions most commonly seen to occur at a freak show." Those looks are what inspired me to learn how to control myself. It was problem after problem, loud noise after loud noise and people looking at me weirdly. And then people knowing what I had and *still* making fun of me. But the natural part of you that makes you different doesn't need to be your defining trait.

I think the poem is an ultimatum saying, "You can give me shit over this, but at the end of the day I'm going to turn you into an awesome poem that makes me sound like a badass [*he laughs*]." I wanted to say something in the poem about the bullying and about the violence.

The music metaphor

Being pushed down a flight of stairs is the most distinct memory I have. I think it was an accident, because they punched me in the arm, and we were on the stairs, and I fell. But I fell down the stairs and they were quiet, and then I started moving and they realized they wouldn't get in trouble because I wasn't dead, and they started laughing. Like it was my fault. So the short story is—they pushed me down a flight of stairs. At the same time, I didn't want to say this has affected me so deeply that they've won.

---

67   On youtube.com search: Jamie Sanders, This Time, Tourettes. As of this date Jamie's video has more than 53,000 views.

I needed to say I've turned it into something good. But how do you turn being pushed down the stairs into something good?

I realized I needed to use the music metaphor. Because I'm ticcing like a metronome. Everything is music. I *feel* rhythms in everything I do. Everything is based around rhythm, around the way something sounds. Slide a door shut—the way that shuts, and the way the final thing clicks into place, affects how my next footstep falls. My next footstep is going to be two beats or one beat and I make a rhythm as I walk in.

I perceive the world in a way other people can't

I realized falling down the stairs, that is a symphony. That is so many sounds. Of me colliding with the ground at Mach 6 [*he laughs*], making a massive noise that leads to them laughing, that leads to me pulling myself to my feet. You know? With my Johnny Bravo keychain dangling and clinking against the side of the wall—it's music. I perceive the world in a way that other people can't. People living their day-to-day life, they don't notice things like that. They don't feel things like that. I feel spasms in my back when I touch the cover of a book I'm about to read because my pinkie scratched it in a certain way, and it's a rhythm. And it's unique to me.

I'm sure someone else with Tourette's will feel something in their own way. It's all about finding your own rhythm and how your spasms are bouncing around your insides, and sometimes they need to come out. But ultimately you're playing music inside yourself all the time. And that's fucking cool.

Carrie's soft Louisiana accent reminds me of a gracious Cajun waltz. Like many in this book, her creativity is irrepressible. She understands that our responsibility is to find what we love and make the most of it. Her view resonates with a Buddhist precept, which urges us to approach each situation with an open mind and compassionate heart, do the best we can, and accept the consequences.

CARRIE
28 years old

I don't want to be in the public eye

I started writing when I was very young. I won a poetry contest and had my first poem published when I was eleven. When I got married and didn't have anything to do after my kids were asleep, I started writing again. It turned into writing novels and short stories.

My book is a novel based in south Louisiana. It's called *Southern Hospitality.*[68] The art team is doing the cover now and I'm excited. It makes it more real every time they give me more information.

I have to host pre-release parties. I'm nervous about those parties. I think that's why I never tried to get published before, because I don't want to be in the public eye. The only reason I'm okay with it now is because I have a cause. It's not just about getting my work out there. It's about helping people. Ten percent of proceeds are going to the TSA. Anything I do for the book will be a platform for the TSA and Tourette's education.

I've got about five other novels[69] I'm sitting on, but I've never tried to do anything with them. I think I was scared to. The only reason I sent this one is my brother-in-law dared me [*she chuckles*].

I had a neurologist and psychiatrist and I loved her. I probably pushed her to her limits because I didn't want to cooperate. I was mad at the world. I appreciate her so much that she's on the guest list for my

---

68   *Southern Hospitality* by Carrie Delatte, was released November 11, 2014. It is available for Kindle, Nook, and iTunes e-readers.

69   Her published novel count is now at four: She added *The Daydreamer's Currency, Coming Up Cajun,* and *Vidalia.* As for the future, in her words: "I've got a list of about twelve titles hanging on the side of our fridge that I'm steadily making my way through."

book-release party. It'll be nice to show her that all the effort she put into helpin' me paid off.

I would not have gone as extreme with medications

I'm the baby of five children and I'm the one and only that had Tourette's. I was seven when the tics started with my eyes blinkin' and my nose twitchin' and opening my jaw really wide, like I was yawning, but quick and forceful. My first grade teacher called my mom and said, "I'm not saying it's Tourette's, but I had another student who went through the same thing."

A light bulb went off in my mom's head because my third cousin on my dad's side has Tourette's. So by the time I was out of first grade I had a diagnosis. My cousin's parents got mom and dad into their first support group.

I wouldn't say my parents had a solid footing with Tourette's. Back then there wasn't a lot of information. I would not have gone as extreme with medications. I know they had no other options, but it's... it's given me issues even to this day. But that's being a parent—you learn as you go.

I was heavily medicated from seven to nineteen, when I stopped everything. When I was growing up I can't say I ever had a hundred percent control over what was going on. Even if I *could* figure it out, I was too zombied-out from medication, or my Tourette's was so bad I couldn't handle anything anyway.

I missed half the school year every year. Either my tics were so bad I couldn't go, or I didn't want to go. I *begged* my parents to let me quit when I turned seventeen. So when I graduated, people were shocked. I took honors English and was on the honor roll.

This is on you

In between junior high and my first year of high school my grandfather was diagnosed with cancer and died within a month. I was close to him... [*softly*] yeah. So things got really rough really fast. That summer I ended up in a hospital for two weeks. They wanted me off the three medications I was on and to start a new medicine.

My doctor told me, "You have a choice. You're gonna let this ruin your life or you're going to figure out how to live a productive and happy life. This is on you. What do *you* want out of life?" Her pep talk did some good [*she laughs*].

I don't know *why*, but between nineteen and two years ago, my tics were relatively calm. I handled them on my own. And when I couldn't, I could handle the situation around me enough to be unmedicated. Then two years ago they got worse, out of nowhere. I started grinding my teeth so hard I was breaking teeth. I had to be put back on medication.

They tried Celexa and that was very bad. I went a little while being scared of medication, then they put me on Risperidol and that helped my tics and anxiety issues a lot. But it was back to how I was as a kid. I could see everything going on around me but I didn't feel active. I decided to stop taking it.

The tics have increased but are manageable. I think they're the worst late at night, once I have homework done with the kids and have them tucked in. That's when I'd normally be writing. But I've got so much going on, with kids and the book being published, I have not had time to write.

Be the best version of yourself that you can be

Like a lot of people with Tourette's, my motto is, 'Never judge a book by its cover.' If you don't know what's goin' on with somebody, you have no right to pass judgment.

I wish non-TSers understood how exhausting tics can be. When my head's twitchin' really bad, I get nauseous. You get headaches, you get neck pains, shoulder pains. It also takes a mental toll, because when it's bad you're more aware of people looking at you, which makes it worse. It's a never-ending cycle—the worse your tics are, the more looks you get, the more you think about it. It's exhausting.

Tourette's is becoming more known, so nowadays people will straight up ask me if I have Tourette's. Some people just don't believe you can't control it. It took me a long time to not worry about them. I try my best to walk away. There are some people you *cannot* help them to understand.

When I was younger I couldn't grasp how people could be so cruel. I hated everything. I was so angry. But over the last decade there's a new light shined on everything. You can't control how people view you, so be the best version of yourself that you can be. If that's not good enough for somebody, then oh well. *You* know you're doing your best.

I feel for those people

The idea of Tourette's out in society and the media is not good. They're quick to make it about one symptom—everybody knows what that is—and people don't associate it with anything but a joke. I had a three-month period where I had to deal with coprolalia. I could not be swearing at school events and things. So when it happened, I pretty much shut myself in until that tic dissipated. I feel for those people.

And seeing kids going through Tourette's is difficult. I just hope they know that's not all life has to offer. I'd tell those kids to hold on a few years and they're gonna see how wonderful things can be.

When you get picked on, when you get laughed at, when you get mocked, it forces you to build character and strength

I think half my strength as a single parent comes from growing up with Tourette's. You have to be stronger than the people who are mentally abusing you. When you get picked on, when you get laughed at, when you get mocked, it forces you to build character and strength. There's that Jeff Foxworthy quote,[70] and I cried when I saw that.

My faith has been a strong support for me. My breaking point came about a year ago, when life as a single mom had gotten difficult. It came down to, "Okay, I understand I'm not married anymore. I understand my ex-husband doesn't want anything to do with my kids."

But I know I need God. Because I cannot do it alone. And the more I built my relationship back up with God—because I had been slacking in recent years [*she chuckles*]—the more I came to terms with everything. The more I was able to forgive *myself* for not always being the best person I could be.

I'm okay with myself. I have things to work on still, but everybody does. When I meet new people, whether they are quick to notice my Tourette's or not, that's my rule of thumb—this is who I am, take it or leave it. I'm doing just fine without you in my life, so if you walk away now it's not going to be that big a difference.

---

70   Foxworthy's statement was about the value of understanding. He said that if the general public understood what it takes to live with Tourette syndrome, people would see Touretters as role models of strength rather than as social outsiders.

―――――――――――――――――――― ❧ ――――――――――――――――――――

The lotus flower, symbol of Buddhist enlightenment, grows with its roots deep in mud, the metaphoric soil of suffering. Thich Nhat Hanh, the noted Vietnamese teacher, has this simple formulation: "No mud, no lotus." Sutie has used dance to transform her suffering into wisdom, and this is how she shares her teaching about Tourette syndrome. She calls it 'redefining the disorder,' which involves accepting it, finding positive qualities in it, and understanding what we, as Touretters, have to give back to the larger community.

SUTIE
33 years old

Who could blame them?

My tics started when I was eight and progressed until I was thirteen, when my parents took me to a neurologist, who diagnosed me with Tourette syndrome. He put me on Haldol. My mom noticed it was making me like a zombie, and didn't help the tics. So she got me right off of that, thankfully.

Since then I haven't been medicated for Tourette syndrome. For the past ten years I've been taking Klonopin, a small dose. It helps anxiety and obsessive-compulsiveness, and the ADD. I take it at bedtime so it calms me down and I can get some rest for another day of battle in my head. Gotta make sure I'm well rested for that [*she laughs*]. Just recently I started on an antidepressant. It helps the anxiety, and I have a lot of anxiety. A lot of people with Tourette's have anxiety, and who could blame them? So much of having TS is you feel out of control.

Life's hard enough

When I was eleven I wanted to become a professional ballerina. I was devoted to the point of obsession. It was part of OCD. If someone played music too loud I'd say, "Please turn the music down because if I lose my hearing I won't be able to hear the music on stage. It'll ruin my dance career." It's absurd, but that's how irrational obsessions are. I was afraid to look at a bright light because God forbid it blinded me and I wouldn't be able to dance on stage.

I was unhealthy, I was isolated. I became anorexic for a couple of years. And I was eleven years old. It shook up my parents, and at fourteen my mom pulled me out of dance class. It was heartbreaking. I threw a fit and didn't want to speak to anybody.

I remember *that*, more than my parents responding to my Tourette's. I remember my dad would say I'd grow out of it. But by the time I was sixteen, and still ticcing, I realized he didn't know what he was talking about. It made me sad because I think his lack of interest was partly his guilt that I had this. He probably felt helpless, so he swept it under the rug. "Why do you have to do that?" he'd say. "Life's hard enough."

I was self-medicating

At elementary school I was pretty good at suppressing the tics. I didn't get bullied or picked on too much. It didn't hinder me from having friendships. Things became different in college, as I began to accept my disorder and was more forthcoming about it with my peers. They were accepting. I even developed a sense of humor about it. I'd be sitting around with friends and I'd do a tic, and we'd laugh together, and they'd try to imitate it. We'd make it sort of fun. That was important to me. Adding humor into it was a positive way to deal with it. It normalized it.

I can guarantee Tourette played a big part in developing my self-image, even today as an adult. Being able to control it and not being bullied was a great help. But when I was a teenager and, until recently, I was self-medicating. At fourteen I stopped dancing and was heartbroken. But the next year I saw *Forrest Gump,* and it changed my life. I wanted to be like Jenny. Off I went to the hippie vintage shops. I found sex, drugs, and rock'n'roll. I became a normal teenager. So now I had a boyfriend. Now I listened to the Grateful Dead. Now I smoked pot. That was the beginning of my big change.

I stepped away from one realm of compulsion into another, which involved hedonism and drugs. Not healthier, but different. It did mellow me out more than dancing. And it worked for years. Not just the pot, but I began drinking too. That, thankfully, didn't really pick up until my twenties. I had my daughter, Della, when I was twenty-three and had post-partum depression. Then I got a divorce. And my father passed away. My drinking went off to the races. And I've been drinking every day for the last ten years of my life.

The hardest challenge

So to be honest, unfortunately I became an alcoholic. And now I'm in AA. It's been one month. What I'm going through now, getting sober, is this new journey I'm embarking on. This is the hardest challenge I've stood up to in my life. Specially because it's my own undertaking. No one forced my hand. I put myself in AA. I didn't like that I'd become a slave to this self-medicating. I saw that it was hurting my body and mental faculties. I wasn't functioning properly anymore.

And to top it off, I was spiritually depraved. I could tell it was gnawing away at my integrity and my spirit. My moral conscience said, "That's enough." So this is a huge thing I'm doing. I'm under so much stress. There are so many days I want to drink again and numb it out for a couple of hours. It's not just the Tourette's, it's the obsessive thinking. It's the thinking! It's alarming that alcohol, the quick fix, ends up being poison.

I learned that my only coping skill ended up being alcohol. I didn't realize how poorly I was handling stress. So I'm learning about myself. It goes all the way back to when I was anorexic, doing ballet, and how unhealthy I was at that point in my life. I never learned healthy coping skills. Whoa! What a realization!

Coping means, for one thing, regulating your emotions. Not acting out of impulse, which is often what I do, and is part of Tourette's. It's about stopping and breathing before I have a knee-jerk reaction. I also could say exercise, journaling, praying. I do believe in God. I'm trying to pray more.

A battle wound, a purple heart

I got my BFA in oil painting. At that point I was very forthcoming about my Tourette's. Almost like I wore it as a badge on my sleeve. Like a battle wound, a purple heart. And not to evoke self-pity, either. It was, "I'm courageous." Kinda like that. "I can own my disability and I'm okay with it."

I was in the middle of my painting thesis, and increasingly frustrated with the materials. Paint was messy and expensive, and I wanted more movement with my art. So I rented a camera and made this strange little video. It didn't even have to do with Tourette's. My painting teacher thought it was interesting and said, "Have you thought about doing a video about your disorder?"

So I did this 7-minute video called *The Twitch Trials*. I wrapped myself in chains and went down into my basement. It was very metaphoric, like, "Oh, I'm in chains! I'm a slave to my disorder!" [*She laughs.*] This was the first rekindling of dance for me. So in the video I'm restricted by chains but still trying to tic, and also incorporating slow, dance-like movement. Then I began layering clips and making them translucent over each other, piling them up. So there are these different versions of me ticcing and dancing. It's kind of dark and weird. I added an audio track to give it this haunted feeling.

BAM

My painting professor thought it was beautiful and suggested I see a video professor. He'd never seen anything like it. I was claiming my disability and manifesting it through video. He became my mentor, and together we made *Twitch Trials #2*. We explored combining my tics and dance. For example, I have the barking tic. So it can become almost a percussion instrument. I made five or six videos, which became my thesis for my degree. And for the final showing of student work, I had this huge wall-mounted screen playing videos and sound [*she laughs*]. And everyone else had their quiet little paintings next to it.

Then my mentor suggested finding trained modern dancers and teaching them some tics and seeing what it would look like putting them into dance combinations. The light bulb went off. Within four months I found dancers, taught them about Tourette's, choreographed a dance piece, hired a musician to compose music, found a venue, promoted the show, and held two performances, each with an audience of eighty-five people. I just—BAM—made it happen. I guess I gave birth to it. I made it happen.

There's a lot to admire about our resilience and strength

That was when my dance troupe, *Band of Artists,*[71] got rolling. It was a renaissance in my life. We were on fire. It was extremely liberating for me as a person. And it had a beautiful effect on my self-image. I went from someone who might feel insecure about themselves, to feeling almost proud to be different. Wanting to share with people what makes this disorder unique, and even beautiful. Giving it new meaning. These are all part of our mission as *Band of Artists*. Redefining this disorder through artistic means.

We want people to go beyond tolerance. Tolerance is a good start, but I want to teach appreciation for people with disabilities, what we do every day. We have something invaluable to give back. People need to know this. Living like this takes stamina. It takes creativity. There's a lot to admire about our resilience and strength. It takes a great deal of strength—physical, emotional, and spiritual strength—to maintain and survive with Tourette syndrome. People ought to understand that and admire that. There's a certain power we have, that we're surviving, let alone being successful.

It's what I manifest through my dance. I use tics with the music—very sharp movements that aren't pretty and soft. And the music is intense. I want to communicate that this is hard work, and it takes a lot of power to move through the world with a disability.

Buy groceries and pump gas

We're all complex human beings, right? And that was the case for me. I loved parties and I had friends. And I was deeply tortured. I still am, on a daily basis. I'm always living with a certain amount of discomfort. And when I go in public, there's always going to be an amount of self-consciousness. Because I know people are looking at me when I'm trying to buy groceries and pump gas. It's a pain in the ass. Because there's always someone looking at you funny and you're like, "Yeah, whatever." There are other times I turn around and say, "I have Tourette's." Then they're apologetic, and then *I'm* apologetic. So it's frustrating. And on top of it, I'm jerking my body so much I give myself a headache sometimes. It's exhausting. It's also mentally draining to have all these urges constantly

---

71   Find Sutie at bandofartists.org and on Facebook at *Band of Artists*.

flooding your mind, distracting you from whatever task has to be done. It's all-encompassing, sometimes, to live with this. And so in the videos, with the chains and the darkness... I feel like I'm sort of enslaved by this disorder.

I want to evolve

I have a sense of humor, and I have a huge heart, and I like to have fun. And you know what? Maybe that saves me. Because I love to party, hence the alcoholism. It was even easier for me to have fun and fit in. But now I can no longer drink successfully. It's holding me back. And spiritually it's holding me back. I can't move ahead and grow as a person and as a spirit. I want to evolve and live to my fullest potential, and contribute that to the world. And I know I can't if I continue down that hedonistic path.

There's definitely something valuable in having Tourette syndrome, as much as it is a huge challenge to live with. The benefit is people with Tourette's almost always have OCD, and those can have their benefits. When an individual with Tourette's decides what they're interested in, they can harness that OCD and make it into almost a hyper-focus. When I really want to get something done it's almost like my disorders help me. I become more determined and more focused than the average person. It doesn't happen all the time, obviously. It's only when we finally figure out what we want to go for, whether a short- or long-term goal.

As a science nerd, I appreciate the creativity of science, and was excited talking with Gary. I love to say "Zero Gradient Synchrotron." As a high-energy physicist, he routinely accelerated protons to near light speed (186,000 miles a second). Fast. And now he does Zumba. Also fast. I like that his response to Tourette's was to roll up his sleeves and get involved with the Tourette Association of America. He's made a difference, and in so doing, he's set an example.

GARY
76 years old

These things don't last long

I was interested in physics even in high school, so when I went to college I knew what I wanted to be. I majored in physics, went to Case Institute of Technology[72] and got my Bachelors Degree in Physics, then got my Masters at Auburn, and my Ph.D. at Ohio State. I did research for my dissertation at Argonne National Laboratory outside of Chicago. My specialty was high-energy physics, so I worked with the particle accelerator we had there, the Zero Gradient Synchrotron. That's where my career was for the next 30 years.

My experiment was to measure how many elementary particles were produced by a high-energy proton beam hitting various targets, like Beryllium. Pions and kaons, these things don't last long. Nanoseconds.

What's really interesting is the Large Hadron Collider over in Switzerland. It's amazing that this huge accelerator is so perfectly aligned that protons, circulating in opposite directions around the superconducting ring, can be made to collide.[73] I know how accelerators function, and it's astounding that it works at all.

I spent a good part of my career working with the Department of Energy, trying to find a place to bury high-level nuclear waste from nuclear power plants. We looked at nine different sites, including salt deposits in Texas, Mississippi, Utah, and Louisiana. DOE ended up picking Yucca

72   Now Case Western Reserve University.
73   The Large Hadron Collider, the single largest machine in the world, is a circle 27 kilometers (17 miles) long. A proton is 0.8768 millionths of a billionth of a meter.

Mountain in Nevada. Unfortunately, after spending billions of dollars, the project was cancelled.

Everything is political. I ended up working on several other DOE projects. The Superconducting Super Collider they were going to build in Texas. After digging the tunnel, and spending a couple of billion dollars, it was cancelled. I worked on a centrifuge facility to enrich uranium. They built the whole plant, operated it for one day to prove it would work—contaminating it—and shut it down. The centrifuges had to be decontaminated. That's another couple of billion dollars. Never operated after that.

Gee, that's me

I wasn't diagnosed until my early 30s. I didn't know what was wrong with me. The doctors said I was just nervous. The local TSA group had gotten an article in the Chicago newspaper and I read it and said, "Gee, that's me." It was a big relief to finally know what was wrong with me. Now it had a name, and I wasn't the only one.

During grade school and high school, I just worked through it. I didn't have much problem with people bothering me. I didn't let it get in the way of anything. So I've not had difficulty with the emotional aspects of Tourette's, not at all. I think part of it is that my tics are a lot worse now than when I was young.

I never took medication, but when I quit smoking, about thirty years ago, my Tourette's got worse. There's been some talk of nicotine[74] helping and that might be true. A couple of times since, when my tics were particularly bad, I tried nicotine patches, and it helped some. You just have to find a better delivery device than cigarettes or vaping.

I also have OCD and can't sit still and do one thing for more than a few minutes at a time. I do have trouble concentrating for long periods. Usually when reading books, I'll read a few pages and get up and move around. With my experiments, I was out in a trailer, mostly by myself, and there were things to do all the time, so I had to concentrate.

I have to get one of those

I'm never without my tics. I'm in a band and I tic when I play. It's a

---

74   See links from tourette.org.

klezmer band and I play hammered dulcimer. We play for parties, bar mitzvahs, weddings, we play Purim and Hannukah celebrations. Most of what we do is free.

I went to a folk festival in the early '90s, and saw this group of people with four or five hammered dulcimers. I'd never seen one and was fascinated. I spent the whole time watching them. I loved the sound. I came back the next year and they were there again, and finally I said, "I have to get one of those." I have two now. I had one, then found another that was bigger, nicer, better sounding, and more expensive too [*he chuckles*]. Music plays an important part of my life. I just love it, and love to play it, and being in the band.

Zumba

I just celebrated my birthday, and since it was the day after Thanksgiving, I had a pumpkin pie instead of a cake. Then I went to Zumba. That's what I do now, I go to Zumba every day. Exercise with dance—that's it. Half my friends are Zumba people. They tried to get together the largest Zumba class in the world for the Guinness Book of Records. We didn't even come close, but it was fun. The only tic I have when I do Zumba is my vocal tic.

My onset with Tourette's was at five years old. I have thirty or forty different tics now, all the time. Some occur in special places, like if I'm sitting in a chair and I can bounce my head back, I'll do that. My one big vocal tic is throat clearing.

Most of my tics I can hide, so people don't see them. A shoulder shrug, or I hit myself, or move my toes. The most noticeable is my vocal tic. It's worse on an airplane when you're sitting next to somebody. People usually don't say anything, or they think I'm sick. If somebody does say something, I'll tell them I have Tourette's.

It's part of who I am

I have lots of friends with Tourette's now through the Tourette Syndrome Association. I've gone to many conventions they put on. I was President of the Illinois chapter before I retired and moved to Arizona. I used to go to schools and give presentations. Usually I would go because one of the kids in the class had Tourette's. I also belong to the Tourette Syndrome

Foundation of Canada.[75] I went to a conference of theirs and joined the Newfoundland chapter. I even spoke on a panel of speakers at one of the Canadian conferences.

Tourette's is part of me. I've learned to live with it. I've ticced all my life and I wouldn't know what it's like not to. It's part of who I am.

Nearly thirty years ago, just as a lark, I went to my first LA Kings hockey game. As I was leaving to attend the game, a friend, big sports fan, said, "This will change your life." Ridiculous! I laughed, went to the arena, and the next morning rushed out to buy season tickets. I get it when Chelsea says hockey is her passion. Her reflexes are Tourette-fast. But TS has taken its toll on her socially and academically. Brilliant on ice, she struggles off ice with her confidence. She's learning to bring her strength as a goalie to her everyday life. And most important, she's learning to love herself instead of searching for approval first from others.

CHELSEA
23 years old

I'm trying to buckle down

I had seizures from around five or six, and after the seizures fizzled out at fifteen, I started with Tourette's. When I was ten, I'd put my hand in the air and wiggle my fingers at the sky. It was kinda weird. I knew I couldn't stop doing it. My mom and my brother tried to make it a silly thing because they didn't want me to feel bad that I couldn't stop. We didn't think too much about it.

In middle school it got worse with vocal noises, and socially it was rough for me through high school. There was a lot of bullying. I had Special Education, but some teachers didn't take time with people like me. I had a hard time learning. I was angry. It was rough and I remember most of it. My social world at school was awful. I cried daily.

---

75   tourette.ca.

It was tough for my mom. But she's really supportive. She tells me all the time that I gotta wake up, I gotta realize what I want. Now I'm trying to buckle down and get my diploma and graduate. I'm trying to get something going for myself.

I thought I was one of the only ones

I have other issues besides Tourette's. I have anxiety. I do have a little depression. I guess I have bad low self-esteem. Yeah. Sometimes I'm too hard on myself. I need to realize I've been through a lot and I've been strong. I'm starting to meet other people online who have Tourette's. I never knew *all* these people had it. My mom found me the Facebook Tourette group.[76] Before this group, I couldn't find any support. I called the Tourette Association, but they didn't have any support groups in my area. So Facebook is a big help. I realized that mine's bad, but there are people who have it way worse. I'm learning from others what they do to help themselves. It's nice to be able to reach out and talk to people. I thought I was one of the only ones. I thought I was a loner.

The pain is just awful. My shoulders, they twitch four hundred times at day at least, and they grind. My neck and my back always hurt. I do a lot of stretching for my pain. I use a stress ball sometimes and that helps. I try to focus on positive things and keep myself busy. If I don't, the Tourette's really acts up. I've tried medical marijuana. It works, but it's not the best thing on your lungs. I know there are edibles, too. But it only works for a few hours. If you don't use it every day, I don't think it helps. So I don't think it's for me. I can't do prescription pain pills. I don't like them. So it's OTC for pain and I'm looking into essential oils. I also know there's deep brain surgery. But I live with Tourette's now. I'm so used to it. I don't know if it'll ever go away.

There are worse things out there

When I go places and my Tourette's acts up, I still have a hard time with the stares. Little kids who look at me and don't understand. It's hard. I almost feel like I'm not human sometimes. But there are worse things out there. I think of people with missing legs, missing arms, terrible things,

---

76   There are various Tourette's groups on Facebook. Simply search "Tourette syndrome."

and I try to tell myself, "You have this, but you can walk, you can see, you're doing pretty good. You just have to let people think what they want."

The confidence, I'm still working on it, but I'm doing better. Before, I used to get upset and angry. I've come home from stores crying. When people see me twitching, sometimes they think I'm cold and I say, "No, I have Tourette syndrome." It's hard to explain it without sounding kinda crazy. It's terrible and not fair because everyone else can control their movements, but we can't.

My reflexes scare me they're so fast

I've been playing ice hockey since I was five years old. Around the time of my seizures. I played all the way up until I was 19. I played at a very high level. I went to Nationals in California.

Once I get into hockey, my Tourette's calms down. It's a comfort place for me. It makes me look like a strong person. Everybody's proud of me for doing it. People don't even notice I have Tourette's. Hockey is something I have such a passion for. I love it. It makes me happy [*she laughs*].

I always thought goalie was a cool position. Playing other positions, I always got beat on the ice [*she chuckles*], so I felt goalie was good for me. It's nerve-racking sometimes. But when it's one of those tight games and I have to keep my team in, and not let in any goals, it teaches me how to overcome things and be strong and believe in myself. I do think my Tourette's has made me faster. My reflexes scare me they're so fast. Yeah, I think my reflexes for a goalie have been better since my Tourette's. It's pretty amazing when I make a huge save. Your heart beats real fast, you know you did good. Another thing is the crowd. I love people watching me. I love the cheers.

I'm going to be coaching at a women's high school. I'm real excited about it. I've always wanted to teach younger people to play the sport, especially goalie, because that's one position you need to take time to learn. My mom put me through so many camps when I was younger. I remember everything [*she chuckles*]. It's cool to see myself grow as an athlete and as a person. I would love to see that happen to other people.

I'm not so closed in

I love art. It calms my Tourette's. It's like hockey. Once I get on the ice I'm calm, and once I sit down to draw or paint, it relaxes me. That's one thing that's big in my life. My mom makes rustic wood signs, she makes watercolors, all kinds of art crafts. We go to festivals and sell our art. Since we've started doing this, it helps me be confident, talking with people and making sales. It helps because I'm not so closed in and feeling like I can't interact with the public. I notice that when I just sit around, I think too much and my anxiety acts up more.

I never took the time to think what school subjects interested me because I was so into hockey. I thought hockey was going to be everything and I didn't need anything else. But I'm interested in social work, helping people, or counseling maybe. Helping people work through their issues. I've always been good at listening. I've always been a compassionate person. I love helping and making people feel good. I always had that in me. I don't like seeing people hurt. So I'm trying to find what I'd like to do because I know I've got to figure it out.

I think you have to judge who you let yourself be with

I recently got out of a pretty bad relationship. He was very non-support-ive. He would always tell me to stop ticcing. He didn't want to take the time to understand. I think my self-image affected the people I chose in relationships. I picked people who accepted me, and most men did because... you know how men are. And they always gave me a hard time about my Tourette's. I finally pulled myself out and realized, "You need to be with someone who supports your Tourette's and supports you as a person."

I need to make more time to love myself first, and figure out who I am, before I jump back into relationships. Since I didn't have a lot of friends, having boyfriends was something I had to have. That was a prob-lem because I never knew what I wanted, you know? So I've been trying to take more time to think what I want to do. I think you have to judge who you let yourself be with. Just because you have Tourette's doesn't mean you have to be with someone who doesn't care for you. It makes you feel like you don't have anybody, and you feel like giving up.

The short part of the stick

I'm trying new things, to be more talkative, meet people and make friends, instead of just boyfriends. I want to have a group of friends that support me. I have friends from hockey, but I don't hang out with any of them. My mom's pushing me more to do that. She wants to see me bond with people who I have confidence with. I want a buddy, a girlfriend to call, to hang out with, to laugh.

Sometimes people spend so much time making other people happy they forget about themselves. I've done that a lot in my life. I think I've given myself the short part of the stick because I always try to make everyone else happy, and I'm last. But you can't make everyone happy [*she laughs*].

I would say to any kid with Tourette's to stay strong. You gotta realize it's not your fault. You were born this way. You can still be successful. I would tell a younger person, "Don't let people get you down. Stay positive about things in your life that make you happy." What's important is to be who you are and not care what people think. Like me, I do sports and things that show I'm a strong person and I'm not incapable.

It was one of my dreams to play college hockey. I knew if I didn't get my school together, I couldn't. I want to play in the NWHL[77] too. But they require a four-year college degree and I can't complete the academics 'cause of Tourette's. It's not fair that I can't play a pro sport. On the men's side there is no college requirement. It's a double standard. You'd think the NWHL would want a strong goaltender, who has Tourette's, who says, "Yes I can," and who could bring notice to the league. It would be fantastic PR. I *have* the talent. I was followed by Wisconsin and other Division-1 schools, but it's the academics. My older brother, he's twenty-five, he played hockey through Juniors, USHL, NAHL, OJHL, and he played college hockey. I love him and he's very supportive of me.

It frustrates me now. There are lots of opportunities I let go by because I was low self-esteem. I thought I could never, ever finish high school. Now that I realize life isn't all about hockey, I know I've got more options. I think I never let myself look at other things.

I'm still playing. I'm in a summer league. We have a game tonight. We're in the playoffs now. I took some time off from hockey because of

77   The professional level of women's hockey is the NWHL, National Women's Hockey League.

that terrible boyfriend. He actually took me away from my sport and made me a whole different person. So I'm coming back and realizing this is who I am, and I need to do the things I love.

CHAPTER NINE

CHANGE

In Buddhism, a fundamental truth is "impermanence," the fact that reality is in constant flux, nothing is fixed, things begin and they end; each end is a beginning. Things change.

In 1979, Argentinian folk singer Mercedes Sosa was exiled by the military junta then in its sixth year conducting its Process of National Reorganization (what the people called The Dirty War). That government eventually killed as many as 30,000 of its own citizens. These were murderous times and the population suffered greatly. As that dictatorship was collapsing in 1982, Mercedes Sosa returned and, at the Teatro Colòn, sang the rousing song *Todo Cambia (Everything Changes)*.

Here are three sets of interviews that illustrate change. The first features a mother and son, the interviews separated by seven years. The last two sets are separated by one year only. Short term, long term, *todo cambia*.

Patience. Hope. Don't give up. These are the lessons of change.

———————————————

I spoke with Sharon and Jad on a sunny day in the California mountains. We sat at a picnic table. They often leaned into one another, exchanging looks and smiles, and sometimes deep grief. Sharon speaks buoyantly with an English accent; Jad's voice is softer but he is expressive nonetheless. This was one of my first interviews for the book, and I was appalled at the suffering they'd endured and encouraged by the hope they were able to harness.

SHARON AND HER SON JAD (13 YEARS OLD)
Kenneth Michael Staebler Tourette Spectrum Camp 2007

Now I know I'm normal

Jad: I started ticcing when I was ten.

Sharon: It was about a year later that the doctors diagnosed it as Tourette's. They thought it was PANDAS.[78]

Jad: It was hard because I would get throat injuries and I had to whisper.

Sharon: Generally, for the last three years, his tics are motion tics, localized in his left shoulder, neck, and leg. He spasms so much, sometimes he's in severe pain

Jad: I felt that I didn't deserve it. I used to think I was from a different planet or something. But now I know I'm normal.

Sharon: Of course you are [*they hug*]. He used to say to me, "Why am I getting punished like this, mom? Why is God doing this to me? I want to control it and I can't. It's taking over who I am." There were times when he couldn't function. He couldn't hold a pencil. He found it hard to walk. [*To Jad*] Your whole body was in pain, wasn't it? And with school and how you felt in society.

Jad: Yeah. I felt like an outcast.

Sharon: Yeah. I said to him, "Well, Jad, God doesn't give us more than we can endure. You will cope with this. There's a reason you have this. It might be to help others." At one point he said, "I'm going to be a doctor and find a cure for Tourette's."

Jad: Yeah.

---

78   Pediatric Autoimmune Neuropsychiatric Disorders Associated with Streptococcal Infections. See Bill, Chapter Four.

Fantastic, brilliant, amazing

Sharon: He told every neurologist this: "I'm going to find a cure." And I said to him, "You'll be an inspiration to other children you meet." But it's not easy. All the parents will tell you. Behind the scenes you cry, but in front of my son I will be strong and say, "We can do this together." And that's how we got through it, and this is where we are today. It's been a hard road, hasn't it?

Jad: Yeah.

Sharon: What was the wish you have that you told me a moment ago?

Jad: That I wish I didn't have it.

Sharon: But what did you want? For three years he's had this wish... [*she laughs*].

Jad: Oh yeah—to meet a kid with Tourette's, but we hadn't found any. But we found this camp, which is filled with Tourette's kids.

Sharon: Which is fantastic, brilliant, amazing. With new friends from day one is...

Jad: Magic.

Sharon: I've sat here and watched him and it's been worth everything. To see him mixing. Because generally, he likes his own company. He likes to be alone a lot.

Jad: Yeah. Here you can be welcome because everybody has Tourette's.

I'm going to cry now

Sharon: Yeah. At camp you can do your tics and it doesn't matter. But at school it's a different story, isn't it?

Jad: Yeah.

Sharon: School's been the biggest challenge. We've changed schools. A lot. I think it's through people not being educated about Tourette's. On his own account he took the video *I Have Tourette's, But Tourette's Doesn't Have Me* to school. And he took *Teaching the Tiger*, which is a book. And he stood up in front of the class and tried to educate the students about Tourette's.

Jad: Yeah.

Sharon: I really admired him for doing that. I never told him to do it.

Jad: The teacher, she said we never had time to watch the video, so only she watched it. But even when I told the kids about my Tourette's, they still made fun of me. So that was kind of hard.

Sharon: He's not at that school anymore. We're at a better school now.
Jad: Yeah.
Sharon: And he's smiling, which is a great thing. Because for the first two years of Tourette's, he wasn't smiling. He was a sad child.
Jad: It was the medicine.
Sharon: That's a very difficult process. At one point, he was so sedated he couldn't walk. It was the wrong medication, too strong. And we've been through depression. I remember distinctively taking him out for lunch, and he sat across from me, and he looked into my eyes... and I'm going to cry now, and I shouldn't... And he said, "I don't want to live anymore, mom. Let me die." That was heartbreaking for a mother to hear. Because the tics were so bad and life was... not worth living for him. The existence of being at home, no school, no life, no friends.

We went another direction

Sharon: I took him off the medication so I could have my son back again. Because I didn't want him to be like that. We went another direction then [*she laughs*]. I was working in a clinic and they offered biofeedback. I found that very effective. And he would sit in a chair for two hours, hooked up to...
Jad: A machine. And it went inside me and saw everything that was wrong. And the first time I went there, they found my Tourette's.
Sharon: I didn't tell her that he had Tourette's because she was a co-worker. I just said I would like my son to have a treatment and see if he likes it. So two minutes into the session Tourette's came up. Biofeedback relaxed him.
Jad: I like swimming, too.
Sharon: And drawing to relax. When his Tourette's is bad, he'll draw. He draws a lot.
Jad: Mainly, when you're in water, your Tourette's stops for mostly every kid.
Sharon: He can have severe Tourette's, like where he's finding it hard to walk, and I'll just put him in water and he'll relax.
Jad: So that's maybe the key [*they laugh*]. Water.
Sharon: And I think also music. And massage.
Jad: Yeah, massage.

Sharon: And you know, anything that can just relax them. Meditation. Yoga. And breathing, you know, all of this could help.

I help them

Jad: When my Tourette's is bad, it feels like my insides are exploding. And it really hurts. I can bang my arm on a table and it starts to bleed and it hurts.

Sharon: He was so much trying to control it in school that his whole left side of his body was black and blue from banging it against the desk. That's when I said, "You can't stay at school. It's not working. We can't do this."

Jad: Yeah.

Sharon: He's passed out a few times, if he bangs his head or something like that.

Jad: My Tourette's, on the positive side, has made me smarter. I'm better skilled in drawing.

Sharon: What do you feel when you see another child with disabilities?

Jad: Yeah, I help them.

Sharon: He wants to go out of his way to help them because he can relate to how they're feeling. You're a good child. You're a good boy.

She's his tough side

Jad: I have friends I've known for years. I told them I had Tourette's and they don't see anything wrong with me. They think I'm a normal person.

Sharon: Now, at school, when they see the Tourette's, do they do anything?

Jad: They don't see it because I try to hold it in. I don't want them to make fun of me.

Sharon: He holds it in at school and when he comes home, he'll have his…

Jad: Breakout.

Sharon: Breakout. Whatever he needs to do just to get it out.

Jad: I have a sister, her name's Ellie. She's eight, she's younger.

Sharon: She is his tough side.

Jad: [*He laughs*]

Sharon: When he'd come from school crying because the boys had teased him, she'd say, "I'm gonna go to that school and I'm gonna tell them that my brother's got Tourette's and they'd better not...," you know. Then you get the other side when, sometimes the Tourette's is bad, so Jad has to hit everything in sight. So he hits her sometimes, and he doesn't mean to. Then she'll feel, "Why do I get *him* as a brother?"

There was a lot of silence

Sharon: When you get diagnosed, not knowing, you're surprised, and shocked, and emotionally distraught. Initially when they tell you Tourette's... Jad thought he was going to die. And I said no, we just need to educate ourselves on this. Because at the time, it was an emergency. I thought they were seizures.

When Jad first got diagnosed with Tourette's, I'll be honest with you, my husband and I couldn't talk for a long time. We were just... we needed time and space to get our heads around what had happened. Because, you know, you go from having a son with nothing, and one day you have someone who, on a day-to-day basis, you don't know what you're dealing with. So we went through a period where there was a lot of silence in our relationship, in the marriage. It took us a while, then we started talking about it, and I had floods of tears. You know, it's your son, it's your baby, it's your life.

[*Jad's been gazing down, serious and reflective. Now he smiles.*]

I was emotional about it, but didn't want Jad to see that either, so I kept it hidden. Then his father and I started opening up, and started talking about it, and we decided that if we're going to get him through this, we've got to be his backbone and his friend, and we need to pull together. And really, it changed our whole life because it brought us together as a family. We needed to be there for Jad. The whole household changed. When he needs quiet time, we have to change the household. But it took my husband longer to accept the condition because... a man and his son, you know. But we accept it now.

Jad: Yeah.

Sharon: It's part of our lives and we don't let it get in our way. We do everything a normal family would do. I think we do *more* because you make the effort because you have a child with Tourette's. We wouldn't be at this camp if he didn't have Tourette's, and we wouldn't have met all these wonderful people.

He's telling all the children and people out there to never give up

Sharon: There's been a fantastic happening in England that has changed a lot of people. There's a show called *Big Brother* and a boy who won it, he had Tourette's.

Jad: He has his own show now. Pete Bennett.

Sharon: And he's getting married, and my mom says it's all over the newspaper and everybody knows about Tourette's now, so that's helped my family understand it more.

Jad: He had it really bad. He had the vocals.

Sharon: Like the swearing Tourette's. What did you think when you saw him?

Jad: People made comments that he was faking it, but he wasn't.

Sharon: But he didn't care, you know. He just was himself on national TV on a weekly basis. And I was saluting him all the way. And I think it made Jad feel better, didn't it?

Jad: Yeah.

Sharon: Because Jad read every article about him.

Jad: That was pretty cool.

Sharon: So there's a message in that. When you see someone like that, it's like he's telling all the children and people out there to never give up. You have to continue, because there is hope.

Jad: He's the role model. I explain Tourette's by talking about all the details, like sometimes I do weird things, so don't judge me or anything, I can't help it. And like, if sometimes I need to be alone, I just have to be alone, and sometimes I have to go home earlier than normally.

Sharon: He wrote a small article—they had to write about themselves—and he put, "I'm a nice boy. I have a good heart. And I would like to be your friend. But don't just judge me because you see my tics." And I thought, "Thumbs up!"

[*They look at each other and laugh.*]

Todo cambia—everything changes. Seven years on, Jad sits across the dining room table from me, a young man, handsome and self-assured. He has a wry, self-effacing smile. Sharon, to my left, retains her verve and enthusiasm for her son and his future. Jad is another Touretter whose isolation, because it was filled with activity he loved, gave him an opportunity to build a career for himself. Jad's fearsome health episodes, the family's quest for answers, and their perseverance have led them to this contented place where mother and child can look at each other and laugh joyfully.

SHARON AND HER SON JAD (20 YEARS OLD)
interviewed in their home 2014

He's not going to survive this one

Sharon: At one point, he hated everything.

Jad: I was fifteen at the time. I went from a hundred fifteen pounds to two hundred.

Sharon: From the meds.

Jad: It was Risperdal. It was horrible.

Sharon: And the tics, they were bad. He didn't want to stay with us… [*she pauses*] he didn't want to be here anymore. I remember he sat across from me at lunch and said, "This is horrible, mom. I can't do this any longer." This was the second time he said that. So I took him off all medications. [*To Jad*] I took you off for one year.

Jad: Yeah.

Sharon: I remember I said, "That's it. We're stopping." I stopped it all. I stopped going to doctors. And I just helped him on my own.

Jad: Right in time.

Sharon: He managed for one year, then came January, and we had to call the ambulance. He's had several episodes in his life where he stops breathing, he passes out, his body goes into like… I can't… his body starts *shaking*, out of control. And I thought, "That's it. He's not going to survive this one." So he had to go back on medications. [*To Jad*] But you did good for that year, and you lost a bit of weight, didn't you?

Jad: Yeah.

You shouldn't be in here

Sharon: There was that doctor, everybody in the waiting room had tics. It was the first time we'd been to a neurologist where I saw everybody with movement disorders. We thought, "This guy knows what he's doing." He said, "I want you to try new meds." So we kept trying new things, as you do, to see what works.

Jad: I asked if I could have Deep Brain Stimulation surgery. Only as a last resort, he said.

Sharon: I remember calling the doctor —after two years being with him—and saying, "We're at maximum capacity on all meds. He's put his foot and hand through walls. This is out of control. You've got to help me." He said, "Your only option is to call a Fifty-One-Fifty.[79]" And that's what we did.

Jad: It was longer than seventy-two hours. I want to say five days. I don't want to go into it too much, but you'd have a room, you'd have a room-mate. You'd share stories and stuff, and then they'd make you go to sleep. A lot of doctors come and talk to you, separate you into groups for activities.

Sharon: No one in there had Tourette's.

Jad: People would ask me, "Why are you in here?" And I'd say, "I have Tourette's." And they'd say, "You shouldn't be in here." There was one kid, fourteen, addicted to heroin, that was bad. I remember one night I could hear him screaming.

It's not a thing to do

Jad: I wasn't a part of it, but I felt empathy. And I did give them quite a slap on the wrist, as well. I said, "You're taking all these drugs, you want to commit suicide, and you have all these reasons. But what about people with cancer? Or people in Africa who can barely eat? You have your problems, but you shouldn't use drugs. Drugs lead only to violence and death and being nothing in your life.

Committing suicide... it's not a thing to do. You say you do it to

79   In California, a 5150 (Fifty-One-Fifty) is a seventy-two-hour involuntary psychiatric hold on a person suspected to have a mental disorder that makes him or her a danger to themselves, a danger to others, and/or gravely disabled. It is three days in a locked psychiatric ward. If medical conditions warrant, the hold can be extended.

yourself, but honestly, it causes so much pain for others. When I think about it now, I wonder, "Why was I thinking of suicide?"

Sharon: Well I know why. You were in a situation…

Jad: I used to go to school and get bullied every day. I stopped talking for a long time. At school, at home, I wouldn't talk.

Sharon: Like a zombie. That was the black, dark place, his bedroom, and he wouldn't come out. And I couldn't get to him. That was the worst time ever for me. I hated it.

Jad: That was middle school.

Sharon: Yeah, thirteen. Then it got bad.[80]

Jad: Eighth grade, that's when I went to home school. I did that until the end of ninth. Then it was getting better.

Sharon: 'Cause that's when you got on Orap.

Jad: Orap—that was a good medicine. That helped me a lot. The thing is, my body got used to it and it stopped working. So then try more meds, guinea pig, basically. Some made me allergic, crazy—

Sharon: Haldol.

Jad: That was it. Haldol. It was bad.

He felt bad he was making us pay all this money

Jad: Right now I'm pretty stable. Recently they found what's been causing my Tourette's. They told me about this thing called PANDAS.[81] We went to a new doctor—this guy, he is literally a genius. He is *the* guy for Tourette's.

Sharon: He knew immediately. He's a neurologist and movement-disorder specialist, but he crosses over into many other things. He has a lot of patients with Tourette's.

Jad: What he found was, when I was young, I used to take a lot of antibiotics.

Sharon: This was in England.

Jad: Now it's caused… your normal level of antibodies is like 200 and mine is 1,200. That's what's causing the nerves in my head to misfire, and causing the movements.

Sharon: And it puts stress on the heart valves as well.

---

80   Just after his 2007 interview for this book.
81   Pediatric Autoimmune Neuropsychiatric Disorder Associated with Streptococcal Infections. See Bill, Chapter Four.

Jad: I did have heart surgery. All my life I've had palpitations and passing out. One day I was at my friend's house and I started shaking. So they took me to the hospital. My heart rate was 200 and they found I had, what, seven holes?

Sharon: Yeah. On the left side of the heart.

Jad: So they filled the holes—

Sharon: They cauterized each one.

Jad: And I haven't had anything after that. It's great [*he laughs*]. But then another problem surfaced. I began to have seizures.

Sharon: But we don't know yet what it is.

Jad: It was eight months ago and I was having them every other day. But now I've been taking some new medicine and that's working, so I'm like, "Let's stay on that!" [*He laughs.*]

Sharon: They're going to do this new treatment for six months.

Jad: Like a blood transfusion, to get my white blood cell count down.

Sharon: Very expensive. Not covered by insurance. Earlier, we ended up with no insurance for four years because nobody would cover him. They said it was pre-existing and they wouldn't cover it. They kicked us off the program. We had to get a lawsuit on them, but we can't talk about it. So Jad was refused any healthcare for four years. It was… expensive. There was one medication, it was $2,800 for a one-month supply. And after two days, he had a bad reaction and we had to throw that medicine in the bin. So he didn't want to see a doctor because he felt bad he was making us pay all this money.

Jad: And I was thinking, "None of this is helping me anyway."

Sharon: And then finally my husband was able to include Jad on his business insurance.

> ### You know what? I have Tourette's.
> ### You got a problem with it? I don't really care.

Jad: My tics are pretty under control right now. It's great [*he laughs*].

Sharon: It's all been terribly difficult. He's cried a lot. I've cried a lot. But it has brought us closer. I think of all these crises we've dealt with, and I feel like we're all really close. We get through milestones, we conquer this or that and we say, "Yeah!"

Jad: I used to feel like an outcast. Now I feel great [*he chuckles*]. I feel like one of the guys, one of the cool, one of the normal kids. I've got some good friends, I'm pretty popular. I would say it changed around the end of high school. Eleventh and twelfth grades. But what was different?

Sharon: I know what it was. [*To Jad*] But you say it.

Jad: I felt I could finally say, "You know what? I have Tourette's. You got a problem with it? I don't really care."

Sharon: That was the first time he'd ever said that. He had confidence. I said to him, "Jad, you're doing your Tourette's out in public." And he said, "Yeah, mom, because I've decided that why should I try to hold it in and hurt *my*self." So now, he said, "I'm just doin' it, mom. And if people look at me, let 'em look." And I thought, "Wow."

Jad: Yeah, I was like, "If you don't like it, that's your problem [*he laughs*]." It was some kind of confidence boost. You mainly… you have to *find* it. I don't know how to explain. When I got to high school, and the tics were a little under control, I started talking to people and making more friends. I kinda reached the point where, "Why is this such a big deal? My friends don't mind, so why should I?"

Sharon: Yeah.

Jad: Something has to boost your confidence. It happens in different ways.

Sharon: I think when we moved to Newport Beach, that was a big step.

Jad: That was a big one.

Sharon: Getting a new home, away from all the darkness.

Jad: Change of scenery. New people. Clean slate, that's what it is.

Find hobbies that distract you

Sharon: We never give up. I always made him feel like we're not going to let this get us down. Things are going to get better. Because you've got to stay positive. If I'm going to be negative, it's going to make him feel worse. I'm always like, "Come on, Jad. We can do this. Anything's possible."

Kids with disabilities, they've got to have advocate parents, who fight and never give up, and always strive. You know, when your child gets diagnosed with Tourette's, you want to stay quiet about it, you don't want to talk because people think you're weird maybe. Then, when you live with it, you decide, "No, it's good to talk." So I feel that I want to meet parents of kids with disabilities. It can only lead to helping the child more. [*To Jad*] I'd love you to meet more kids with Tourette's, to say, "It's going to get better."

Jad: Yeah. I would tell them I've been through it. I'd say, "Find hobbies that distract you." Or I'd say, "Don't do that, it only makes it worse." Like homeschool. That was a huge mistake [*he sighs*]. I confined myself. You don't have confidence because you're not socializing. You're just staying in the house, like a prison.

Do something to get out of the house and socialize

Jad: The problem, of course, is I couldn't socialize because of Tourette's.
Sharon: The more he stayed home—
Jad: The worse it got.
Sharon: Everything was closing in. All he knew was the Tourette's and the more he hated it the more it came. It was not good for him. I should have—
Jad: And if you do homeschooling, always find a social life, like a club or a sport or *something*. So even if you're homeschooled, you know that later on you can hang out with friends. Do something to get out of the house and socialize. That is the main thing. For me, it was my interest in comic books and collectibles and video games and selling those. People might be like, "Oh, it's video games," but if that's what you like to do, it'll still help you. A focus, so you're not focusing on your Tourette's. Anything you like that replaces thinking about Tourette's.

    I started my business around sixteen, when I had collectibles I'd sell on eBay for a couple of dollars, nothing major. But I got to know people at places like Comic-Con[82]. It expanded to where I'd try to get an eBay page with hundreds of items, that had a hundred percent positive ratings. It grew to the point where it wasn't just collectibles.
Sharon: One lady contacted him and said, "This has been in my shed."
Jad: Yeah, she brought me a signed picture of *Star Wars*, the whole cast from the fourth one, and wow—that's like my thing!
Sharon: [*She laughs.*]
Jad: It got bigger and bigger, and this last week I paid $400 for a booth at a convention. The first day, in three hours, I made $1,500. I met people who wanted to get me into other areas. I was supposed to go on Wednesday to a business meeting, full on, suit and tie, everything [*he laughs*]. It got cancelled last minute, but I definitely would like to do

---

82   A multi-genre entertainment and comic convention held annually in San Diego, CA.

that. It's weird how things work. Sixteen, little business, and then it gets bigger and bigger [*he chuckles*]. Yeah, following your passions.

What did they call you in high school?

Sharon: You see, everything happens for a reason, that's my belief. He's in the house for homeschooling and the four walls are feeling like a prison. But what came out of that was, "Hmmm… I'll start working on the computer." And then he was saying, "I'm going to do a business, mom." If he had been in a school environment, he might not have started that business because he wouldn't have had the time.

Jad: Exactly. Like I said, you have to find something you like. Me? Before the business it was drawing, swimming, comic books. Now… it's the same thing [*he laughs*].

Sharon: And now he wants his own store.

Jad: I do want to set up my website.

Sharon: That's business sense. And the girls, they love him [*she laughs*]. What did they call you in high school? Tell.

Jad: [*He hesitates, chuckles*] Ladies man.

[*They laugh again.*]

Jad: When I was in middle school, there was no hope for me getting a girlfriend. Depression, number one. And then the Tourette's. But I got to high school and started working out, losing weight. More confidence and, you know, I didn't care about Tourette's anymore, and that's when it began. So I could finally have a girlfriend. [*He laughs.*] It's great.

Small steps

Jad: My tics were a lot less in high school, and right now it's the best it's ever been. Junior, senior year you could tell I had tics, but people would never notice unless you told them. That was the Orap.

Sharon: I found a small school that was on a farm. It was not a traditional school. He could leave the classroom if he needed to walk and get fresh air. They really accommodated us. Kids were different there. More accepting. And the teachers were cool. And that's when he changed.

Jad: These were kids like me that couldn't go to normal high schools. There were only, what, maybe a hundred students. Everyone knew everyone, we were just a big group, all friends, like a neighborhood.

That was the one thing, though—the academics were not very good [*he chuckles*].

Sharon: You know what? I was looking at it like this—do I worry about academics, when he's been in such a dark place that he doesn't want to live anymore? Or do I put him in some sunshine with people his own age, and forget the academics. Or do I worry about the academics and destroy him even more, with bullies and people where he will not be accepted? So you have to make a decision as a parent, and I made that decision.

Jad: Even if it's for a little while, because I did leave after two years.

Sharon: It was a transition. And that's what you've got to think about.

Jad: Then you can go to regular school. I graduated from a regular high school.

Sharon: So you just have to do transitions. Small steps.

Jad: That's what it is, exactly. Small steps. But once you take them, you get results.

We're all born naked

Sharon: Tourette kids are very intelligent. I think they have that quality about them, I don't know what it is, but it's special, it's different.

Like how he treats other people. We started realizing that yes, he's got Tourette's, it's made him the person he is, [*to Jad*] and I'm so proud of who you are because I know you will be an amazing person in society. Society needs more people like you because you are compassionate and caring. That's how he is. He will do anything for anybody. And every time I drive, [*to Jad*] what do you always say to me? He says, "Mom, roll down the window and give that homeless person some money." This is him.

Jad: What I said to my mom was, if every person gave that one man even fifty cents or a dollar, he would not be homeless.

Sharon: It makes you feel good inside. Giving. If you can, of course. It doesn't have to be money. Give your time, be a good listener, volunteer. You know, we're all humans, we're all born naked. And then, if God blesses you with stuff, you need to pass this on.

To me Maria embodies compassion, and her story demonstrates it both in this interview and the one following, which took place a year later. Under the most trying circumstances she withholds harsh judgment. She credits her Tourette's for this reflex. Yes, she feels legitimate anger, and she defends her rights when others might falter. In this interview she looks to a bright future, one she will make through her own intelligence and hard work. She has built character; she is poised. She wants her unfolding life to matter. I believe it does already by her example of perseverance, courage, and a heart that encompasses friends and foes alike.

MARIA
18 years old
2014

I thought I had a brain tumor

As I grew up and into myself—I mean, I'm still growing up—I put a lot of emphasis on my appearance. I can't control people's first impressions of me because... I bark and do other animal sounds, I say weird things, and I do awful body movements. The one thing I *can* control is the way people view me. And even though I'm a little bit different, I'm still sophisticated, I'm still beautiful, and I'm out there.

I live in the Midwest, in a suburb. Growing up, I got bullied a lot because I was very smart. I had a lot of trouble finding myself because there was no one I could relate to. My family was very conscientious of the lifestyle we lead. It's all about doing the best *you* can do, making a positive impact on society.

My Tourette's came on freshman year of high school. I started having shivers up my spine, they increased in frequency, and pretty soon I was moving my head, jerking, and blinking uncontrollably. My vocal tics used to be really awkward sex sounds, like weird moaning. It was *awful*. It was horrible and embarrassing. I didn't know what was wrong with me. For over a year, I was freaking out because I thought I had a brain tumor.

I wallowed and felt sorry for myself for a couple of months. Then, a friend told me about a girl who meowed when she sneezed. I thought,

"Wow, wouldn't that be great, instead of these awful sex sounds." So I worked hard and changed my tics to noises I could control. Now my default sound is a bark. It's pretty great. I can do impressions of Beagles, Chihuahuas, Cocker Spaniels, sometimes I can even pull out a Great Dane.

This is who I was

My regular doctors said, "Maybe it'll go away." They sent me to a neurologist, who didn't want to diagnose Tourette's because my tics weren't "incapacitating" enough. I was diagnosed with a tic disorder, severe depression, anxiety, ADHD, restless legs syndrome, insomnia, a couple of other things. Over the course of two years, I was on about twenty different medications. Yeah. And none of my doctors collaborated. None of them talked to *me* about what was going on. And I was too naïve to ask good questions.

So I went around for half my sophomore year telling people I had a tic disorder and they were thinking, "You can control it." Later on, I found out I'd had Tourette's the whole time. I was crushed. All my classmates thought I was doing it for attention. I lost a lot of friends and didn't know what to do with myself.

So my junior year I finally figured out this is what I had. This is who I was. I started telling everybody that the best way to respond was to laugh at me or make a joke. I would say funny things. If a teacher asked, "What is the meaning to life?" I might tic, "Herpes viral infection." But it was still really difficult.

Laughter releases tension

I decided to go to community college a year early. But in every class it was the same thing. Stand up, say who I am, this is what I do, and it's okay to laugh at me. There are pros and cons with this strategy, but I didn't see a way around it. I can't control what people say behind my back, but I can control the initial response. More than anything, laughter releases tension. So I would like to think I opened up emotional space for people to be more themselves. That's one of the reasons I'm glad I have TS. Because it brings people together. Ultimately, it's not a laughing matter, but it's kind of the only way you can deal with it. There are days when I definitely wish

I didn't have Tourette's. Just be a normal kid and not have to worry about looks, absurdities, and making a scene. But I've also started a lot of good conversations.

I like to think people like me for *me*. Does that make sense? So many people have horrible experiences with Tourette's, and I feel guilty because my experiences... well, it's definitely been difficult, but a lot of them haven't been awful. That's an advantage. There are so many kids and adults who never learn to love themselves, just because they're different.

When I understood it myself, I could explain it better to them

My dad has Tourette's as well, undiagnosed. We've talked about it a little bit. He has throat clearing, nose twitching, eye blinking... it's very, very mild, but it's there. When my parents went to the neurologist with me, they were concerned because... I think a large part of it was, they were going through a divorce and didn't know how to handle me, on top of everything else. They thought I was doing it for attention. "You're doing this because you want us to stay together," was how I interpreted their reaction. It was a horrible, horrible experience because they didn't believe I couldn't control myself. And I had some stupid neurologist misinforming them.

My parents love me unconditionally, but they wanted me to cut the shit, stop what I was doing. And, of course, I couldn't. The last few months, they've started to see. Part of it was, when I understood it myself, I could explain it better to them. Some things we're still battling, like I feel I have components of OCD, but they don't believe that.

TS forces me to put myself in other people's shoes, and not judge them

Tourette's *has* had an effect on my life, but it's made me who I am today. I think I'm a good person with a unique perspective. TS forces me to put myself in other people's shoes, and not judge them. I'm a compassionate person, but TS took that to a different level. I really respect people who have disabilities. It was interesting for me to put Tourette's in comparison with things like autism. We're both prisoners, in a sense. I realized I wish people would see the person I am inside this struggling form.

My Tourette's is obviously inhibiting, but more than anything, what affects me is my depression. It's hard because, for a while, I had to choose between managing my depression with meds, and exacerbating my tics with them. Overall I have a pretty positive view of myself, and if I have tics, I can put them in perspective. But it's ten times harder with depression. I would give anything to get rid of my horrible mood issues. It's funny how I want to get rid of this silent aspect of me and keep the loud, obnoxious part.

I don't handle bad days very well because I can't go on medication anymore. I had horrible reactions. After months with medication, I called it quits and stopped cold turkey. So I can only manage my depression through... I don't even know *how* to manage it. There are obviously things like eat good food and exercise. But when it comes down to it, I just have to take it day by day and see if I can rationalize what I'm feeling.

I don't want to do something because it's easy. I want my life to matter

For my graduation party, for example, I invited like 450 people. I expected *maybe* two hundred people. But, discounting my family, eighteen people came. Just eighteen. So I've got all this food, and all this hype and nobody comes. [*She pauses*] And it was really hard. Yeah, it's superficial, and people were probably at work, or they forgot, or it didn't matter. But for me, it was a big day. A day where I finally got to say, "I made it through hell. I survived, and I'm going to accomplish something with my life! Come celebrate this with me!" Barely anybody cared enough t o show.

There are a lot of people who told me I made an impact on their lives, and because of me, they looked at life a little differently. And those people didn't come. It just happened in June, and I have a hard time putting that in perspective. It's like, "I spent so much time trying to relate to you people, and trying to make sense of what is wrong with me [*her voice falters*], and keep up in school, and do a good job, and make friends, and be a good person." I don't know what more I could have done. It's silly, because it's just one day. And I'm sure, if people knew how much it meant to me, they would have come. So, I don't know...

With my future, I always struggle, thinking do I play it safe or do I take that risk? I'm afraid to make the wrong choice. I don't want to do something just because it's easy. I want my life to matter. And if there's one thing I don't want for myself, it's to *not* be extraordinary, to be part of life and not live.

The fact is, I am very intelligent and whatever I do, I'll be good at. I could become an awesome doctor or scientist. But I don't want that. What do I want? [*A long pause*] I don't know. What does my heart tell me? I don't know that, either.

I feel sometimes I could suppress my tics enough to where they would disappear. But I wouldn't feel like me without them. Tourette's is a large part of what makes me interesting. And the last thing I want is to be just another person.

Todo cambia—everything changes. It is one year later. Maria is as strong, creative, and resilient as they come, but no woman should endure what she has suffered. No woman. But here she is—in an environment that ought to be supportive and thrilling—grappling with despair and fear. And yet, Maria hopes. She hopes for relief. She hopes for a kinder, more rewarding future. She hopes for change.

MARIA
19 years old
2015

I've always been creative and spontaneous

I started doing improv in high school. I was in a theater group where we did it. That was my first experience with improv, and it was the most incredible thing. I never knew how they did it until I started, and it turned out I had a knack for it. Then I saw this college improv group and was floored. They were so funny, and they really had a connection with each other. I wanted to be a part of it. So when I got here to university my freshman year, last year, I auditioned for their short- form and long-form improv groups. I got into both.

I've always been creative and spontaneous. When I was growing up I used to put on skits for my mom, and grandma, and friends. Sometimes you fall into things in your life, and improv is one of those things. It's great too because when I'm performing, I don't have tics. It's been a great chance for me to meet people and not so much be judged for Tourette's. I get judged on my humor and who I am as a person.

I'd be happy to work with you

Most definitely I've been judged for my Tourette's at college. This was a surprise to me. Coming in after high school, I had high hopes. I was a lot more myself than I am today. I had so many dreams of what it could be. And then that year happened, and this year is happening, and it's honestly been, in terms of Tourette's, it's been the worst time of my life. Yeah.

I would get up on the first day of class and say, "Hi, my name is Maria, I have Tourette syndrome. This is what Tourette's is and this is what you can expect from me in class. My preference is if I say something funny, feel free to laugh, as long as you're not laughing at me. If you have questions or concerns, I'd be happy to work with you."

So I was not nervous about doing that the first day. I was confident and I felt good about it. I thought I was going to have a great time breaking the ice. The roommate I have now, one of my best friends, we met because after I stood up that first day, she sat by me and we got to talking, and now we live together.

But there was also a lot of criticism and judgment and a lot of hate I was not anticipating, in particular from my teachers. I emailed all my teachers before the first day of school and let them know the situation, gave them my letter from the campus Disability Resource Center[83], and let them know what they can expect from me. My first semester last year I had a teacher, he met with me before class and was like, "Oh, I think this is going to work out fine. You seem like a very bright student and I'm excited to have you in my class." Then every single time I would make a sound—which are opera notes and scales at this point, and a lot of commentary, basically whatever is in my subconscious gets blurted out—whenever I would have a tic he would give me this death-glare. Or he'd say, "Okay, Maria, settle down." Stuff like that. I had a lot of people coming up to me after class saying, "I can't believe he's doing this. You

---

83   Check to see if your college or university has a Disability Resource Center.

don't deserve this." They thought I should contact Disability Services and get him some training. I felt kind of bad for the guy because this was his first time teaching at university, and it would be unfair of me to call him out. I felt he was doing the best he could.

Tourette's! Sorry!

For the first semester I had a really great view of myself. I was confident going forward. But then things started getting worse. I lived in a dorm in a single room. It was hard to meet people. I was the person who knocked on every door and most people in the building knew me, several hundred people. But I couldn't go anywhere without being called out for my Tourette's. I would go into the dining room, for example, and most people don't know me, and my tics were a complete surprise. I'd make an opera noise and everyone would turn at me and stare. I mean, I'm used to that, right? But then there were people who would come up and say, "Would you stop that? This isn't funny. You're looking for attention." I'd explain that I had Tourette's and they'd just walk away. I'd do my best, you know, like, "Tourette's! Sorry!" or I'd ignore them. But it got harder to do. I'd go to do laundry and I'd have people come up to me when I was ticcing and they'd start swearing at me, they would tell me I wasn't welcome there, they would say I should go home because this was a college and it didn't have time for kids. They thought I was being immature. I have to have some sympathy for them, for what they thought I was doing. But the way they approached me was terrible. I was like, "Excuse me, the only one who gets to swear in this scenario is me, so would you kindly fuck off."

But it kept getting worse. Over winter break I had a friend commit suicide. They had just graduated and just turned twenty years old. I was out of the country so I didn't get to say goodbye or go to the funeral. So I get back into second semester and the person I was dating first semester, we broke up. And then I was struggling with depression, clinical depression, and it was a bad episode of it. I was on new medication which was making me pass out, so over break I stopped it. But I was having a terrible withdrawal from it, which escalated my depression. At school I kept trudging through, even though I didn't have anyone to talk to. The few friends I did have, no one wanted to talk about hard stuff. So I'm living alone, I have a bunch of acquaintances but no close friends, I'm getting bullied everywhere I go for my Tourette's. And then it really starts happening.

I didn't feel safe

[*A long pause.*] I... was actually... I was raped twice and sexually assaulted twice. I have not reported them at this time. It's complicated. It's very difficult. So this affected the way I could attend class. I was in a class, there were maybe three hundred people there, and the entire time I'm making a lot of tics, a lot of commentary. The teacher was a very kind person, but the people in the class were not. They would look at me and walk out of the lecture. There were people making fun of me the whole time.

There's an app for universities where people can post different things going on. It's supposed to be anonymous. But people severely started cyber-bullying me on there. They'd put, "This specific class, this is the girl with Tourette's." They'd say, "I can't believe she did this." I felt so vulnerable and I didn't feel safe.

There's nothing I can do about Tourette's, right? I physically cannot stop my body and there are people talking all about me on social media. I could not bring myself to go to class. I emailed my professors and told them I'd recently had a lot of sexual crimes committed against me and I'm doing my best to deal with it, but I couldn't make it out of bed today, or I feel judged and like nobody wants me around in class.

Most of my teachers were okay with that, they were helping me however they could. But university policy is you have to advocate for yourself. And that's hard to do when you feel powerless. So unless you have a personal assistant in your back pocket, you have to schedule all these different things, and it's overwhelming when you're already behind on coursework and emotionally drained.

I had this one teacher, when I sent the email saying I had a bunch of sexual crimes committed against me, when she answered she didn't even get my name right. She sent an email back saying, "Mary, your absence today is still not accepted." I was crushed. These are the people who are paid to be my mentors. The same lady, she thought I was very disruptive in her class. She wanted me to drop out or she would put a failing grade on my permanent transcript. If I withdrew I would have to tell my parents. They're helping me with college and it would be unacceptable for me to withdraw from a course. And I was in no way, shape, or form ready to tell them what happened to me.

I felt like such a failure. I've never failed a class in my life. I've only ever gotten As and maybe one or two Bs. And that this teacher wanted me out so badly she's willing to do that at such a terrible time in my life? Dropping her course was excruciatingly painful. It was more painful than anything I'd endured because it felt like a personal mistake. The other things I couldn't control, but I should have been able to control getting credit for this course. I couldn't do that. I did end up having to drop out of that class. I didn't tell my parents. I couldn't.

So it was a really shitty time. There were people making fun of me in class and my teachers didn't want me there. It hurt my trust in people and it hurt my self-esteem and it made me feel like, for the first time *ever*, that this thing I wasn't too ashamed of, Tourette's, I felt like I should hide it. So…

This is unacceptable

Yeah, it was really hard. There was a day, first year, when I went to hang out with my now-roommate, and she was having a party. I was hanging out with her because I still very recently didn't feel safe. There was this man there, and he was very, very intoxicated, and he came up to me and gave me a hug and just *squeezed so hard* I could barely breathe. I kept telling him, "Stop. Stop. Stop," and he wouldn't stop. And I freaked out. I had a total panic attack and ran home. It was a huge trigger.

I'm on my way home, I'm almost there, and I start ticcing. And these guys start making the sounds back at me through their window, and mocking me, and yelling profanities at me, and I *lost* it. I started screaming at them, "I have Tourette's! You guys are so mean! Stop it!" That made it worse because they kept doing it even more. So I ran into the building and I got the security guard, saying, "This is unacceptable. I have a disability and this is what they're doing. You need to find them and hold them accountable." I walked out with the security guard and pointed him in the direction of the window I thought it was coming from, and all of a sudden it just hit me, and I was so sad. I couldn't believe I had acted this way, that the events in my life had so much power over me. I started sobbing, uncontrolled.

All of a sudden I saw someone from my high school, who was also at the university. This was the girl who, in high school, told me to kill myself. Yep. That was her response to me. I did not want her to see me in this state so I hid in the bushes, I just ducked into them. Turns out she was a student security monitor, so I had to get out. And I'm trying to stop crying and I can't. It was horribly embarrassing. So finally she left and I went up to my room. But I couldn't get my key into the lock, my hands were shaking so hard. I dropped my keys, then fell in the middle of the hallway and just cried. I couldn't get into my room, I couldn't go anywhere. So I ran back downstairs and hid in the bushes again. I felt very alone.

Apparently the security guard had called the cops. So they arrive, they see this girl hiding in the bushes and they're saying to me, "You have to get out, you have to get out." I was petrified because, even though I did nothing wrong, you know, it's the cops, they're shining lights, looking at you in the bushes and you're thinking, "Oh, crap, what did I do?" So I ran out of the bushes, I'm trying to just get back into my building, but they ran after me and tackled me to the ground and they put me in handcuffs. They brought me to their car, where everyone can see. It was terrible. They're saying, "What did you do? How much have you had to drink tonight?" And I'm saying, "I didn't do anything. It's all because these guys were yelling at me, at my Tourette's." So they let me go and I got an email the next day saying, in so many words, "We're sorry we did this. Please don't sue us." I was arrested, tackled, and put in handcuffs because I was harassed for my Tourette's. It is probably the most embarrassing thing that has happened to me to date. And frightening. I was very, very scared.

I hate being labeled by Tourette's

Ever since then, it's been a downhill spiral. I have a hard time connecting with people; I don't trust anybody anymore. My first day of classes second year was pretty standard, I got up in front of everyone and said the same old speech. It's the twentieth time I've said this speech now. But it's terrible because one of the classes I'm in, the majority of students are from the lecture where they were bullying me online. I'm afraid of everybody. I don't feel safe on campus. I don't feel like there's anybody I can trust. It's gotten so bad I no longer feel comfortable ticcing in my classes. I'm suppressing and it's terrible. I get home and the distress of holding them in all day comes out and I start screaming my tics. And my roommates hate it. They freak out, they jump. They're like, "Gosh, Maria, stop it." They don't say it, but it's there. And it's just... it sucks.

You know, my first interview was more about me, it wasn't about Tourette's. This is who I am, this is what I hope to do, oh, and I have

Tourette's. Now this second one is a real statement, like, "Oh, life happens. And here I am." I hate being labeled by Tourette's. It is so shitty that *the* reason people know me is for Tourette's. So I don't even want to associate myself with it.

I went to my first Tourette support group on campus and it was a big letdown. I got there and there were three other people. The first two were other students, who ran the meeting, but they had very mild tics, very manageable Tourette's. In the meeting, I was ticcing profusely and they were not. All of a sudden this guy walks in, who it seemed like he had a lot of problems, but I don't know if he actually had tics. It seemed more he had OCD. So I have a tic and suddenly he throws his hands up, covers his ears, and starts bitching me out for ticcing. And I'm thinking, "This is a Tourette's support group?" But there is a support group I'm going to this Tuesday for the sexual assaults, and I'm hoping to maybe find some connections there, people who do understand.

The truth is

I thought about transferring, but I'm going to graduate after next fall semester, so it's not worth it. I came in with forty-eight credits and after this semester I'll only have thirty-four left. I'm creating my own major, so I have areas of focus in communications, psychology, and global studies. Once I graduate I'd like to do a lot of things. I'd like to be a paleontologist and dig up some dinosaur bones. I'd like to be a wine sommelier. I'm working on a thesis on human nature I'd like to publish and use to reform ideas we hold about capitalism, and change the way we govern our societies. I still am planning on acting. I was actually in my first feature film over the summer. An independent film, and I was the lead. And I got a call from ABC, so that's exciting. They're doing a documentary series called *Insight,* and they do reenactments.

This morning I woke up and gave myself the goal to just get through the day. No homework attached, no find-something-to-be-happy-about, it was just make it through. It's sad because the confidence I had in myself, the assurance of who I was, really doesn't seem to be there anymore.

I know that in the future, at least I hope in the future, things will change for the better, and that I'll learn how to trust again. I hope that I'll regain some of the confidence I had in the beginning. But I don't believe I'm going to find any of those things while I'm in college. I'm going to have to get out of this environment before I can achieve the goals I have for myself.

This isn't a story that says, "Hey, everything's sad, nothing is ever good." I've met some awesome people and I've learned a lot. But I'd be lying if I said things have gotten any easier. I'd be lying if I told you that. I *was* happy. [*A long pause*] So, you know, Tourette's sucks. Life sucks. And I'm just surviving. I was thinking the other day, I was thinking about if I would ever get over this. If I would ever feel safe again or ever feel like I could trust anybody again. It's taken already a year of my life trying to deal with this and I feel like I've gotten further behind than forward. I don't know if I can see a place, at least now, where I'm ever over this or where I'm comfortable again.

Even with my tics, I don't know if I'm ever going to get my confidence back with those. I've begun to accept that I'll probably have Tourette's for the rest of my life and I've begun to accept that there's not a whole lot I can do about it. Even though I've been trying CBIT and medications, nothing seems to work for me. And I just... I get more discouraged every day. I have hopes for the future, I *hope* that things get better, I *hope* I'm able to have a successful life, but the truth is I'm going to be graduating shortly after I turn twenty. And I have *no* idea what I want to do. Everything I have in my toolbox of hopes is something I don't think I could get to in the blink of an eye. To be a wine sommelier takes years, if not decades of perfecting the art. And I wouldn't even be able to legally drink wine until I'm twenty-one [*she chuckles*]. It's frustrating because I'm going to be doing the great expedition of life after college on my own. All my friends will still be in school. So I have a feeling the next few years are going to be the hardest of my life. And this has already been so difficult. I don't know if I'm going to be able to handle it.

This, elsie's interview, was my most difficult to recover from emotionally. I was brokenhearted by her suffering. I was enraged at the cruelties of life. Yet here she was sharing her story with me, laughing at times, her voice tentative and plaintive at others. Finding her way to the next day. I admired her greatly. Her second interview follows this one, and with that, my admiration for elsie grew.

elsie
(she prefers her name lower case)
58 years old
2014

I became a master hider

Ever since I was very small I've been intuitive. I don't do it on purpose, but I feel I can see what's inside people. I see people's pain because that's what I know.

I remember third grade, sitting in class and kids are telling me, "Shut up. Shut up." I was making noises, I guess. I've had periods of time where I could not take one breath without making noises, to the point where I couldn't eat.

I became a master hider, and now I know why. I went through every possible type of abuse from my mother, my father, and my evil grandmother. I do not use that word lightly. Emotional, physical, sexual abuse.

There was no one who knew I had TS, not my family, not any doctor. At school I was teased and bullied and laughed at, until high school. Then I became a hippie and I got hormones, and I started raging back at my mother, who was one of my major abusers. I could fight back.

I ran from the East Coast, from my family. California is the furthest you can go without getting into the ocean [*she chuckles*]. But I made a life here, I guess. I raised a special needs kid here.

I was a chameleon

I was a chameleon. I went to college and would do what anyone suggested, because I had no identity of my own. Someone said, "You like animals. Be a vet." I said, "Okay," and spent a year in pre-vet. I had all these pre-med students around, so I switched to pre-med. I was accepted to pharmacy school, contingent on passing organic chemistry. Because of the stress, I dropped the class the day before the final exam.

I was accepted into nursing school, went for a quarter and hated it. Back then you had to wear those stupid hats. So I got my Bachelor's in psychology, with which you could do absolutely nothing [*she chuckles*].

I worked off and on but didn't know what to do. Someone said, "Why don't you go back to nursing school?" I said, "Okay." My son was two months old when I started. I graduated valedictorian of my class. So I worked in nursing and liked my job.

But I was in a car accident and my life ended as I knew it. I had back surgery and was recovering for two years.

Oprah diagnosed me

I don't remember about tics because I've blacked out much of my life. I was running to doctors and psychiatrists and didn't know what was wrong with me. I'd have rage attacks, I'd have these 'whiteouts,' where I was watching myself do things. I couldn't stop. Afterwards I'd feel remorseful. I cried a lot.

I remember watching an Oprah program and she had this Orthodox Jewish couple from New York, and he would bark like a dog all night. They were trying to throw him out of the neighborhood. And that's the first time I heard the word Tourette's. I was so excited. I called my brother and said, "Guess what we have! It has a name!" So basically Oprah diagnosed me.

I was paranoid about having things on my medical record, so I went to Mexico to get Haldol. I'm supersensitive to medication and tiny doses worked wonders. I was taking pediatric doses, eighths of a tablet. I remember the first time, within half an hour, my whole body relaxed.

I went to a neurologist and said, "I have Tourette's!" I wanted to get Haldol from him. I had a cold at the time and was coughing, and he said, "Oh, you're coughing. That's a vocal tic. Here's some Haldol." It was awesome, until the Haldol stopped working years later.

Clonipin backfired on me and I couldn't get off of it. After two and a half years, I'm almost off now. I'm trying to get off meds completely and let my body recover, and it's hell. These meds are toxic. But what do you do? My body was so painful I *had* to do something. Plus the shame was killing me. Which is the lesser of the evils? I had to make it stop. And now I can't, and it sucks.

I'm terminally unique

Coming off the meds, all my tics came out with a vengeance—I couldn't go out in public, I couldn't eat or sleep, I couldn't function. Tics have destroyed my neck, my wrist, and my fingers. Right now, vocal tics are secondary to physical tics, and it's nice they alternate, so I can get a break. But I've lost some function in my hands; they get numb. I'm tightening up my legs in bed so I can't sleep or relax.

I'm the one who seems to've gotten the worst case of TS in my family. And because I'm female, it's even more shameful. I feel like guys can almost get away with it. It's because of the double standard in this culture. If women are not perfect, they're ugly. If you're scrunching up your face and twisting your body, you're ugly. If men do it, it's just weird. Weird men can get by in this world, but disgusting women, all contorted and twisted, don't get by too well.

I spent my whole life trying to belong and fit in. I'm terminally unique. I hate feeling like that all the time.

The T-word

The thing I hate most is being dependent on someone, because I can't stand not being in control. Yeah, I have OCD, but how much of it is because every ounce of control was taken from me mentally and physically? I never had control in my life.

The only thing you can control, because you can't control people, is your environment. My environment is very important to me. I know I have sensory issues, now that I've read up on it. There are times I can't stand my hair touching me. I've tried to rip it out. Sometimes I can't stand being touched. And I have hypervigilance and startle response from my past abuse. I can't filter stuff the way 'normal' people can.

I'm not crazy. You know? Everything I went through has been confirmed by my family. I know it all happened. I know it wasn't my fault. But I still feel the Tourette's is my fault. I do. I have trouble saying the word, the T-word. I'll say, "I have tics." I'll say, "TS." It's still a secret.

I can't let anybody see me. I've risked telling a few people, but I say it like, "I'm going to tell you my deepest, darkest secret." I struggle with so much shame around my Tourette's. I made it my entire identity.

Tourette's has me

There was a program on TV, it showed how people made a life for themselves despite Tourette's. It was *I Have Tourette's, But Tourette's Doesn't Have Me*. Well, you know what? Tourette's has me. It has ruined my life.

Recently I've been raging at God for not listening to me. You can get angry as hell at my God because God can take it. What brought me to a spiritual relationship with a Higher Power is 12-step programs, like Al-Anon. That program helped me more in my life than anything. I also started SIA—Survivors of Incest Anonymous. But I'm sick now and can't get to meetings. Fortunately there are phone meetings.

You live in a different world when you have a bad case of Tourette's. It is a different world. They say so many kids grow out of their tics, but there are those of us that our Tourette's has gotten worse as we get older.

They saved me

Sometimes I just have to write a poem. I feel like it comes through me. It absolutely helps with my emotions. It puts my feelings out there. Sometimes I literally have to run to the computer to write something down.

And I post a lot on Facebook. I would literally spend all day with TS groups, and they saved me from wanting to kill everything inside me. I was so isolated. In the extreme group[84] I can say anything I want, I can get it all out. Those groups changed my life.

---

84 There was a Facebook group for people with severe Tourette syndrome. It no longer exists.

———————————— ∿ ————————————

Todo cambia—everything changes. Creativity and self-awareness brought relief. Elsie now spells her name this way. Notable for me is her discovery of bodywork and its healing connection with Tourette syndrome. I took my own experiments with bodywork to an extreme, while Elsie's progress was moderate, and more successful. Cleansing her body of medications, as so many others have said, also was pivotal in her new clarity of mind and spirit. As devastated as I was by our first interview, by healing herself she also healed me.

ELSIE
59 years old
2015

This is my spiritual awakening

I've been going through hell for three or four years. The last interview feels like a long time ago. But now... how do you put this in words? I have reconnected with my spirituality, and that's what's getting me through. A spiritual reawakening. Also what helped is getting off all the meds, and getting properly rediagnosed.

I was rediagnosed with complex post-traumatic stress disorder and dissociative identity disorder. Multiple personalities from severe trauma. Yeah. So all that *and* the pain of getting off meds. I had a hard time with that. I wanted to die every day. I don't know if I still feel that. [*A pause.*] I want to go home. Back to where I came from [*she laughs*]. To God. I wanna go home, oh yeah. This is my spiritual reawakening.

I started having flashbacks of things I had blocked out

My cousin popped into my life and triggered memories of particular types of abuse from my childhood. So it got worse. Oh yeah—I fought for my life. My TS Facebook group kept me alive many, many nights. I also joined a couple of closed support groups on Facebook. I'm a member of a Survivors of Incest Anonymous phone bridge.

We're not just talking about Tourette's, obviously. March, a year ago, I remember the night, I started having flashbacks of things I had blocked out. And my Tourette's is very wrapped up with my abuse. This is why there was an incredible amount of hiding and shame and embarrassment. Because my father, who gave me my Tourette's, was one of my primary perpetrators. He died last Saturday night. And no—I didn't go to his funeral.

I'm home

People with Tourette's do not relax their body ever. They'd say to me, "Sit still and relax," and I'd say, "Are you kidding me?" [*She chuckles.*] Tics can really trash your body.

The flashbacks, and the chronic pain from my tics, everything together reached a crisis point. I did all the self-help stuff I could and realized I needed to do something for my body. People were saying, "Yoga, yoga, yoga." I don't like yoga. It's like, be in weird positions and relax? What's *that* mean? But I found this thing called kundalini yoga on Meetup[1]. So I went to a kundalini yoga workshop and it changed my life. Just one class and I said, "I'm home."

Also on Meetup[85], I saw this Healing Fair. I couldn't walk well and hadn't left my apartment for months, but I went. There was a psychic channeler. She was interesting. She sat with me, took my hands, and the first thing she said was, "All I want to do is cry right now." And I thought, "Think how *I* feel [*she chuckles*]." Then there was the massage therapist, that was cool. But the third person, she did Reiki[86] and energy healing.

I had cried out to God, "Help me," and I think that's what happened

This Reiki woman was a survivor of the killing fields in Laos. And I'm a survivor of the most horrendous abuse that I don't need to talk about. I thought, "Maybe this lady will understand." Well, whatever she did really helped me. It was weird. But weird or not, I don't freakin' care. And she wrote down a lady's name in Long Beach and said, "Go see her."

I had cried out to God, "Help me," and I think that's what happened. So I went to see this woman in Long Beach. Call it the realm of energy

85   Meetup.com is an online social-networking portal that facilitates offline group meetings.
86   Reiki is a Japanese bodywork technique for stress reduction and relaxation that also promotes healing.

healing, which is not new on the planet. She helped me release a lot of negative energy from my body. All non-verbal stuff. Talking about Tourette's 'til you're blue in the face doesn't help. Tourette's is a form of body trauma. It's something you're living with. You want to crawl out of your freakin' body. My God! This woman took the pain out of my leg ninety-five percent in one two-hour session. I swear.

Between kundalini yoga, the Reiki woman, and this woman in Long Beach, it changed my entire life. I'm not saying I'm done with pain. And I have a long road to go dealing with my abuse. I still dissociate, but a lot of my trauma has been neutralized.

I now have an experience of possibilities, of hope, of things that can change

I now have an experience of possibilities, of hope, of things that can change. There's a way you can separate suffering from physical pain, and release it. I didn't understand that. Now I do. I am healing my own body.

Massage and self-massage help me, especially accupressure and compression. I found arthritic gloves, and they help a lot, and I wear them to sleep every night. It's very soothing. I like IMAK gloves because they're soft and don't have seams. I also wear wrist splints at night. And ice helps with pain. Ice is my best freakin' friend. Other things that help for pain are rub-in creams. Some of them are cooling and some are hot ones. You gotta experiment. I like Tiger Balm.

Active meditation, like tai chi, works for me too. It all goes back to energy. Regular meditation, where you sit and don't move—are you kidding? It drives me crazy. So things like walking meditation, where you're focusing but you're moving, that's what works for me. Anything that's relaxing and distracting, but it's going to be different for everybody.

Something else that soothes me so much is mantra music.[87] You know when you're OCD and you wake up with the *stupidest* lyric from the *stupidest* song in your head—for days? Now I have mantra music in my head and it soothes me.

Also the healing of what they call a gong bath.[88] It *soothes* me. It's all on YouTube. I have it playing all day in the background in the house. I never get tired of it. So you're either gonna go around for days singing

87   Search youtube.com for *mantra music.*
88   Search youtube.com for *gong bath* and *sound healing.*

something ridiculous like, "Don't worry, be happy," or you can listen to this music and it brings your nerves down. It's really cool with headphones.

I guess I don't need to know why *anymore*

Sometimes I feel God dropped me here on my head and said, "Deal with it." But I guess I don't need to know *why* anymore. We're all traumatized, just by being on this freakin' planet. This world needs to be fixed and Tourette's is under that umbrella. Back to basics—teaching tolerance.

I wish someone had told me, "So what that you make horrible faces, and twist and contort your body. You're still beautiful." Hiding it has caused me great physical and mental and emotional pain. What helped me most was being believed and validated. We have to validate these kids, whatever they're experiencing, and help them with it.

Tourette's and the associated disorders suck, but that does not mean the world owes us. It sucks. Deal with it. Many kids get teased and bullied, even *without* disabilities. Tell kids they are okay the way they are. Teach them coping and survival skills for a harsh world, because one day you will not be there to protect them. Love them unconditionally, listen to them, encourage them to be the best they can be. Find out what's special about your child. Don't make it that the specialness is just Tourette's. We're not special *because* of Tourette's—we just have it.

The white elephant in the room

For parents, don't make a problem where there isn't one. Your child's tics may be mild. I relate to severe cases, like mine. It pisses me off when I hear parents making a big deal of their child's TS, if it's an average case. Tourette's is not their life, okay? Deal with the specifics of it and teach your kid coping skills.

It reminds me of Brad Cohen's story.[89] Walking into class, proactive, saying, "This is what I have. This is not something I do voluntarily. I still want friends, I'm still a nice person, I still have the same needs everyone else does."

Talk about Tourette's with your kid. Don't make it the white elephant in the room. I was the queen of not talking about Tourette's. I mean, it was wrapped up in abuse too. Of course I hid. Of course I isolated. I had no

---

89   bradcohentourettefoundation.com.

one telling me what was going on. But I don't care anymore what people think. I'm too old to care [*she chuckles*]. But by saying I'm too old to care, I don't want it to seem like there's no hope for an eleven-year old, and they think they have to wait.

Let your kids scream, rant, be angry, even at God—He can take it. Holding it in makes the TS worse. Provide them with a connection to a Higher Power. Teach them they were not plopped here and abandoned. Healing is possible, even if the tics stay. I am doing it.

CHAPTER TEN

ALTERNATIVE TREATMENTS

Most of us expect modern pharmacology to target medication precisely. It's a bias we hold about Western medicine—it's supposed to *work*. For those with Tourette's, however, we can't escape the distressing sense that conventional medicine treats us with a sledgehammer. Each person responds differently to each med, so there's a hit-and-miss component to finding proper treatment. And whatever relief we get is often countered by side effects that diminish quality of life or adversely affect health. Who wants to gain a hundred pounds? Who wants to be reduced to a "zombie?"

Current research breakthroughs do hold promise for developing better medications, but until then, adults and families grappling with Tourette's and its comorbid conditions will continue to seek alternative methods of relief.

And consequently, many Touretters have become creative in their treatment. Some options are risky and involve Deep Brain Stimulation surgery. Others are less radical and less expensive. In this chapter you'll hear from people who've found viable alternatives to pills.

Carlie has been incredibly proactive in managing her medications (convention-
al and alternative) and ultimately seeking Deep Brain Stimulation(DBS)[90]
surgery. Her story illustrates the tangle of comorbid symptoms we often deal
with; once DBS removed her tics, she still wasn't out of the woods. Since our
conversation, she graduated college and is working at a small software compa-
ny. She says her coworkers "have no clue" about her Tourette's. All is well with
her DBS, although her tics have increased somewhat due to her new, nine-to-
five schedule, and she plans to get minor adjustments to her neurostimulation
device.

CARLIE
28 years old

I have to have that

The way I learned about DBS was I saw Jeff[91] on Oprah Winfrey. In
the clip they showed, he couldn't speak a regular sentence. He couldn't
drink out of a glass because he would squeeze it and break it. He couldn't
walk normally without jumping. But he went out on stage and was like a
normal person.

For me there was no thought process. It was, "I have to have that."
'Cause even though I was doing well in college, it was a struggle with the
tics. I was starting to realize there were going to be huge obstacles in life
getting a job and living on my own.

I had some tics that were disturbing. I would stomp my foot, which
shook our whole house, so I knew an apartment would never work out.
And I was doing a number on my body. I had foot injuries, I was injuring
property.

I feel it's part of Tourette's that when I get my mind on something,
I'm full-on until it happens. My mom always said it was 'dig my heels in'

---

90   A medical procedure involving implantation of a "brain pacemaker" for
      treatment of movement disorders.
91   Jeff Matovic is the first person to have his Tourette Syndrome controlled
      through deep brain stimulation. Much of his media coverage is available
      online. His story is chronicled in *Ticked: A Medical Miracle, a Friendship, and
      the Weird World of Tourette Syndrome* by James A. Fussell and Jeff Matovik.

type of stubbornness. For two years I went to my neurologist every two months and mentioned DBS, and he'd say, 'No, it's too new.' I asked him one day in March of 2006. I don't know if he just wanted to shut me up [*she chuckles*], but he said, "I can give you a referral."

I still think, "How is this possible?" It's such a gift

It took six months to get a consult. I went to the Lahey Clinic, where they did DBS for Parkinson's, but I was the first they did for Tourette's. They told me it was experimental. I didn't care. Jeff said in an interview, "Is it the quality of life you want to live?" 'Cause like him, I had exhausted all medications and the tics kept getting worse.

The first step was videotaping me to see my tics. Then I went for testing, and psychological testing, and on December 20th, I had the surgery.

Results were immediate. I didn't have any tics at all. They told me it was probably because of swelling around the brain. This was before they powered on the device. But then, at a month or six weeks, the tics came back. That's when the doctors switched my device on. They said it can take quite a bit of time to find the right setting. It took probably a year for the doctors to find settings where my tics were ninety-five to ninety-eight percent absent. And to this day they have been.

It's surreal. I still think, "How is this possible?" It's such a gift. I'm going to cry just talking about it [*she stifles tears*].

I can't

When I'm stumbling over my words or looking for a word, I think it could be the brain surgery. I feel my articulation skills used to be better. That's frustrating for me.

During my surgery an air embolism produced symptoms identical to a stroke. When I first noticed, I wanted to say, "I can't speak." All I was able to get out was, "I can't." After about thirty seconds, they understood and said, "Try to move your right arm," and I couldn't. My whole right side of my body was paralyzed. They were like, "Oh, shit." They took me for a CT and by the time I got back to the OR things had started to resolve. But I think maybe it's a residual of that.

I've been sensitive to medication my whole life

Anxiety, depression, the mood swings, that all came up from under-neath once the tics were out of the way. I had a panic attack because I forgot to fill my Luvox, which had pretty much eradicated my debil-itating OCD. At the ER they gave me Klonopin, take it as needed. I didn't know you can become dependent on it, that you can have severe panic attacks when you withdraw from it or even between doses, which leads you to take more. I told my psychiatrist that my panic attacks were getting worse and instead of 'take as needed,' he put me on a regular dose.

I felt I had completely lost *me*—my memory was gone, my compre-hension absolutely was shot. And my inhibitions were nil. I was afraid to say anything to anyone. It wasn't until later I thought the meds were the problem 'cause every time I went to the doctor, he put me on more Klonopin.

I've been sensitive to medication my whole life. I started tapering off Klonopin under my doctor's supervision. When the tablets got too small, I crushed them, got a drug scale and filled empty capsules, until July of 2013, when I came off Klonopin. And the past year has been the best I've had in a long time.

It was like I woke up from a dream

When I was diagnosed with Tourette's at six, they put me on Clonidine, and it's the only one I remain on today for Tourette's. But my tics were bad enough they wanted to try anything and everything.

I started having behavioral issues. Some of it was Tourette's but I *know* some of it was the medication. There were suicide attempts both times I was on Klonopin. As a child, it was an act that could have resulted in my death. I suppose you could call it a loud cry for help.

At that time I had been moved to a collaborative school, all sorts of kids with behavioral issues. So I was going to school, you know, just a regular day, in my school cab, and I decided I was going to jump out of the vehicle. I think I said something to the driver beforehand so he slowed down, but yeah, I did jump.

That put me in the psychiatric hospital. I was twelve. I was there a month, until my parents came to the conclusion they couldn't manage me at home. I went to a residential school for children with behavior issues. My new psychologist weaned me off all medication. It was like I woke up from a dream. That whole eight- to eleven-years old period is foggy. I chalk it up to all the medication.

After the residential program, I started at a small high school for children with learning disabilities. It was fantastic. The Clearway School in Newton, Massachusetts. I owe a lot to them. In tenth grade I'd spend half day in a regular school, integrating me to prepare for college.

I graduated from Clearway and went to community college, majored in computer information systems. I made the Dean's List, I joined Phi Theta Kappa, which is Phi Beta Kappa for two-year colleges. I graduated with a 3.92, highest honors. That was very... it was... I can't even think of a word to describe how I felt.

Good old-fashioned fun

Learning my mind and body and its triggers is number one, and I'm still learning. I know I need to be aware. For panic attacks, I've discovered a few herbs, like valerian root, that help. I also found homeopathic pills that have valerian, hops, chamomile, and lemon balm. I always keep those handy in my bag.

I've been out meeting people although there is still some anxiety. Because of my quirks, I feel it's harder to get people to accept me. But I know anyone who doesn't accept me doesn't deserve to be my friend. I feel like *I* would want to be my friend [*she chuckles*]. I'm probably one of the most loyal, generous, nonjudgmental people you could know. And I think my empathy comes from everything I've been through.

I feel blessed with such good parents, who were able to deal with my problems and make sure I learned life skills. I'm so lucky I had all the resources, because I never, ever would have come close to this far.

I feel I've earned some good old-fashioned fun. Definitely. I'm attending University of Massachusetts, Boston, and will graduate this May with my B.S. in Information Technology/Computer Forensics.

I say to myself that this last year of school is not going to be about grades, because I have a three-point-five. So this last year I want to have fun. I feel I've earned it. 'Cause when I graduate I'm gonna need a job. I'm going to need to be professional.

One more person knows

I've never met anyone with Tourette's or any other disability who isn't tough as nails. I was worried that when I got the surgery, and the tics go away, is everything that makes me *me* going to go away too? Growing up with TS played a large role in shaping me into the person I am. Particularly making me more of an empath, giving me humility, helping me understand how important it is *not* to judge people. Also making me embrace my 'quirkiness' as part of who I am.

Tics don't happen often now, but when they do, and people stare or comment, I have to remind myself it's ignorance. Most people aren't jerks. But it upsets me more than it ever did. If I've had a stressful day and know whatever I say isn't going to be nice, I keep my mouth shut. Yeah, if it's a situation where I can tell someone, I'll tell them. And that other part of me is thinking, "I shouldn't have to tell." But there's the other part of me that knows that to tell them is to educate them and that means one more person knows.

Kevin strikes me as All-American: fifth-generation in a small town, serves his community as a firefighter, loves Fourth of July parades and muscle cars. Growing up in the accepting arms of a family and community can mean the difference between self-love and self-loathing. So much depends on luck. I like how he holds that in perspective and, despite Tourette syndrome, has learned to appreciate what he has.

KEVIN
33 years old

Hey, Kev!

I've been a paramedic for eight years and a firefighter for six. I always wanted to be a firefighter. I enjoyed helping people. With one of my first medications, Haldol, I had an anaphalactic shock. I passed out and remember coming to in the ambulance and thinking, "That's pretty cool." Now, when I do that for someone, I think, "Yep. I know how you feel." That compassion for your patients, it comes from a deep place.

You never know what's going to happen. Yesterday we delivered a baby girl in someone's house. It was my first one in the field. We've had all kinds of medicals, traumas, accidents, people losing limbs. I was on duty the day of the Boston bombing. I was on the ambulance and we got mobilized. They put a strike force together in case something else happened. Luckily nothing ever did. That was scary.

Then there's the Fourth of July parade. I love that. I'm part of the honor guard so we carry the flags. Seeing the whole town out and everyone's shouting, "Hey, Kev!" It's pretty nice. I'm fifth-generation here in town, so everyone knows who I am.

That's good and it's bad. I go to someone's house, they see me and they can relax. The downside is I see people I know, who are in bad shape. It's more emotional. My first call was the father of a high school friend. But you gotta do what you gotta do.

We all live on the same street, my whole family. I couldn't have done it without my mother and father, and my grandparents and my brother. They're always there for me. My father, he's an old-school guy. You know, you cut yourself, put some dirt in it and walk it off [*he laughs*]. He's been a big influence on me. A great, caring guy. My mother's more like me, more an outwardly caring person.

I always wanted to serve

I started showing signs of TS when I was in second grade, but wasn't diagnosed until I was fourteen. Tics would come and go and for a couple of years they were gone.

In high school I was lucky because I was always the biggest. And in junior high I was the kid with a beard [*he laughs*]. I didn't get ridiculed as much. I was active in sports and had good friends. But it was tough for me to even *go* to school. I did my tests well, but I struggled just to get there and stay in class. I developed a phobia to school.

Once I got on meds it was a downfall. I was just going through the motions I was so drugged up. When I got out of high school, I thought, "I'm done with meds."

Growing up, I wanted to be in the military. I always wanted to serve.

I signed up in high school and went to training, but when they figured out I had Tourette syndrome, I got an entry-level discharge. But I'm still serving people. That's why I love what I do. Growing up, when anyone needed a hand, I was always the friend to call. I still am.

I need a steady hand with the pin-striping

My father and his brother built muscle cars. He grew up painting cars and I grew up watching him. And my father was the art teacher at high school. So I grew up with a wrench in one hand and a paintbrush in the other.

I went to college, got an art-and-design degree to fine-tune the techniques I already had. I specialized in hand painting signs, gold leafing, custom cars, motorcycles, helmets. I like to do flames. Flames are always good. I like the old '50s-style pin striping and that's my area of expertise.

I do that as a side job and it helps with the tics. I need a steady hand with the pin striping. It was a good ego boost and got me more comfortable with who I am. Confidence is a huge thing. Something I was good at that I shouldn't be able to do. I'm shaking so much I can't have a cup of coffee, but pin striping? It's nothin' [*he chuckles*]. If I'm painting, I won't make a sound. I'm in my zone. Or when I'm working on a patient. I get in that different mindset.

I still race motocross, dirt bikes, and that's a great outlet for me. To hammer on the throttle and get the aggression out. I don't do as much as I used to 'cause now it takes a lot longer to get up when I fall [*he chuckles*]. But when I was younger, there'd be a new 100-foot jump—who's gonna do it first? "Let Kev. He'll do it [*he laughs*]."

I always thought I would go to college and play lacrosse. Then the Tourette's came really bad, and the medicine, and that folded those plans but, oh, well. I still play lacrosse in adult leagues. I love it. And I'm very fortunate to be able to say I love my job. I still love getting in the truck and runnin' out the door to some call. I'm that kid who never grew up.

I decided to turn it off

When I was fourteen, my dad had an operation and needed a home nurse. Carlie's[92] mother is a home-travelling nurse and so she saw me tic.

---

92   See Carlie's interview in this chapter.

Next thing you know I was at the doctor's and yep, Tourette's. Then skip to a couple of years ago, Carlie had DBS[93] surgery and she had success with it.

So when my vocal tics came back in force and I was at the fire station, it made things difficult. Swearing—I never did that before, it's good times [*he chuckles*]. I'd exhausted my medication options and so the DBS became a possibility. I thought, "Can't hurt to try," so I went to Carlie's doctor.

I did the DBS surgery about a year and a half ago. I wasn't too concerned about the severity of the operation 'cause I see that stuff all the time. I was in a good mood, more excited than nervous. After the surgery they turned the device on and things were looking good for the first month. Then the tics came back. I was going back and forth to the hospital every other week to change settings and nothing was working.

The last time I went back to my doctor, six months ago, I was there all day and they ran me through the gauntlet. They went through every lead and every setting and when I walked out of there I felt like I got the crap kicked out of me.

So I decided to turn it off and see how things go. That's where I am now. Let's see if my body calms down by itself. Who knows? Good days, bad days. Next week I'm going back to discuss more setting options. Give it another whirl.

The failure wasn't a let down. I went through it with the mindset, 'If it works great. If it doesn't, I still am who I am. I've still got a good life.'

I'm finally at that stage where I know who I am and I'm comfortable in my own skin

In my early twenties there were dark days, dealing with the tics. But I went to school, got my life in order. Now I've got the job, I've got my house, I'm finally at that stage where I know who I am and I'm comfortable in my own skin.

Going out in public, honestly it's become a little difficult with the vocal tics being what they are. But I try not to let it get in the way of my life. There are places where I'm more comfortable, like a bar-type atmosphere, because it's loud. I pick and choose. Some days I stay home and watch TV. But for me it's always been, "Don't hibernate. You gotta go out and enjoy life."

---

93   Deep Brain Stimulation surgery. See tourette.org for details.

I try to stay positive, have a good outlook. It could be worse. That's always been my go-to. I'm still walkin', talkin', can still do what I enjoy. I see people a lot worse than I can imagine being.

In my mid-teens, I had to spend the night in the hospital for testing. In the bed next to me was a boy, a lot younger, and he was hooked up to machines and people were coming in and crying. I'm thinking, "That kid's not gonna come out of here."

And I realized, "I got nothin' to complain about. Yeah, I got TS, it sucks, but this kid's a lot worse than I am." That put things in perspective for me at a young age. That's helped me through the tough times.

Kayley's cautionary tale is about the medical profession and how important it is for parents and patients to educate themselves for their own protection. It doesn't matter how prestigious the institution or how assertive the doctor. Her story also tells of the dedication and compassion of doctors and institutions intervening to make DBS possible for her. And finally it's about Mack, her service dog, who is seventy-five pounds of love and caring and the best thing that's happened to her. Be engaged in life, says Kayley, as she climbs up the next hill to see the vista from the top.

KAYLEY
20 years old

Something snapped in my brain

The Yale Global Tic Severity scale goes from zero being no tics and one hundred being as severe as it possibly can get. I was a ninety-five out of a hundred. Yeah. I was nine when I was diagnosed. Around thirteen I was diagnosed with Asperger's, which was about the time my OCD started becoming horrific. I had hidden it for years, until it got so bad I couldn't function. They were violent images, or guilty feelings like, "What if I hurt somebody?" They would loop around and around, and the more scared I got, the worse it would get. I would try to argue my way out of the thought cycle, "This isn't real," but every time it would come back, "What if it is?" And it would never, never end.

So I was started on Luvox. I did not respond well to it. On December 15, 2008—I know the exact date, which is strange—something snapped in my brain. I was in band class, trying to play a song for a test, and my arms started doing a shaky thing. They sent me home because I couldn't hold a pencil, and that was the last day I was at school for more than a year.

Within two days I was swearing, I was jerking on the floor, I was doing twisty postures. It mushroomed. None of the doctors could say why. In fact, my tics had been mild to moderate until then. Before my tic exacerbation, OCD was the big issue. When they hit, my tics stayed severe up until I had Deep Brain Stimulation surgery last year.

A paradoxical reaction

Among the first medications I tried was Fluphenazine. It was recommended by a well-regarded neurologist after Risperdal and a couple of other medications failed. The first day or two went well. The third day I woke up and something didn't feel right. Eating lunch, my head turned to the side and wouldn't go straight again. My back started tensing up too, so I called my mom. She tried to get me to relax, but it didn't help.

My back bowed and my arms bent, and my hands and toes clenched up. My mouth clenched up funny, and my tongue twisted so it was hard to speak and hard to swallow. Even my eyes pulled back in my head, so it hurt to try to look at anything. My dad came home from work and carried me to the car. When we got to the ER, I could barely speak. They asked me if I was "usually like this," and that terrified me. I kept thinking, "Wait—there are people usually like this? Is this going to go away?" They gave me an IV of Benadryl and Cogentin, and after about 20 minutes my body finally relaxed. It was such a relief. They told me it was an acute dystonic reaction.

Another time I went to the ER for a bad reaction to Ativan. The triage nurse saw me screaming and ticcing, she called security, and they came and tackled me. I was fighting them, because it hurt, and I was terrified and half out of my mind from the Ativan. They put me in four-point restraints and gave me more Ativan. Apparently that's the drug of choice for sedation [*she sighs*].

I started fighting the restraints, screaming, trying to tic because the urge building up was physically painful. I was having a paradoxical reaction to Ativan, in which the opposite of the normal response occurs. My parents warned them I couldn't have Fluphenazine, so they gave me Prolixin. I passed out. They said I was a danger to myself and held me in their overflow psych ward for thirty hours. They didn't let me go until a neurologist came down and said, "Oh, yeah, that's Tourette's."

The day after I was discharged, I started having muscle spasms again, very similar to my reaction to Fluphenazine. My mom looked up Prolixin—it's another name for Fluphenazine.

Eventually I got in with a habit reversal therapy specialist. The therapist kept saying if I just tried *harder* I could stop ticcing. Yes, she said that. This was a prestigious university hospital [*she laughs*]. It just goes to show, it doesn't matter if they're big names or experts. It depends on if they believe you.

The most important thing you can do for yourself is be engaged in life

It was pretty clear meds weren't going to work. We'd heard about service dogs, and thought that might help. So we applied and were approved, but it was a year wait. The dog was a puppy and had to be raised and trained.

I had done the first year of high school on hospital-homebound[94]. However, we saw John Leckman at Yale, *the* expert on Tourette's, who said the most important thing you can do for yourself is be engaged in life. So we tried to get me back into high school, but they didn't want me. I swore and yelled racial slurs, I would convulse and fall out of my wheelchair. It took the better part of a semester, and what *really* did it was when we went to the newspaper [*she chuckles*]. Suddenly the school was, "Yes, yes, yes, we'll let you back in."

Being allowed to return to school thrilled me, because I felt my rights were being violated. At the same time, I was terrified because I had no idea how people were going to respond to the things I said. You know, there are *fights* in high school. My coprolalia was awful, especially the racial slurs. I just wanted to disappear into the floor. Early on, hearing myself say the things I said, I could barely take it. I had never been one to bring attention to myself, so you can imagine being in public, yelling things I'd never say voluntarily. It was devastating. I spent a lot of time hating myself, hating what my body did to me.

---

94   An accommodation that allowed her, for medical reasons, to work at home.

However, the school assigned me an attendant, who went to every class with me. She was a godsend. I couldn't take notes because I was ticcing, so she did that for me. The whole high school was educated about Tourette's. I was also in honors classes and I think that helped, because of the maturity of the students.

The single best thing

That summer, I started a new medication, Dronabinol, which is THC. Strangely, that helped with only one tic, that I would squat down while walking. It's why I needed the wheelchair. After the first dose, that went away and I was able to walk again.

Then it was time to get my service dog. I went to a two-week training boot camp for me and Mack,[95] who is a Golden Retriever. He is the single best thing that ever happened to me. I can say that even now, after DBS. We knew that deep pressure, like a bear hug or weighted blanket, helped my convulsions. Mack weighs seventy-five pounds, so we hoped he could do that for me. The first time he lay on me, my attack lasted twenty minutes, which was shorter than most attacks. Within the two weeks of training, as soon as he lay down on top of me, my movements would stop.

I had expected the dog to be wonderful and amazing, but Mack was so much more. Not only was I walking, but I now had an 'Off' button for my attacks. Everyone at school was amazed at how well I was doing. Instead of hauling me off to an office where I could convulse without disrupting anything, now I could get Mack to lie on me, and even stay in class. This was my junior year, and it passed pretty well.

Most of what Mack does is deep pressure, but sometimes I had him take away an object I might hit myself with, or retrieve something that I'd thrown across the room. Even when I was without the wheelchair, sometimes I was unsteady due to tics, so he did 'bracing,' which is he stands beside me and lets me lean on him.

The first person in history

I decided to try to go to college. I've been extremely interested in neuroscience and Tourette's and psychology and the brain. So I went and [*she*

---

95   Kayley can be reached through a Facebook group. Search DBS, Tourette's, and Service dogs and request to join the group.

pauses], it did not go well. I did stick it out but I'm not sure that was a good decision. There were classes I was forced out of because I was too noisy. So I asked my neurologist about DBS. She said I should just try to live my life and deal with it. I'm thinking, "What?! They're kicking me out of college."

An online friend, who'd had DBS at NYU, suggested I call them. I was terrified they'd say no, because at this point DBS was all I had. I was beyond desperate. I felt I didn't have a life. NYU said yes. So I'm probably the first person in history who was happy to find out they were going to have invasive brain surgery [*she laughs*].

I was anticipating the insurance would be the most difficult hurdle. The operation can cost as much as $250,000 and insurance doesn't cover it for Tourette's. But my surgeon and nurse coordinator got them to pay for all of it. I have no idea how they did it. They are amazing people, very compassionate.

Is that what makes me tic?

The surgery is done in two stages. They put the leads in your brain and then connect batteries to it. They put the batteries either in the chest or, mine are in my abdomen. I usually don't know they're there, but one of them sits closer to the surface, and my hand will bump it and I'll think, "Eww, there's a battery."

I didn't sleep at all the night before the operation. I wasn't afraid it wouldn't work, but I was afraid of the pain afterwards. So I'm in pre-op, and they say, "Oh, by the way, we want to do this conscious-sedated." I knew they did that for DBS, but I thought for TS they drugged you up so you were out of it. They felt, for my case, they'd get better results if I was conscious during the operation [*she chuckles*]. And I *was* awake.

There's this giant, horrible device they bolt your skull into, and I was like, "You're going to knock me out for that, right?" They said, "Yes." Then we got another scan, they sedated me for the initial incisions, and the next thing I heard, it's time for a test stimulation.

I heard this really strange… it sounded like a radio on static. I knew, because I'd read everything I could find about the surgery, that this was the probes picking up electrical signals of my brain. And there were these screechy noises, and I noticed they coincided with my tics. I thought, "Is that what makes me tic?"

Everyone was so nice. It made the whole I'm-awake-for-brain-surgery thing a lot easier than it sounds [*she laughs*]. I have to say the worst part was when they were done, they have to close the incisions, and they used this big compression bandage. They had to keep wrapping and wrapping and that *hurt*.

I want to go up that hill

I slept for the first week after surgery. The second week I was awake enough to be moving. I walked around Manhattan with my mom, catching cabs, with the giant brain surgery bandage on my head [*she chuckles*].

I still had tics, but they weren't as violent, and they were shorter. I was walking. I felt incredibly free. We went to Central Park and there were all these people standing at the top of a hill, as if there was something to look at. I said, "Mom, I want to go up that hill." And she said, "You're crazy? You just had brain surgery." I was disappointed because I felt so fantastic.

After a week, they turned the batteries on, and went through the whole range of stimulation to make sure everything was working. Because I lived so far away, they gave me a remote control and told me to increase my setting every few weeks.

At three months, I flew back to New York for a follow-up. I flew by myself, the first time without anyone to meet me at the airport. The night before my appointment, I had an attack in Manhattan [*she chuckles*] and ended up having the Rescue Squad called. But after that second adjustment, things seemed to be more stable.

The complications with DBS are numerous, but severe ones are rare. One of the most common is it just doesn't work. There's device breakage, where people with tics hit themselves and damage the battery or the leads. I've talked with people who couldn't stop ticcing and messing with the battery. Another big issue is infection, which seems to be a problem with Tourette's patients, from tic movements or picking at wounds. The other big drawback to DBS for people with TS is people tend to think it's a cure. DBS is not a cure for Tourette syndrome.

I went into the operation feeling even a thirty-percent improvement would be good. If I still needed a wheelchair, I was gonna be happy if I can go to school and live a normal life. I got a lot more than that, obviously [*she laughs*]. I'm very lucky.

My new normal

I'm now doing really, really well. My body is my own again, no longer controlled by Tourette's. As incredible as DBS has been for me, it didn't happen overnight. Early on in the process of programming my stimulators last year, I was having fluctuations. Despite the periodic attacks, I wanted to do something with my time, so I got a seasonal job as a cashier. The store was amazing. They loved Mack, gave him his own little nametag, which I put on his harness. They did everything they could to help me. That was my first experience of somebody, who owes me nothing, going out of their way to help me.

Ideally, I would like to be a psychiatrist or neurologist. However, me and math, me and chemistry, we don't get along. Although it may be different if I can actually *stay* in class [*she chuckles*]. So I'm thinking I might become a psychologist. But all my friends on the DBS support group said I needed to take a year and figure out what my new normal is.

I have this awesome doctor now, who has been there for us. She doesn't have all the answers, she's not a big name, she's not a researcher, but she's *there*, and she believes me when I say, "This drug did this to me." She's been my lifeline. So ideally, I would like to be *that* doctor for someone. When I was going through all the worst of it, the horrible parts, I felt there could be no reason for it. Since then, I think if I can make my life matter, I'm going to do it.

I spoke with Lynn and Andrew via Skype. Andrew wore a sports jersey, and when I asked him about it, he slyly turned to show me the name on the back: Howard[96]. So much love and energy was exchanged between mother and son during our interview. To me, the two of them represented their entire family dynamic of working together and supporting one another to deal with Andrew's Tourette's.

LYNN AND HER SON ANDREW (11 YEARS OLD)

Why are the Cheerios hurting me?

Lynn: I am amazed by my son, absolutely amazed. Andrew has four diagnoses—ADHD, OCD, anxiety, and Tourette's. Each of those play against each other.

Andrew: The first thing was, we figured out I had OCD. When I was younger, she was reading to me the book *The Ants Go Marching*, and she realized I was touching the page in a funny way.

Lynn: He was adamant about not turning the page until he could touch all the ants with both hands.

Andrew: Yeah. And then, when I got a little older, I got a new tic. I would do something inside the joints of my arms and legs that would hurt, like a burning pain.

Lynn: He'd be eating Cheerios and ask, "Why are the Cheerios hurting me?" He was attributing his discomfort to anything that was right in front of him. We had him hospitalized at NYU and he had MRIs and CAT scans. We kept asking, "What's wrong with our kid?"

In our family, my father had bipolar disorder, and I had some OCD behaviors and anxiety when I was younger. I used to walk down the streets of Manhattan reading license plates. But I attributed it to a stressful home life and that I was trying to establish order. Not quite—I think it was in my blood [*she laughs*]. But that's why I had that feeling from Andrew when we read the book about the ants. I looked at him and had a sense it was that same thing.

---

96   Tim Howard, the champion pro soccer goalie, who has Tourette syndrome. In 2014 he set the World Cup record of sixteen saves in a single match.

I know to say to him, "Use your tools"

Lynn: So we went from doctor to doctor, telling what we could of his story.

Andrew: We had many temporary doctors. We kept trying.

Lynn: You're right. Andrew would have panicky times when he couldn't tell if he was awake or asleep. He would pinch the back of his hand to the point of bleeding, trying to wake himself up.

Then, when he was around five, he had a full-blown meltdown in public, what I think of as a panic attack. I used to have those. He was screaming, "I gotta get out of here! Where are you, where are you?!" It was just so sad to watch.

Someone came up to me and said, "Can I call you tomorrow?" I had known her for a very long time, but had no idea what she did as a profession. Well, she ran an anxiety disorders clinic. So that was when we started down a path with a really great doctor who does CBIT and CBT.[97]

We needed to learn. And we always said, in doctors' offices, what Andrew says carries weight. We all have to be honest and we have to stick together. The doctors have to help me and my husband, as well as Andrew's three brothers, understand what's going on. Where do we accommodate and where does accommodation cause dysfunction? Where do Andrew's boundaries differ from those of his three brothers? When he has anxieties now, I know to say to him, "Use your tools," rather than crawling into bed with him until he's so exhausted he falls asleep. So [*to Andrew*], what do you do for anxiety?

Andrew: Well, pretty recently, when I was at school playing soccer with my friends, I felt some anxiety coming along. It was pretty bad, and I just remembered, "Try to keep calm, try to think of something else. Keep doing what I'm doing." I tried to push the thought out of my head and be as calm as possible. I try not to get too deep into the thought of anxiety.

Lynn: After years of working with the same doctor—

Andrew: I just thought what made sense to do.

---

97   Cognitive Behavioral Intervention for Tics. See tourette.org for details. CBT is Cognitive Behavioral Therapy.

'The Balance Monster'

Lynn: What language do you use for OCD?

Andrew: Oh, yeah. I would call it 'The Balance Monster.' I have to balance something out. So I would touch my car with one hand, if I accidentally bumped it or something, and I would be like, "Oh, gotta stop, do it with my other hand." I think it was the same thing with *The Ants Go Marching*. I would touch it with one hand and then have to touch it with the other.

Lynn: What did Doctor Meagan have you do for that?

Andrew: Touch it as many times with one hand as I can, then hold back my other one.

Lynn: Exposure therapy.

Andrew: I haven't had that in a like a year, so I'd say it works pretty well.

Lynn: You think so?

Andrew: Yeah. Remember? I didn't complain about it.

Lynn: You haven't had the urges? I wonder if it's because you worked so hard on your tools, you have them so front and center, that you stop it before it becomes an issue.

Andrew: Yes.

Lynn: That's pretty impressive.

Andrew: It's so small right now. It really doesn't get in the way at all.

Lynn: This is all CBT therapy in that same clinic we initially went to and this one doctor who's been amazing for us. She's trained in all the things that happen to be Andrew's challenges. She just keeps rolling out her next basket of goods every time Andrew comes in with something.

We're in a perfect place to say we can handle it

Andrew: And... my tics. How do I handle them? Well, it's really boring, but it works [*he chuckles*]. So this is true, I had a head-shaking tic, so the competing response is where I'd do the opposite until the urge goes away.

Lynn: Whenever Andrew has a new tic, the doctor talks to him about the feeling and they find something that counters it.

Andrew: There's one, a blinking tic, where she'd have me do a slow, controlled blink. That would be different than blinking fast. Or like today, I had a sniffling tic and I would do a normal breath, just breathe.

Lynn: Now he's on 27 mg of Concerta for the ADHD, and he is on 1 mg of Intuniv at night. You know, it's hard to say what cocktail, or what *part* of the cocktail, works. Andrew is trying so many different things, sometimes it's hard to say what works. Is it his willingness to use his tools, is it the meds, is it the clinical study?

Andrew: Tell about that.

Lynn: I will. But for what works, I don't know. I don't think any of us knows. Some of these tools develop over time. We've learned, as parents and siblings, how to better help Andrew. How not to say, "Stop ticcing," or "What are you doing?"

We're adding and adding tools and resources and haven't stopped to think, "Should we take anything away?" I would be nervous to do that, since things are working. Andrew has this terrible time with sleep sometimes. It puts us back ten steps, because things erupt when you're under-slept. I don't know that we're ever in a place to say we found the answer, but I know we're in a perfect place to say we can handle it.

We're all on the same page as a family

Lynn: We've learned how to better parent him. It's not even about parenting. It's how to support him. If we're watching a movie and Andrew's compelled to do reporting, which is continually repeating what was said, it can make us crazy [*they chuckle*]. So we say to him, "Use your competing responses." It's hard sometimes, but we've come to a point in our family where Andrew is like, "All right, all right, I get it." No one's offended by it, no one's upset by it, and we're all on the same page as a family.

What's interesting is, we needed it as much as Andrew did. We needed to know where to accommodate, where you ignore. If Andrew says, "My arm is sore," I can ask him, "Is that because of a tic?"

Andrew: Wait, wait, wait. Actually, you shouldn't ask if it's a tic, you should just ask, "What happened?" Because if you bring up the thought of a tic, that goes to my head and I go, "Oh, yeah, tic," and it becomes a tic.

Lynn: Yeah. So somehow we're trying to get it. He'd say, "You're not supposed to ask me, mom." And I'd say, "Okay, okay."

Andrew: It would happen over and over [*he laughs*].

Lynn: Until I learned.

It's just crazy how things happen

Andrew: Now tell about how you actually found the clinical study.

Lynn: Andrew loves to play sports. About a year and a half ago, I was at a soccer game, and I was watching him on the field. He'd been having some terrible tics for a long time, and I stood on the sidelines and I cried. I said to a friend, "I can't stand here and watch Andrew tic anymore. I just can't." A parent, who was sitting right in front of me, said, "Did you say tics? Who's your son?" I said, "The guy over there looking over his shoulder." 'Cause he had a tic of looking back over his shoulder and couldn't keep his eye on the ball [*they both laugh*]. We laugh about this now. And he said, "I was at a benefit last night for this organization Tic Toc Stop.[98] Would you like me to put you in touch with them?" And I said, well, first of all, "Who *are* you?" and "Yes, please." So within twenty-four hours I was in touch with them, and it turned out they were starting a clinical study. It's just crazy how things happen.

Andrew: The clinical study was the mouthpiece.[99]

Lynn: We had to go through this process where they had to figure out what size oral orthotic they were going to make for him.

Andrew: They videotaped me a bunch of times. The first time was just me and I was not supposed to hold back any of my tics. Let them go if they were there. And there were forty tics. After that, they put three tongue depressors in my mouth to bite down on. And I had twenty-six tics. The urges are going way down. So then they tried four tongue depressors on each side and it was twenty-eight tics. Then they tried five and it was like thirty-something. So we realized three was a good amount. And they made the mouthpiece that size.

Lynn: We had to go back every weekend for a while, and now it's been about ten weeks.

Andrew: My tics got less right away. I just felt relief, like, "Here it is." Yep.

Lynn: They go down even with him not wearing it. I don't understand.

Andrew: I think it helps me, like, get in a groove.

Lynn: He says he doesn't have as many urges, even when he takes it out.

---

98   tictocstop.com.
99   The mouth orthotic for tics. Search "orthotic" at tourette.org.

I love that people try things

Lynn: My biggest fear was Andrew would go down the path of self-medicating.

Andrew: What does that mean?

Lynn: Drugs and alcohol.

Andrew: No! Never.

Lynn: But I think you get into a place where it's really hard, and that's why all I want is to give him tools. I love that people try things. It's important to stay as open as you can, because you never know whether it's going to be chemistry or a soccer sideline that will give you an answer. Just embrace it as something that's part of your life. I always say to Andrew, "You deserve to be at the same starting line as everyone else in the morning." That's it. You shouldn't be ten steps back. We go in, we meet with his teachers—

Andrew: At the beginning of the year you talk to them. They never seem judgey about it.

Lynn: He's going to middle school next year. We don't want to change life's rules to accommodate Andrew's challenges. If the teacher sees something, that means Andrew needs another tool. Rather than say, "You have to excuse this because, because, because."

We live in Westchester and it's so much about getting ahead. It's an affluent community where, if you can somehow sneak something in for your kid, parents will do it. We're doing absolutely the opposite. We're trying to keep Andrew on track and labeling it, calling it what it is, and just being open to *try* things. We have four other kids in our family. I don't know how any other one of them would have done in this situation—

Andrew: Three other kids.

Lynn: Yes, three [*she chuckles*], four total. But this guy, he's been such a partner in this, always on the same page. It's been very hard for us at times, but he's always willing to try something new. He'll go and explain to anybody. He's going into middle school and he went in front of the principal, the social worker, and the guidance counselor, around a conference room table, and talked about it. They kept saying, "What can we do for you?" And we kept saying, "Nothing. Just know. Just be our partners." We don't want untimed tests, we don't want any accommodations. If there's a challenge, text me, call me, email me. And we'll figure out what we, all of us, need to do to help him. Andrew doesn't deserve a free ticket in life. He deserves a regular life.

Andrew: I might need a homework pass sometimes. [*He chuckles*] I'm joking. I just really don't like homework. Why do you need to do work outside of school?

He's better than all of us!

Andrew: I don't know why I started playing hockey. I just thought it would be fun. I was three years old when I thought of it [*he chuckles*] and I started skating. It was actually before. When I was younger, they didn't give you positions, and now I'm a forward, right wing or left wing. 'Cause my coach knows I'm the best [*he laughs*].

Lynn: But he went an entire year when he couldn't keep his eyes on the puck because his tic was he was always looking over his shoulder. But he stuck to it. You know, I get really proud. I think, "This is a kid who is incredibly resilient." And although this is difficult, he's got life skills that are gonna see him through whatever arises. It's funny because my mom, who's an eighty-four-year-old Jewish woman from Manhattan, says, "How's my Andrew?" all the time. And I say, "Ma, he's better than all of us!" [*She laughs.*] "We should all have his skills. Stop worrying about him."

————————— ❦ —————————

In Chapter Five, Shayna spoke about the salutary effects of Tourette syndrome camps. Here she tells about her experience with a service dog to help with her tics. She's well informed on the legal aspects of service dogs, and it was important to her that people understand the differences between service dogs, emotional-support animals, and therapy animals.

SHAYNA
24 years old

There are so many tasks a dog can be trained to do to improve my life

A new development has recently blossomed in my life with Tourette syndrome. My friends have service dogs for Tourette syndrome and I've benefitted greatly from the privilege of using their service dogs. I'm in the process of obtaining my own.

I have a hugging tic and also sensory issues. The only way to keep them from spiraling is for somebody to give me a tight hug. I have to be the one who initiates it. If I don't allow myself to have a big hug, and I try to suppress that tic, it's going to lead into tic attacks. I rely on my parents for hugs. I'm not in school anymore, but I relied on classmates and friends. If I'm in public, I'm kinda stuck. My concern is that one day my involuntary hugging will 'land' on someone who'll respond very negatively. My hope is that one day I can have a service dog available to me at all times. The service dog would then complete that cycle for me because I can initiate that big hug.

Some other ways a service dog can help with tics is support for tics that impede mobility, alerting the person with tics to an oncoming attack or unconscious self-injurious behaviors. They can also guide someone away from triggering environments to a quieter safe environment.

There are so many tasks a dog can be trained to do to improve my life. I've applied for one and have been accepted.[100] I filled out a prelimi-

———————————

100   Shayna is slated to be partnered with her service dog in summer 2016. Her website is shaynapulley.webs.com (best viewed on PC or Mac, not mobile devices).

nary application online and that led to them sending me reference forms. I had one filled out by my doctor, one by a professor, and one by a friend who was formerly a mental-health worker. Also I had a classmate who frequently had to help me at school, and my friend I went to a Tourette camp with.

I honestly can't wait until that blanket can walk itself

I have many other conditions, and most of them benefit from something called 'deep pressure.' One way to accomplish this is with my weighted blanket, which is deep pressure therapy. It's difficult to travel with my weighted blanket because it's sixteen pounds, and I take it on planes. The only time I even have it in public is when I'm travelling by air and I honestly can't wait until that blanket can walk itself [*she chuckles*]. The service dog can help by performing deep-pressure therapy, which means I lie on the floor and the dog lies with its full weight pressing down on me. The act of the dog performing deep pressure therapy is so much more effective than a weighted blanket at alleviating my symptoms.

In America, service animals perform tasks a disabled person cannot effectively do for themselves. Businesses can ask what task the service animal has been trained to perform, to ensure it is a service animal as defined by the Americans with Disabilities Act. They can't ask for details about a person's disability.

There are emotional-support animals, but they are not allowed in most public places. Emotional-support animals are not task trained. And therapy animals are simply animals that go into nursing homes or other institutions, but they have zero legal rights.

My decision to seek a service dog was based on my need for an animal to be trained in tasks to assist me throughout the day. Some people may find that a pet offering just emotional support at home is enough for them. For me, this hasn't been the case.

Jodi is one of several folks here who credited their Tourette-induced isolation for successful endeavors. Without the focused time alone, Jodi would not have found her particular artistic outlet. Her story is also a cautionary tale of careless physicians, because she is among those who were not informed of drug side effects and now suffer serious consequences. With Sabbath, her service-dog companion, and supported by her family and community, she moves through each day, fully aware of the strength it takes to live a full life with Tourette syndrome.

JODI
47 years old

I'm sure I'm going crazy

Here in Saskatchewan, we're so rural I have a three-and-a-half-hour drive just to get to a doctor's appointment. It seems that's all I do out here, travel back and forth, but hopefully that'll end one of these days. Sometimes you do feel so very all alone, especially in an area like where I live, where there aren't a lot of people, never mind a lot of people with Tourette's.

Not every day is an up day. I still have down days with Tourette's, with depression, with secluding myself. My message to people is—it sucks, yeah, but it sucks for everybody. We all have our crosses to bear. This is ours, with Tourette's.

In the initial stages of my Tourette's, they didn't know what it was. My parents divorced when I was six, and I felt it was blamed on me, on the Tourette's. I would pinch people, I would poke people, I would flap my arms and smash the heel of my hand into my nose. I broke my nose a couple of times doing that. They couldn't deal with me.

As I was growing up, my family was involved with government officials throughout the world. I lived in twenty-one countries, which meant I went to fourteen different schools. You learn to not get close to anybody. You learn to leave. You never reveal yourself with your Tourette's. Sitting in class, I'd flail my arm, so I would pretend I had a shoulder ache or something. By the time I reached my teens, I was depressed and had other issues. I was quite high-functioning, but I had learned to hide.

In my early twenties, I said to my mom, "I'm sure I'm going crazy." There was something wrong with me and I had to find out what. If I am insane, let me know. They sent me to a neurologist, who said, "You have Tourette syndrome. It's quite obvious." I laughed, "No, I don't have that. I don't swear." But in fact, I did have it.

I looked at myself in my pajamas

My kids accept my Tourette's, as does my community. My son lives in town and helps if I need it. My family teases me about my TS, we joke about it, but we do realize it's a serious thing. It's a tough life.

I have opportunities others don't, but even with that, I suffer from confinement. I never know when I'm going to flail my arms, when I'm going to knock a stand of blueberries all over the grocery floor. I started staying home more and more, to the point where I wouldn't leave my house for weeks on end. You know, that's not a life. Simply not a life [*she sighs*].

What got me out of this cycle of isolation was the threat to my marriage. I'm lucky enough to have a husband who helps me through. He runs a pipe-fitting company and works in an oil-drilling camp in northern British Columbia. He's away for three weeks, home for one. We want a life together, we want to travel and do things. I realized that I still had half my life to live, not half my life to *exist*. I wanted to live for those remaining years, not sit in my house with the TV on. I looked at myself in my pajamas, sitting in the house for *another* day, phoning to have groceries delivered because I couldn't even get out of the house to do that. I got angry. Angry at Tourette syndrome. You get to that, "Why me? Why did I get this?" Well, who knows why? It's yours, so let's get on with it.

He's one-hundred-seventy-pounds worth of dog

I decided to look into a service dog. I'd seen them for other things, so why couldn't this work for me? I found a breeder in Ohio who was willing to donate a Great Dane puppy to me. When I got Sabbath, training and certification were up to me. He's being trained by Assistance Dogs International to be certified for public access. He learns how I react, how my muscle tensions express, and I learn how he reacts to me.

Sabbath's tasks are to "alert" and "pin." That means he will alert me to an upcoming grand-motion tic. He leans against me with a lot of weight—he's one-hundred-seventy-pounds worth of dog. I can sometimes recognize the tic beginning, but not always. I get kind of a grabbing sensation in my stomach and all of a sudden up go my arms. There's something in the muscles, in the chemicals given off by my body, that Sabbath can sense. Once he detects I'm going to have a grand-motion tic, he pins me, using his head and body to guide me against a solid object. He'll push me up against a wall, for example, so I'm away from harming others or myself. He can take my arm in his mouth, gently, and he's able to hold it down.

I consider myself an advocate for Tourette syndrome. The Tourette Syndrome Foundation of Canada posted a story I wrote[101] about my life and about Sabbath. He was also in Modern Dog Magazine,[102] where they did an issue on service dogs. And he was in Abilities Magazine.[103] I try to get the word out about what TS really is. It's not easy, but you can lead a good life, a very rewarding life. I've married, I've had children, I work as an artist and make a decent living. Granted, I might not want to work as a receptionist [*she chuckles*], but there are many things I can do.

Some kind of street junkie

When I leave my house without Sabbath, and I'm throwing my head around and flailing my arms, I know people are looking at me, like, "What is wrong with her?" And even if they're not, that's what I *think* they're thinking of me. That is the part that made me turn into a recluse. Exactly that. And you do get depressed then.

What I find the hardest is the embarrassment of it. Yesterday, for example, I went to the hospital to have a twenty-four-hour heart monitor removed. I was throwing my head back and gasping, making grimaces, and I could tell the lady checking me in was thinking something was mentally wrong with me. Like my facets aren't quite polished [*she laughs*]. And that's it—I do feel polished, as a human being. I have a decent education, I speak four languages fluently, and I'm considering learning either Hindi or Tagalog. Yet those people look at me like I'm some kind of street junkie.

I almost wonder, if I didn't have TS, would I be as accomplished as I am? Without the isolation Tourette syndrome forced me into, would

---

101   www.tourette.ca.
102   moderndogmagazine.com in the December 2014 issue.
103   www.abilities.ca January 2015 issue.

I have put the time and effort into it? I spent hours and hours teaching myself languages and art. So in that regard, I do consider it a blessing.

A gift of a few hours

I'm a digital artist and I work from home. It requires very fine motor skills. When I'm doing things like that, I find it controls the Tourette's. When I do art I don't have tics and twitches. It's calm and soothing. So not only am I doing something nice for somebody else, it also gives me a gift of a few hours where I focus on art and don't worry about the rest of it.

I love my art. I do pet portraits, mainly. The reason is because I lost one of my Great Danes and it was devastating. Every photo I had was him standing in front of the garbage can in the kitchen or something like that [*she chuckles*]. So I taught myself to digitally edit that picture. People saw that and started asking me to edit pictures of their pets who'd died. So now, for $40, I give people something that's nice to remember their pets.[104] People get a digital file and they can print it any way they want.

Together we can deal with that

My mother-in-law is a nurse, my father-in-law is a doctor, and they're very supportive of me with TS. The problem is, I have to be honest with them about what I'm feeling. If I'm telling them everything's okay, they can't help me. But if I say, "I'm having difficulty getting out of the house again," together we can deal with that. I think that's key, learning to be honest about what's going on. It's not always easy, because you get so used to hiding your entire life. I think honesty plays a huge role in not getting depressed. If I'm not voicing that I'm having issues, my support network can't help me.

Right now I don't take medication for my Tourette syndrome. I do take Elavil for depression. Previously I took Haldol and Xanax. The Haldol I got off of because of its propensity for tardive dyskinesia. A lot of the meds for Tourette's have such wicked-bad side effects that I'm no longer willing to put myself through that. And now, at the age of forty-seven, I'm in stage 1 of liver failure from the Haldol.

Am I ticked off about it? Absolutely. Do I feel resentment? Absolutely. I'm resentful that there weren't better options available. Haldol was the

104 *Fur Real Pet Portraits* on Facebook.

only medication I was offered. And I was never told about side effects. They never, ever mentioned tardive dyskinesia or liver damage. Yeah.

People do not appreciate the strength it takes or us to make it through the day

I've never felt depressed enough to take my own life, but I have thought, "People would be happier if they didn't have to deal with me." I think a lot of us do feel that way. I never seriously attempted anything. Instead, I chose to get Sabbath.

If I'd had more information about what it was like for other people, I might have been able to avoid some of the depression. If I had not felt so all alone, and so weird and messed up and such an oddball, I think it would have been different for me. I've succeeded in life, but those successes have not come without struggle.

People do not appreciate the strength it takes for us to make it through the day. Even my husband, as supportive as he is, sometimes forgets that there is anything wrong with me. Well, not "wrong." That's in air quotes [*she chuckles*]. I am quite high- functioning and he'll forget that I have *issues*, if you will. He gets frustrated and will say something, and I think, "If you only knew what it took for me to get this task done." And then you get angry at them because they just don't *see* it, they don't *get* it. It's different for someone with a more visible disability. And that's why the dog helps in that regard. People see me alone and they don't recognize how difficult it is for me to get through the day. They see me with the dog, in his service vest, and they think, "Oh, that person has a medical issue."

Rachel is creating her life through mindfulness and meditation. She's honing what is sure to be a keen sense of self, rooted in acceptance of Tourette syndrome. She, her husband, and their four-year old boy share in a natural way of life that provides them clean food, a quiet environment, and lots of rabbits. I like how Rachel brings mindfulness to her day, and the sanctuary from stress it gives her.

RACHEL
35 years old

We're far from pioneers

Nutrition helps, absolutely, with my Tourette's. I say that with guilt, because I know what I shouldn't have. They say, "Quit the food you want most, because it's what you shouldn't have." Espresso is my nemesis. I've found certain food additives, like MSG, also create a reaction for my Tourette's. Sugar increases my stress levels and makes things more difficult.

Nutrition's important for us and our little guy. I like to make healthy choices as much as possible. So it surprises me, because I am a city girl, that we raise our own meat. It's not cows, it's rabbits. We started with three last May and have about forty-five now. My husband bought the equipment and we do the processing ourselves. We did make an attempt at tanning the animals, to use all parts of the rabbits, but... it didn't work out [*she laughs*]. We're far from pioneers.

I've opened to the possibility of a bigger, broader meaning to life

I feel Tourette's is about trying to find balance. I've come to terms with that through meditation, more than anything else. For a long time I tried to micromanage my symptoms. I blamed myself for being so complicated. So I had to do a lot of inner work to release preconceived ideas about what life is.

Those ideas come from the isolation of the Tourette's experience. Now, as an adult, I would also identify as someone with Asperger's. It wasn't on my radar as an adolescent, but I didn't have good comprehension of my experience because I was heavily medicated. I had a lot of clarity once I stopped taking meds.

Before that, I found a way into the world of people by mimicking their behavior. I might have been more comfortable withdrawing, but I didn't do that. Instead, I passed. Rather than doing what I was most comfortable with, I did what was expected of me. You know, wanting to be perceived as... the 'N word'—Normal [*she laughs*].

It's a puzzle I kept trying to solve. I was trying not to be perceived as what I knew I was—completely different. I had a hope that someday I would fit in. But I've opened to the possibility of a bigger, broader meaning to life. I'm on the path to reconciling myself with my difference. I've only gained any sense of who I am in the last five or six years. And that was because what I learned through my bachelor of social work prompted me to stop the meds. That's my feeling about it. Yeah.

I found my way to meditation out of necessity

My tics were worse when I was medicated. After the initial withdrawal, my tics faded to the background, and what was most challenging was facing things I hadn't before. The physical challenges were incredible and led to overwhelm and exhaustion. I would have electric shocks as I went to sleep, over and over again. I had just graduated, just started my new career, and was very stressed. I would be in my office, but it wasn't a familiar space. Or familiar and unfamiliar at the same time.

I found my way to meditation out of necessity, to find quiet where I could process things. A social worker suggested I check out the work by Jon Kabat-Zinn on mindfulness. He's a pioneer for mindfulness practice from the perspective of stress reduction. I took an eight-week course and I've been trying to create space to use mindfulness in more situations.

Mindfulness is seeing things happen, but not being attached to them. I've learned there's more to "right now" than being caught up in what happens. I can observe circumstances, rather than try to achieve a desired outcome. Mindfulness gives me a step back, toward who I really am. It led me to a perspective that was more manageable. What it does for Tourette's is, it doesn't allow an accumulation of stress. I equate tics with stress, and I'm letting go of things that would cause more ticcing.

It's like your mind gets a little cleaner

I used to feel responsible for someone else's dissatisfaction. I'd get caught in self-deprecation. There's this freight train and it's on a path and it needs to *get there*. So mindfulness helps me detach from outcomes, to see that it's just two people with two different ways of seeing something. It's like your mind gets a little cleaner.

As a young adult, I became quite a pleaser [*she laughs*]. I *want* to help people. But when I got my social work degree, I had to understand what that meant. I started to learn about being isolated and how I coped with it. I started asking questions about what I *want* to be rather than all the things I was *trying* to be.

So I took a couple of years to focus on healing, and at the same time, to reflect on my journey. During that time, I also did a lot of reading that helped me understand social work in a much more profound way. In fact, I was my first client.

What it was, and *is*, is me needing space. I'm new to myself. I need to know myself. I'm giving myself the gift of time to be a mom and get past this adjustment. To have space to make good choices. Putting space between what I thought I was going to do and where I am now.

Simply my hands on the steering wheel

Mindfulness for me is more of a walking meditation, because with my little guy it's very difficult to find dedicated time to sit quietly. I *do* sit,[105] and love that time, but mindfulness now is cultivating ongoing awareness as I walk through my day. I think that is the most beneficial for me from a Tourette's standpoint. Whenever there's stillness, it's a cue for me to recognize mindfulness. Sometimes it's simply my hands on the steering wheel.

If my little guy becomes very active, it can get quite wearing. I try to shift my attention from wanting the noise to stop, to putting my attention on the noise. I can master my surroundings because I'm not trying to find silence when silence is not there. It's about when to give up control. Acknowledging what the moment contains. This approach is helpful.

---

105   Meditation when one is sitting in a chair or on a cushion.

Your challenge is to know who you are

TS is not something you invented, it's a part of your physiology, and yet you exist in a world that doesn't tic. I have a lot of guilt for having Tourette's. I somehow ended up with this thing and I've gotta get it in check. People don't believe you can't control yourself. So you tend to blame yourself for not being able to do what everyone else can do. If people around you are staring, you become very aware you have it. So your challenge is to know who you are.

Mindfulness was my first tiny step to hearing my inner voice, which was begging me to slow down. It was push, push, push. Be, be, be. Do, do, do. And what I really needed was let go of ideas about what I should be. Give myself time to find out who I was. Learn to love myself. The whole world shifted and changed. It feels like being lost and found all at the same time.

In chapter one of his book *Far from the Tree*,[106] Andrew Solomon talks about identity, which is what a group of people believe about themselves. That experience of not being sure you fit in. In society, you're expected to not have the movements, not have the noises. You're in a world with a whole bunch of people who don't have Tourette's, and you *do*. You have a thing that makes living much more difficult. You don't want to abstain from life, you need to live life, but the challenges are great.

If I can create, then I am *someone*

Creativity was the vibe I was riding. It was the first thing I saw in myself. Previous to going off the meds, I felt unhuman. I can't grasp how I went from being that person, to following some gut feeling that I needed to stop taking Risperdal, and then liberating a part of me.

My creativity expresses itself a lot in my environment and the things I like. As time went on, I started to write.[107] It comes out in the work I do. I have an interesting way of bringing two separate things together to make something new. It's a creative act to create my life.

Right now I'm doing freelance social media work for small business-es. I enjoy the writing part, content development, and strategy. It's quite

---

106   Andrew Solomon, *Far from the Tree: Parents, Children and the Search for Identity.*

107   Rachel's blog is at herstoryofmadness.com.

fulfilling. It's like the writing I did in the nonprofit sector, but it's easier to turn off at the end of the day.

My ability to create completely debunked this idea that I was excluded from humanity. If I can create, then I *am* someone. It was a revelation—you *can't* be nothing, because you can create things. You can find stuff in nothing.

Coprolalia—who thinks up this stuff? Like a Greek mythological revenge-of-the-gods narrative, you are cursed to endure a life of blurting all things ugly and inappropriate. It's no wonder the media clings to coprolalia as the most entertaining and prevalent Tourette symptom even though rough-ly only ten-percent of Touretters have it. Joanne laughs about it, and she's learned that educating people, as difficult as it sometimes can be, is the best medicine.

JOANNE
53 years old

I meditate on my own almost daily

You have to have a sense of humor about Tourette's. Even when things are difficult. I celebrate and practice Judaism, but have gotten a lot of strength from Buddhist teachings and Native American wisdom. It's a process. Ten or fifteen years ago, I started on a more spiritual path and those teachings have helped me a lot.

I started doing personal growth and self-help work, my spiritual beliefs evolved, and that's when I started to meditate. I meditate on my own almost daily. I find it helps keep stress levels down and keep my mind calmer. I tend to do it more in the evening, and I spend a few moments in the morning setting an intention for the day. And I meditate in short spurts throughout the day.

I know when I relax my body, the tics will decrease. There's definitely a correlation. When we're revved up, not only do our brains work faster, but our tics get worse, we get more stressed, and there's that vicious cycle.

Blubber

I used to speak for the Tourette Syndrome Association at national conferences and ran the National Adult Issues Committee for a few years. I also ran the Massachusettes chapter for many years. I cowrote, with Sue Levi-Pearl,[108] the coprolalia guide and I wrote a housing guide for adults with Tourette's.

I'm proud I had the opportunity to do TV and radio appearances back when Tourette's wasn't understood. I've heard from people who said, "I saw you on TV, and that's when I understood what my son had." Or they saw the Sally Jesse Raphael Show. People remember Jack Klugman did the Quincy episode many years ago. There were people that got proper diagnoses because of those shows.

What was very exciting, I consulted on the set of *Awakenings*, with Robin Williams. Four days with Robin and Oliver Sacks was an incredible experience. I had a little part in the movie but it ended up on the cutting room floor. I think now in one scene you see a clip of the side of my shoulder [*she laughs*]. It was amazing. We were making jokes with Robin about Tourette syndrome on the set. He really understood and related to those of us with Tourette's. His loss recently was heartbreaking.[109] He was very compassionate. A heart of gold.

Oliver has great respect for people with Tourette's. I remember being at the Bronx Zoo with him, and one of the first exhibits was a pool with seals swimming around. A seal swam up to me and I had a tic, I said, "Blubber. Blubber." He thought that was fascinating and quizzed me on why the first thing that came to mind was blubber [*she laughs*].

Three times a week for the next four years

My tics started in fourth grade. My first tic was blinking and it went to sniffing and throat clearing. My mother was a nurse and had the sense I couldn't control what I was doing.

---

108   Sue Levi-Pearl is a founding member of Tourette Syndrome Association and was liaison with medical and scientific programs.
109   Robin Williams committed suicide in 2014. Oliver Sacks died in 2015.

I took ballet lessons and learned to do a 'plié. At that time I had a tic where I would touch my chin to different things. I'd be sitting at the dinner table and put my chin in my plate, or touch my chin to my dresser or my elbow.

I remember taking ice skating lessons too, and we had to go from one end of the ice to the other—I was nine or ten years old—and while I was skating down the ice [*she chuckles*] I bent down and did a plié and then touched my chin to the ice. I remember one parent said to my mother, "What on earth is your daughter doing?" I wasn't diagnosed yet and my mother honestly didn't know. That was a pretty complex tic [*she laughs*].

We went from one doctor to another until a psychiatrist said, "Bring her to me three times a week for the next four years and I might be able to cure her."

At that point, my uncle, a psychiatrist at Yale, said we should see the doctors at the Child Study Center there. At the initial visit they said, "This is a classic case of Tourette's." I was thirteen. That was in 1974. The TSA was just getting started. I still work with James Leckman[110] and am involved in some of their research studies with Tourette's.

Am I loveable?

It was isolating at school and with friendships. A teacher told me if I didn't stop sniffing no one would like me [*she chuckles*]. Certainly there was a lot of teasing. That got worse through high school, which was a nightmare. The principal of the public school suggested that I go to private high school, and that made a huge difference.

I was always very self-conscious. I felt misunderstood. I wasn't popular. I was seldom involved with groups. There's the conversation you have with yourself about, "Am I acceptable? Am I loveable?" I felt that more in my twenties, where I was getting into relationships that weren't the best for me but, "He accepts my Tourette's."

I don't have to apologize

I often felt I had to apologize for my tics, or for who I was, or how I

110　James Leckman M.D., is a child psychiatrist and psychoanalyst and the Neison Harris Professor of Child Psychiatry, Psychiatry, Psychology and Pediatrics at the Yale School of Medicine, recognized for his research in Tourette syndrome and obsessive–compulsive disorder.

made people feel. When I went to graduate school for social work, my friends said, "Joanne, you don't have to apologize. We understand." That's something I struggle with to this day. I don't have to apologize.

I think I was the only person who couldn't wait to turn thirty, because in my twenties my tics were *so* severe. In my thirties and forties the tics subsided a good deal. I feel blessed I don't have to cope with what I coped with all those years.

I'd be walking down the street yelling the N-word at the top of my lungs. You can't hide that. I remember getting on an airplane with a friend. We were going to a Tourette syndrome conference. Flying was always difficult. You had to explain it to the airline, and go through security, then explain it to the stewardess so they could make an announcement.

On the plane, there were two seats left, right in front of us, and the last two men to get on the plane were Black. And we're thinking, "Oh, no." We explained it, they were lovely gentlemen, and very accepting. My friend had a tic of punching the seat in front of him, and I was having the N-word tic [*she laughs*]. Those poor men.

Attitude is the real disability

I think intuition and insight into other people is more honed in those of us with Tourette's. We relate to the underdog and to people's pain. I've worked with kids with Tourette's whose parents tell me, "He cares about everybody." I think a lot of us are highly sensitive about the whole human experience.

Tourette's is probably the reason I went into psychology and social work. The helping professions. There are a lot of people with Tourette's doing that. I went on to get my masters degree in social work, so the rest is history, as they say [*she chuckles*].

Years ago I said, "Attitude is the real disability." It's important for us to feel good about ourselves and to understand there won't always be acceptance and understanding in society. In the past twenty years, disability awareness has become more prevalent, but Tourette's is still difficult to understand for the average person.

Certainly there's a lot of anger with Tourette's

It's easy to blame people for the way they respond. Sadly, I know people with Tourette's, for whom it's one struggle after another. You want to say to them, "You're doing this to yourself, to an extent." They demand more from the way people treat them. They want to put it out as society's problem. They're not *wrong*, but then it becomes a self-fulfilling prophecy. If you go out there being angry at the world and expecting the world to treat you right, those are not situations where people end up having good experiences.

Certainly there's a lot of anger with Tourette's. I've dealt with it. I've been very angry, at God or society or my teachers or an employer who couldn't accept my tics. At some point that anger is not healthy.

I might not want to apologize for my tics, but I'm the first to say, "I have Tourette's." These days, thankfully, most people have heard of it. But if you go in with a chip on your shoulder, there's that constant external and internal fight. Not only with yourself, but with society. I am grateful that my family and friends, as well as colleagues and providers, have always been supportive, caring, and accepting of me.

Craig was outside supervising construction on his house when we spoke. He's a big man and his deep voice suits him. Occasionally he'd interrupt our conversation with an instruction or suggestion to a worker. Even at his size he gets stares when he tics, and his heart breaks thinking of the same thing happening to small children. He describes the crippling effects of tic storms, how biofeedback keeps him on an even keel, and how the South welcomed him with open arms.

CRAIG
55 years old

It's a cool old house

I put myself through college working construction in San Diego. I've been workin' on stuff all my life. I was raised you don't go buy a part, you fix it. My dad and my granddad built Parnelli Jones'[111] first race car. My dad,

---

111 Parnelli Jones was a celebrated racing driver and successful racecar owner.

because of me being a child, turned down a NASCAR ride with Penske[112]. He was gonna drive for them, but he didn't want to be on the road all the time.

I'm building my house now here in Georgia. It's a rebuild, really. It's a cool old house. The first part of it was built in 1945 and—I didn't see this when I bought it—it's had seven additions over the years. It was built, then another layer of walls was put on, and floors. And then another layer of walls. So I'm peeling off all this antique hardwood, okay [*he chuckles*]? I'm getting enough wood out of this house to pay for the house and do all the repairs. Just in recovered wood.

Building things helps me relax. If I can concentrate into what I'm building, I am overall pretty good with the tics. I fish a lot, and that helps. I live three miles from a great big lake. My best friend lives on the lake and has a very nice boat and we go at least a couple of times a week. It's been some years since I played guitar but, especially out in California, I was playing hours a day. My fingers aren't working so well these days, so I can't pull it off anymore.

As soon as the strobe light hit

When I got sick with Tourette's, it was right at my thirty-third birthday. Yeah, it's pretty weird. Over the years I never met anybody like me. It took me about ten years to get diagnosed. Nobody knew what to call it, how to treat it. This was twenty years ago.

Dealing with it when it came on, it was difficult, man. My background at the time was biomedical engineering. I worked for the Bayer Corporation and this was in 1992. How it started was one day I felt like I had a low-level flu. Next day I felt a little worse, just wanted to lay there and not do nothin' and I stayed home. The next morning I woke up and was hurting down my left arm. I thought, "Wow, I'm having a heart attack." So I went to a cardiologist who said, "Something's definitely wrong, but your heart's fine." They put me to the hospital, where they gave me an EEG and put the strobe light on me. As soon as the strobe light hit I had a grand mal seizure.

He is most famous for his achievements at the Indianapolis 500. In 1962, he became the first driver to qualify at over 150 mph.

112   Penske was the biggest owner in American racing at the time.

They started treating me for epilepsy, okay? That was reasonable. Went through a whole host of drugs. One doctor gave me a drug called Reglan. It has a side effect of giving you tardive dyskinesia.[113] So that doctor gave me TD. The doctors were just lookin' at me—you know, I was too old for it to be Tourette's. And this went on for years. All kinds of drugs and horrible medicines. One after the other. Horrible meds. Because nothing was working.

You just keep on swimmin'

I recently learned off a Tourette's website about tic storms. I've been having tic storms since the get-go. They misdiagnosed them all these years. A tic storm is… it's often misdiagnosed as a grand mal seizure. The major difference is that the patient experiencing said tic storm remains awake. And they hurt, okay? The pain is horrific. These poor kids who have to go through this, my God. It's ugly. For the first year, I was having fifty to a hundred a day. I lost the ability to write. One day I woke up and couldn't speak. I only knew one hand signal and it's not politically correct [*he laughs*].

We ended up driving to Baylor University in Texas and seeing a doctor there who diagnosed me with Tourette's. He'd never seen anything like this, somebody coming down with TS at my age. Adult onset—what are you talking about?

So this doctor put me on an experimental medication, Tetrabenazine, and that did help somewhat. The only problem was twice a year I had to go to Texas to get it. And because it was not approved in the United States, I had to pay for it. Well, after a while I just couldn't afford it. But keep on truckin', you know? You just keep on swimin'.

This dismissive and greater-than-thou attitude so many doctors have, as far as I'm concerned, it is disgusting

Then, right before Christmas, I joined Facebook and started reading what other people were having to deal with. A good example is that from the get-go I've been complaining that most of my Tourette's is on my left side. And I posted a question to a bunch of Touretters, "Does anybody have it

---

113   A difficult-to-treat and often incurable disorder resulting in involuntary, repetitive body movements.

more on one side versus the other?" Within fifteen minutes there was a whole bunch of people who said, "Yeah."

And why didn't somebody tell me that there was such a thing as tics at night? I can't tell you how many times I've woke up in the morning feeling like somebody beat the fool out of me. It used to be there was no such things as tics at night. Well, I got a clue for you—there is. This dismissive and greater-than-thou attitude so many doctors have, as far as I'm concerned, it is disgusting. You are not a lick better than me. And vice versa. Just because you have more education doesn't make you any better.

Not too mad, not too sad, not too glad

My TS is fairly severe and I've tried every medicine in the world and nothing works. You've got to find your own way. Controlling it with my own mind and my attitude has been a big part of surviving this. Does biofeedback work for me? Yes, because I do it every day. I've already mastered those techniques. If it was a youngster, oh, yeah, absolutely. Teach them to control it with their mind and not the doctors' poisons.

The great advantage of biofeedback is teaching you to control this with your mind. I have discovered that my attitude, my mood, a lot of things, affect my TS. I have to maintain myself on a very even keel. Not too mad, not too sad, not too glad, not too anything. That is the advantage to biofeedback.

Basically you're playing a game with your mind. It's concentration. What you're learning to do is control the tics. It teaches you to slow your mind. It's almost a meditation, where you learn to calm your mind, you learn to control your body's reaction to the stimulus. As you proceed, you learn to control the tics somewhat better. But it also truly depends on the severity of the TS. Mild, moderate TS, I'd say, oh yeah, get your kid in there. With my severity I can only control it so far. I have never found to where it hurt the situation. It has only helped. The way I see it, it is an advantage to everyone, to varying degrees.

Cutting glass

When I got sick, I had this artistic ability come up out of nowhere. Part of it I had to train myself, mostly in color. I had lost the ability to write.

I couldn't even write my name. I taught myself to write again—and this is kinda crazy—by cutting glass. Cutting stained glass is a very similar muscle movement to writing. I did it for a *long* time, okay? We sold a lot of pieces. Hundreds. We have sold stained glass throughout the United States, north to south. Coast to coast in Canada, in Japan, Brazil, and as far south as Melbourne, Australia.

That breaks my heart

I get noticed pretty much everywhere I go, okay? I'm a big man. But being a Touretter, I still get stares, and at my size. So *what* in the world does a child have to go through? That breaks my heart. Physically and emotionally they have to go through the same thing that I have a difficult time with. But they have to deal with it through the eyes of a young, inexperienced person.

I've learned a tremendous amount of compassion from my Tourette's. Oh, dear God, yes. I'm sure pretty much everybody with Tourette's has said that same thing. Compassion was not even in my vocabulary, especially before Leslie and I got married. What I found is that people in Georgia, in the South, are much nicer about Tourette's than people in Southern California. Leslie's family are just naturally compassionate, soft-spoken people. I finally got myself to where I could pack up my truck and move my family to Georgia, where I knew they'd accept me. And they did. We went back out to California because my dad had brain disease. We just wanted to come home to Georgia the whole time. Leslie's momma got sick and passed away and we came home and we're trying to figure out how to put our world back together again. One more time. Now we're back in Georgia, exactly where we want to be, and I'm not movin' for nothin'.

The attention of a single interested adult can change the course of a child's life. Samantha speaks with a slight accent from her native Queens, New York, of her highly dysfunctional home life. Traumatized parents inflicting their own history on their child. Yet for a brief moment each week, Samantha had love from an unlikely source. Tenderness for an hour a week built her resilience and helped her survive. We make a difference when we take the time to bend down, look a child in the eyes, and acknowledge them with love.

SAMANTHA
58 years old

I don't believe in meds

I have a unique perspective of my diagnosis and I chose a very holistic lifestyle. My husband is a chiropractor, he's a homeopath, and this is the route I believe works for me. I don't believe in the meds.

Homeopathy is all natural remedies. It's not chemicals, it's not drugs. For my severe panic disorder I have a remedy called Aconite. I've had some panic attacks that are so severe I have been screaming, crying, throwing things. You're so afraid of the panic attack that the fear fuels it. When the panic sets in, I take two or three tablets and generally it takes care of it. Sometimes I have to take five or six doses. It helps me get through these episodes. I also have in the room with me now a service dog, and she works with me with panic.

Apex Energetics has expensive but good products and one of them is Neuroflam. It takes down swelling of the brain. If I don't take that every morning, I could go off the handle at any minute. My vocalizations increase, I'm a nervous ball of energy. It keeps my system in check. I still have flares, and on highly stressful days I'll take additional doses. But it helps me function on a more normal level. And it's all natural.

This nice lady

You know, people, they do meds and that's fine. This is the route I have chosen. Do I take medication when I need to? Of course I do. But this is what works for me. And I'm relatively high functioning. No, I don't drive and I'm not good in crowds. I do tend to isolate like most of us. But considering, I lead a fairly normal life.

I was diagnosed only ten years ago. I later found out that my parents knew about the diagnosis, but didn't tell me. When I was a girl, my father owned a small store, and a woman came in and she had the whole thing, the cursing, the motions, the whole bit. She's this nice lady with this little girl, younger than I was, and my father would say, "That's a dollar seventy-two," and she'd say, "Of course, you motherfucker. Here's a dollar. Let me get the rest from home, you cocksucker."

I asked my father what was wrong with her. He explained that she had Tourette's. It wasn't until three years ago I realized, wait a minute—how did my father, an immigrant from Poland, know about this disorder? The answer is, I was diagnosed by the family doctor and my parents never told me.

The worst day of my life and the best day of my life

I was diagnosed by my husband shortly after we met. He said, "I need to talk to you." I thought he was breaking up with me. Typical female, right? He'd noticed all my motions and guttural sounds and OCD and depression. He sat me down and said, "You have Tourette's." And what flashed into my mind was this woman, when I was nine years old, walking through Queens doing all these motions, and I'm like, "I am *not* her."

It was the worst day of my life and the best day of my life. I fought him on it, but he showed me a list of twenty-one symptoms, and I had eighteen. I went into a deep depression. Then, as I came to terms with it, I realized it wasn't that people didn't *like* me. Maybe they didn't know how to react. And I didn't know how to educate them.

They would send me notes

I remember as a child I used to do a lot of leg thumping. I also remember people and kids shied away from me. I was never good with groups so there was a lot of isolation. I was mercilessly bullied in junior high school. There was a group of girls who would send me notes with swastikas—I'm Jewish. My mother actually went to school for that, which if you knew my mother, it's shocking she did anything.

I had older parents. My father fled the Nazis. The rest of his family was wiped out, burned in their homes or gone to the camps. My mother came from an abusive household. We were highly dysfunctional. The dynamic was my brother was violent to me and my parents looked the other way. My mother doted on my brother because he was a Jewish boy and also because he was the 'normal' one. Having a child with a disability upset mom. They did the only thing possible. They hid it from me.

The mother of my heart

My mother had an Irish cleaning lady, Hazel, and Hazel would come to the house once a week, and she was my safe haven. For years. She was who I could speak to, she was who I could be myself with... I mean, she was my mom. Not by birth, not genetically, but Hazel Brady was my mom. And that's who I sat down and talked to about all the girl stuff, and this boy doesn't like me, or this and that. She didn't know about the diagnosis, but she was my safe haven. And I'm very, very grateful to her memory and that she was a part of my life. I only saw her for about an hour or two a week. She is the mother of my heart.

I didn't do anything wrong

I try to reach out to people, and I've made it my mission since I've been diagnosed. I've gotta make it easier for kids and people coming up behind me, because I had it *so* hard. They're not gonna do to you what was done to me.

I am my husband's office manager. I'm very open about what I have. I'll talk to anybody. It's a matter of reaching out. I don't know what I do special except that I don't hide. I'm not ashamed to say I have Tourette's. Because I didn't do anything wrong. Tourette's just happened to me. It was not due to anything I *did*. So why should I be ashamed of it? Is somebody ashamed because they have diabetes? And I don't judge. Absolutely not. As Touretters we've been judged all our lives. I know the pain of being judged. So no. No. Be it Christian, Muslim, Jewish, I don't care. Be good to people.

I cannot have a more loving, understanding husband. The compassion he shows in his practice, it's such an honor. But for me, it's like there's this lack of self-worth. You're a pretender, you don't belong. My husband's always telling me, "You have a right to be here."

I'm more self-accepting now, but on the same note, it's like, "Don't get too comfortable." You know? It's all the years of being told by my mother, you can't, you can't, you can't. Always being the outsider. It's hard to accept that I *do* have a loving family, I *do* have two amazing stepsons. I do have two grandsons that will never know another paternal grandmother than me. And yet it's always—don't get too comfortable, don't get too close. It could be pulled out from under you any second.

At work, I have a strong sense of worth 'cause I'm damn good at what I do. I have a private office, so I can close the door when the Tourette's acts up. Everybody knows I have Tourette's and they say, "Oh, that's just Sammy." But outside work it's difficult.

I always said I just want to breathe. I want to be able to go to a dinner party of friends and sit there and feel like I belong. I want to be able to go to a family function and say, "I belong." And not only say it, but *believe* it.

I think disability is between the ears

The general public has it wrong about some things. They feel we can control the motions. One of the biggest misconceptions is they think we're stupid. Some of the smartest people I know, I've met through the Tourette's community. Highly creative, highly intelligent, really amazing people.

You know, we *all* have limitations, these happen to be mine. It's how we *deal* with them. I think disability is between the ears. Technically I am partially disabled. And I accept that. But is it going to stop me from working and having a fulfilling career, or having a good marriage, or doing things I love?

When my stepson got married, he asked me to do the mother-son dance with him. I don't dance, and really, in front of a hundred people? He said to me, "How will you feel if you start ticcing?" I looked at him and said, "If I blow, I blow. It's their problem."

I refuse to be that

I have a friend with either Lyme Disease or MS, we're not sure which. And she was so hell bent on being an invalid that she turned into one. She could have been helped, she could be living a full life. But now she's about ninety-two pounds and laying in a bed and she never leaves her room. People say to me, "You don't know what it's like."

Are you nuts? Do you know how hard it is to get out of bed every morning? Do you know how hard it is to not fall? Because I have severe balance problems from all the ticcing. I'm in constant pain because even when my husband works on me and puts everything back in order, within three minutes I'm gonna knock it out. Stepping into a room with the panic and anxiety and the motions and smacking people—"Sorry, didn't mean to do that." I understand it more than you do!

I feel sorry for myself once in a while. I curl up in a ball and don't go out for two days. Everybody does. But I won't do it for more than a day or two. You know? It's hard to judge one level of illness against another, but I'm not going to become that person. I refuse to be that. Yes, I isolate myself and I don't go out with the girls, or things like that. But I have things that keep me occupied and keep me busy. What can I tell ya?

Suppressing tics to ease social tension is a powerful temptation. But suppression causes tensions all its own and distances Touretters from who they truly are. Caught in this dilemma, Brynne was able to find her way out and accept her Tourette's. Growing up in a homeopathic household taught her to value unconventional remedies and she has used them to good effect. The range of her interests (from bibliophile to rock climber!) shows what many successful Touretters display: verve for life and an appreciation of the joy available in each moment.

BRYNNE
25 years old

An incident in dance class

My onset began when I was five, but my tics didn't become full-blown until about seven, when I began to get shaking tics in the torso and arms.

I went to my mom and we talked about it and thankfully, she had an idea of what it was. I was diagnosed with full-blown Tourette's within a year.

Honestly, for me as a child, it wasn't difficult. I had a great support system—my mom, dad, and sister. Mom explained everything to me very clearly and succinctly. I had no problem with it because it was not presented to me as a negative thing or something that would debilitate my life.

Once I got older, however, and out into the world, my viewpoint changed. My view of the outside world, its lack of understanding and knowledge about Tourette's, began when I was eleven years old. I had an incident in dance class. In performance, you're required to stand a certain distance apart, and I was standing where I was supposed to be. After seeing me tic, a girl asked me to move over.

That hit me hard because up until then, I didn't care if anyone saw me ticcing. I wasn't bothered that other people saw or heard—my vocal tics were very, very loud. That led to a downward spiral, for several years, of learning to suppress my tics. I began to feel self-conscious and aware of people's reactions and stares. So I learned to suppress everything but my very basic facial tics.

My first panic attack due to suppression

In high school, I had my first panic attack due to anxiety caused by suppression. I remember sitting in geometry class and I had this sudden, overwhelming urge to have motor tics all over. But the thought of everyone seeing them, and what they might think, was even more overwhelming. I became very anxious and began to have all the symptoms of a panic attack. It's a very unpleasant experience.

I'd seen a panic attack before, so I knew a little bit what to do, but at the same time, I was a teenager and embarrassed. I asked the teacher if I could stand up, which I did, trying to regulate my breathing. A friend stood by me, asking if I was okay, which was nice. That led to me relying on medication for my anxiety disorder, which did work. I started on a low dose of Xanax, because it was mild and low on side effects, and it helps to this day.

The worse the tics got, somehow the easier it got

In college, I saw a counselor who helped me stop suppressing my tics, because I couldn't express them even if I *wanted* to. That goes to show you how powerful peer pressure and social anxiety can be. Suppressing my tics took almost the whole of my consciousness. The only expressing I did were a few facial grimaces and eye crossings. Other than that everything else was in there, but I couldn't let it out. Initially, it was hard adjusting to it letting them out. There were days when I came home crying because the stress of trying to express was overwhelming. I wanted to tic so bad, but wasn't able to.

To practice letting them out, I would do little tics that weren't noticeable in front of people. Eventually my tics became full-blown [*she chuckles*]. I started experiencing all the tics I had in the beginning. That was an adjustment process, because the tics came all at once and continued waxing and waning.

But the worse the tics got, somehow the easier it got. There was less social anxiety and more of me accepting my tics. It was a relief, once I came back into myself as a person with Tourette's. I felt like me again. I could let my tics out. I've always felt that my Tourette's was a part of me. It was a relief, honestly.

I'm thankful to that college counselor to this day. I worked for two semesters to become comfortable with ticcing in public and around my classmates. Being able to express my tics again, and being able to feel okay with that, means everything to me.

When I suppress my tics I feel like I'm denying myself

I feel like that part of myself was hidden from me. I wasn't able to access it. Once I was able to, I started feeling comfortable with myself. Each different place I expressed my tics was a challenge. Sometimes it still is. It was a challenge to express my tics at school, jobs, my favorite places, like the bookstore.

I started with motor tics, but the hardest was my vocal tics, especially when I began saying random phrases. I'd always had vocal tics that involve sounds, but I'd never had phrases. I definitely have a good case of echolalia. My vocal tics are still pretty loud [*she chuckles*].

Now when I suppress my tics I feel like I'm denying myself. I feel I'm doing myself a disservice. And in a roundabout way, I feel I'm doing the people around me a disservice, because I'm very big on creating awareness.

I feel happy, like I am being the person I was meant to be. And I feel freer, you know? There's a big sense of freedom there.

A whole different story

We stayed away from drugs for my tics, partially because the side effects outweigh the benefits. The only medicinal things I've taken for tics involve homemade tinctures and homeopathic remedies.

My mom, even as a child, spent years studying homeopathy and herbalism and putting together certain nervines. Nervines are a tincture that contains one or more herbs that will calm the nervous system. I've seen them at vitamin stores. She's made nervines for me with kava, skull-cap, and valerian, which is a great one for bad Tourette's or panic disorder. It's important to know the dosage for each person because everyone's different, and it should be age appropriate as well. There also are some good books[114] out there that point you in the right direction.

I've tried different devices to stop my tics and I do not like those. I feel trapped somehow. Devices to calm my nervous system, that's a whole different story. I've used weighted blankets, for example, and they're fantastic. They were originally created for children who have autism, because of the heightened sensitivity of their nervous system. Those of us who have Tourette's have a similar issue. I've used the weighted blanket when my tics were so bad I couldn't hold still if my life depended on it. It actually does help calm the nervous system and help me feel not so rattled. It's a great therapeutic aid.

I use noise-cancelling headphones too. I'm a big fan of those. If stimulus is too intense, I combine contoured earplugs with the noise cancelling headphones. Also, sunglasses. When going into large stores, I cannot emphasize enough the value of wearing sunglasses and noise-cancelling headphones [*she chuckles*]. It really cuts down on that sensory overload you can get from being in a crowded, brightly lit place.

I'm also in a study for a mouth orthotic[115] for Tourette syndrome. They're theorizing that the trigeminal nerve, that runs up the jawline into

114   For example, *Homeopathy: The Modern Prescriber* by Henrietta Wells; *Weiner's Herbal: The Guide to Herbal Medicine* by Michael Weiner; *Herbal Remedies for Children's Health* by Rosemary Gladstar.

115   See tourette.org.

the brain, is inflamed due to misalignment during early development. It's this misalignment that's causing the misfiring in the brain, which causes tics. The idea is the orthotic will reduce that inflammation and reduce the severity of the tics.

Knowing I'm in control of each movement

I spend my days taking care of my dogs and reading, and I'm always learning. In good weather I enjoy bike riding and rock climbing. I've loved climbing since I was little. When we went on vacation, when I was little, my parents would always make sure there was a place for me to climb, whether it was trees, a climbing wall, or rock climbing in the mountains.

I enjoy a lot of things about climbing. I enjoy the focus it takes to calculate which handhold to take next. My tics disappear. I like the feeling of knowing my limits, and knowing I'm in control of each movement. It's like solving a puzzle, only better, because I'm part of that puzzle. I like the physical exertion too, the feeling of accomplishment when I've reached the end of a new climb.

I don't ever get scared. Sometimes I get nervous with a new climb, but I think that shows I'm a thinking person. It's part of the experience, and pushing past those nerves is just another part of completing the challenge.

Another thing that helps my tics, because I focus, is Zentangle.[116] It's a form of art that is designed to relax you, because of the concentration required, as in Zen. It's a lot of fun.

I initially studied corporate communication, but that's just a stepping-stone. I'm very eclectic in my interests. I would love to study psychology, library science, and deaf culture and sign language. I love helping people, and being able to get out there and inform them. I would love to give lectures. And then, of course, I love journalism. I love writing. At present I am focusing on my blog,[117] and my personal reading and poetry writing.

I am a bibliophile at heart. Bookstores are my favorite place, my home away from home. My books are organized by author last name [*she chuckles*]. That's how much of a book nerd I am. I'm always building my literary collection and I just bought a 1913 edition of *Wind in the Willows*.

---

116   zentangle.com.
117   totestourettes.blogspot.com.

CHAPTER ELEVEN

FAITH

Perhaps the most natural, and urgent, question an individual with TS will ask is, "Why me?" I believe we must step over this question in our lives. There is no answer. It simply is. We must accept our Tourette's and move on. One way to think about it is, "I am who God made me." Each individual must discover a purpose (or more than one!) in life. This is an act of faith: faith in our talents and abilities and interests; faith in our strength and tenacity; faith that we are part of a spirit greater than ourselves. Ultimately we are not alone, as these interviews demonstrate.

A prolific cartoonist, Fish has a gift for finding humor in his Tourette's, despite the severity of his symptoms. I was struck by his gentleness and generosity of spirit, qualities he learned through hard experience. A man of deep faith, he found his way to love through God and the ever-present support of his wife. He understands the power of belief, both its limiting qualities and its infinite possibilities. Here is a man who truly has transformed suffering into wisdom.

FISH
38 years old

The Odd Squad

Most of my tics when I was a kid were as simple as rubbing my nose a lot or scratching in my ear or wiping the corners of my mouth. I never thought twice about it.

Every once in a while, I would have bouts where I couldn't stop saying something. I remember jumping on my bed when I was maybe five, yelling, "Fill it to the rim with Brim!" over and over. I was still saying this three days later. But I didn't realize there was anything unusual.

I had more trouble with issues like temper, and obsessing over one thing, and trouble making friends and reading social cues. The things that make Tourette's and autism so similar. So for most of my school days, I was stuck with one or two kids who couldn't make friends themselves. We were the Odd Squad. I was always lumped with the outcasts.

Spikes and chains

Then around high school time, my rage kicked in with the Tourette's and I got really mean. Suddenly I realized I fit in well with the bad guys in school. I learned that if social interaction is a foreign language, the language between hoodlums was easy to understand. With the newfound rage, I could become popular and have people not only like me, but follow me and do what I say. I finally thought I had it all figured out. So I became one of the baddest, meanest guys in town [*he chuckles*] and had just about everybody in town afraid of me.

This was before anybody in Arkansas had heard about Goth. I had the long, black trench coat, a long Mohawk, and spikes and chains. I grew my fingernails long and cut 'em to points and painted them black. Anything to look intimidating and make people afraid of me.

At that point I thought I was a god. I felt better about myself than I ever had in my life. I'd always felt less-than, always felt scared and intimidated. And now, I could make people react how I wanted. People did what I said because they were afraid to do otherwise. It was childish, and it was selfish, but at the time I was on cloud nine. It's not my proudest moment.

The joys of growing up in a small town

My mom took it personally. My parents got divorced when I was ten so… [*he sighs*] she felt every problem I had was because of that. Mom always took it that she had failed somehow. For years I would get bouts of tics for a month or two, and sometimes I'd get really bad and I'd be out of school. The tics would make doctors and my mom think, "He's faking it for attention." That became the diagnosis—I was acting out because my parents got divorced. I would question myself when I was alone, sitting there ticcing, "Who's sympathy am I trying to get when I'm here by myself?" It was confusing.

I had taken on this mantle of being as offensive as I could be. Lack of impulse control was great. I could tell people whatever I thought and it fit into this new persona I built. When it was late and I was tired I would shake some, I would twitch and jerk but nobody ever saw that. The talking to myself was unusual, but I was always creative. I had been drawing all my life and trying to write and come up with stories.

My mom married my step-dad and he lived in a nice neighborhood. And when I got so mean and everybody was afraid of me, we would get the cops called on me just for walking down the street. The joys of growing up in a small town.

When I was a bad guy all the girls loved me. It never ceased to amaze me. All the girls who before wouldn't give me the time of day, they were telling everybody how they'd slept with me. It was ridiculous [*he laughs*].

I was going to change my life

I ended up moving away for a while. I lived in Louisiana and Mississippi and tried to figure out who was I going to be. I decided I was going to change my life. I was gonna buckle down and follow the rules. So I went from absolutely not caring what people thought, to working hard to be as good a person as I could be.

And it was hard. It took me years to learn how to control that temper. For the longest time, I was focusing on keeping control of myself and not overreacting. After a few years, it got a little easier, and eventually it became second nature.

My mom and brother ordered every set of self-help tapes that were gonna help you win friends and be successful in life, and we listened to all of them. The same things kept coming up. Repeating something until it becomes a reality, things like that. I had already seen that work. I had terribly low self-esteem and thought I was the ugliest person in the world because that's what everybody in school kept telling me. But around junior high I started looking myself in the mirror and saying, "God, you're beautiful!" over and over [*he laughs*]. I ended up with a *grossly* overestimated view of how beautiful I was [*he laughs again*]. But it worked. So I knew there was power in what you say, and what you decide you're going to do. I used those things to try and contain my temper.

Kristen

But all this time I felt broken. I was inherently a failure as a person. Why couldn't I control my temper? That was one of the things that was such a relief when I got diagnosed with Tourette's when I was thirty. My life suddenly made sense. I wasn't broken. It's not a failure of my will or my character. It's a failure in the wiring of my brain. I can't help it, but I can work around it. It was incredibly freeing for me.

I straightened myself out and started college. I went to a tech school, studying graphic design, 3-D animation particularly. By this time, I'd had enough of bad relationships, so I sat down and wrote a list of what I wanted in a wife. I wanted somebody who had goals, somebody smart, who was driven, who had plans for their life. Somebody who was honest. Anyway, I met somebody [*he laughs*]. And we've been married almost eighteen years now. Kristen.

She's been such a good partner along the way. She's always jumped in and rolled up her sleeves when times got hard. When my tics got really severe and we got the diagnosis of Tourette syndrome, I don't know a woman that would've stayed besides her. She takes the commitment we made, you know, till death do us part, sickness or health, richer or poorer—she takes it seriously. And I'm grateful for that.

But the doctor said

From the time we got married, from about twenty-one on, my health started slowly getting worse and worse. For the longest time we thought all the tics must be related to my heart problem. We treated that aggressively and nothing helped the tics much. Finally it got so bad I was losing the use of one side of my body. I was convinced I was having mini-strokes. And it just got worse and worse. My arms were starting to flail around, my legs were starting to kick, I was grunting and gasping for breath all the time.

I was seeing a neurologist, but he wrote it off as I was faking it and looking for attention. I remember when Tourette syndrome came up, he stated very clearly that I didn't swear. And unless I swore, I couldn't have Tourette's. He's the neurologist, so I assumed he was right.

Oddly enough, a local weatherman, Ed Buckner, did a TV special, and he said that he had Tourette syndrome, very mild. He had a guy sitting there jerkin' and flailin' and skakin' and movin', and all my friends called me and said, "There's this guy on TV that looks just like you, and he's got Tourette's." And I was like, "But I don't have Tourette's. I don't swear." I watched it, and one of the things they said is not everybody with Tourette's swears. And I was like, "But the doctor said…"

So we went to another neurologist and as soon as he walked in he asked me, "When were you diagnosed with Tourette syndrome?" And I was like, "I wasn't." And he said, "Trust me, you have Tourette's." He sent me to a movement disorder specialist, and when she walked in the door she said, "When were you diagnosed with Tourette's?" And I was like, "I'm guessing today."

Wrong impulses come out too

Suddenly my whole life made sense. I found out about the rage, and realized I wasn't this violent, broken person. It didn't make it easier that by this time I'd lost mobility and my ability to take care of myself. At this point my arms, legs, neck, torso, everything was constantly shaking, flailing, jerking, swinging around. I remember one night trying to eat a hot dog, and I beat the fool out of myself with that hot dog. I had ketchup and mustard all over my face and my hair. It was tough. I would switch quickly from bouts of flailing to suddenly I can't move my arm or my leg. Facial tics constantly, a lot of eye tics. My irises will even go in and out of focus and start ticcing. My eyes will start shaking back and forth and it makes it incredibly hard to read or draw.

I have lot of trouble breathing. The muscles in my throat close up and I've gotta push as hard as I can to get air out and gasp in air. I couldn't walk without crutches. My dad brought a wheelchair from my grandma's that he'd push me around in. I basically would lay on the couch shaking all day, and my wife would feed me and bathe me. It really, really frustrated me.

After I got diagnosed with Tourette's, they started me on all the medicines. They tried me on a combination of Primidone—I'd been on that for a while and it helped some—and they tried Guanfacine on top of that. That helped a lot and they kinda cancelled out each other's side effects. So most days I can walk around on a cane twenty, thirty feet, maybe a hundred feet, if I'm lucky. I can sit in my recliner or lay in bed and pretty much not tic, but as soon as I try to sit up or stand, I start to tic. It's like the more impulses I'm sending out to stay upright, the more wrong impulses come out too. The only reason I'm able to have this conversation right now is because I took an extra pill, and I've been laying in my bed in a dark room this whole time. But as soon as I stand up, the race is on. Can I make it to the bathroom and back before I can't see anymore? Can I make it to the kitchen to fix a soda and back without dropping it?

If I'm having a good day, I can get up in the morning, make it into the living room, I can wake the kids up for school, sit in my chair and bark out orders to keep them on track to get to school on time. One of my sons will fix me a drink or get me a honey bun so I can put something in my stomach to take my pills. And if it's a really good day, after they go to school, maybe I can go into the kitchen and fix myself a bowl of cereal. I take a nap around eleven, get up when my wife gets home. If it's a *really* good day, I can make it back into the living room that afternoon and spend the evening with my family, maybe make it to church. But that's about it.

I can still draw [*he sighs*]. Some. I never know when it's going to be a day when I can or a month when I can't. It's impossible to go back to full time work. I've had to resign myself to working on projects I can do for myself, mostly stuff I give away [*he chuckles*].

Our words have power, and if we decide we're broken, then we're broken. If we decide we still have a lot to offer the world, then we do

I ran across a young guy, he's nineteen, he blinks a lot and he'll have a bout of coprolalia a couple of times a month. He feels there's no hope of ever getting married, or having kids, or having a life because he's this broken freak. Why? Because his dad told him he was broken when they found out he had Tourette's. And that was that.

And I was like, "Man! Do you have any idea how good you've got it? You can walk. You can see. I mean, oh, if I could *walk*? You would never see me again, I'd be goin' so fast. There are so many things I would be out there doing. I desperately miss being able to ride my bike. I desperately miss being out on the water in the canoe I built with my kids. Be paddling across the water, looking at ducks, and watching turtles come out of the water. Oh, *man*.

Our words have power, and if we decide we're broken, then we're broken. If we decide we still have a lot to offer the world, then we do. That's why I've wanted to start a Tourette's youth group here in Arkansas. I want to reach kids before they get so hurt, and let 'em know, "You're gonna be all right. You can do whatever you want to do." I'm in pretty rough shape but I have a wonderful wife, I have three wonderful boys, I've got an amazing group of friends and church family. I'm a lucky guy. I still get to do some things I love to do. I get to play drums at church. I don't have to be able to see to do that. I get to lead classes and teach at church. I do what I can do and don't dwell on things that I can't.

Anything He showed me to be true

I spent my whole life thinking that God was a lie, and Christianity was fairy tales and nonsense for foolish people that needed to make sense out of a world they couldn't understand. When I pressed people about why they believed in God, it usually boiled down to, "The Bible says so," or "Momma said so." That wasn't good enough for me.

I was driving around drunk with a friend one night in college, and we got to telling stories about the times we almost died. I talked about the time I was in the back of a truck that flipped three times and my head smacked the grass inches from the sidewalk. You know, all the different car wrecks I'd been in. Fires I had accidentally started and should have burned up in. Time after time I should have died and didn't.

And I realized my belief in random chance... there was no way I could flip a coin so many times and get it to come up heads. That was the turning point. Me and my buddy stopped on a dirt road somewhere, and we got out of the car drunk, and we prayed for forgiveness and for being foolish not realizing that God was watching out for us. I realized there was something bigger than me in the universe. I swore on that day that I would seek Him as best I could, and anything He showed me to be true I would grab hold of and hold on to for the rest of my life.

Albert's parents each responded differently to his diagnosis: his mother chose denial, his father fell to guilt. Still and all, they supported him enough that he had the confidence to become a pediatric neurologist. His strength now comes from his faith, his loving wife, and his determination to assuage the suffering of his patients. And yet, despite his accomplishments, and like so many Touretters, he struggles to fully accept himself as he is.

ALBERT
40 years old

He was a cool guy

My first recollection is tics all in my face, blinking and grimacing, extending my jaw. It definitely bothered me. It was in the summertime, allergy season, so people thought it might be that. But it continued in school and, of course, kids made fun of me. My parents went to my pediatrician, who said it sounded like Tourette syndrome. When I first got diagnosed, my doctor said, "It'll probably go away when he gets older." Almost like it wasn't a big deal. I was nine years old then.

I was an only child until was nine. My parents kinda babied me. One of the first moments that bothered me, I was in my mom's bed, doing some movements, and she scolded me. Of course, she didn't know what was going on. I'll never forget—even though I love my mom to death, she's my biggest supporter—it hurt me and I started crying and went into my room. My mom was in denial, thinking the TS would go away, even up through my college years.

My history teacher scolded me in class, "Stop doing that." And I said, "Okay, I'll try," but I knew I couldn't. That upset me because he was a cool guy. I admired him and it hurt when he admonished me like that. When you're young, you think you're a bad boy for doing these things. So my self-esteem started going down the drain. Even now today, to be honest, even though I've outwardly accomplished a lot, my self-esteem has never been very high. I'm very critical of myself.

Will you be my friend?

My family is Chinese-American. My parents emigrated to the United States in the '60s. They came to America to have a better life, of course. I was born the same year my dad got his Ph.D., so it was a good year for him. I was born in South Detroit. Looking back, my parents always wanted the best for me. They sent me to private schools, got me the best education. Academics were a priority.

I remember having a pretty enjoyable childhood before I got diagnosed. You know, spelling bees, recess, all that stuff. Somewhere in third or fourth grade I started having symptoms, then that summer it got unleashed. At some point, middle school maybe, the vocal tics made it more difficult. I used to sniffle. Some kid asked, "Are you doing Lamaze breathing?" I had no idea—what the heck are you talking about? [*He chuckles.*] But it became, "Hey, Lamaze Boy."

I think I was always a likeable kid. I've always had friends, went to birthday parties. But I became more self-conscious after this. I wouldn't say I was socially ostracized. But I used to ask everyone I met a question. I think it was an OCD thing as well. I'd ask, "Will you be my friend?" That was a big thing I said, maybe because I was trying to get accepted. It made me socially awkward. It went away after about a year.

I cut myself

In sixth grade, I did my first science project. I read an article about that surgeon who had Tourette syndrome and wanted to study it. In junior high, I thought being a doctor would be cool, maybe find a cure for Tourette's, thinking, "I'm going to solve this mystery and make people better." My dad influenced me a lot, saying, "You should be a doctor, son." And seeing my child neurologist—even though he gave me medications that didn't work, I respected him. He was a compassionate guy. Having him as a role model solidified that I wanted to be a child neurologist.

My parents were my strongest advocates through school, and wanted the best for me. I have to give them all the credit for helping me get through those early years with Tourette's. That's why I tried so hard to choose the right path and do well in school. It was a source of pride for them.

My Tourette's was especially hard on my dad. Shortly after I got diagnosed, he cut himself on purpose. Like he wanted to punish himself for giving this to me. I saw him, he had a Swiss Army knife next to him, and I remember seeing him turn, seeing the blood, and he was crying. He said, "I cut myself." He must have told me later why he did it. But that image of blood on his finger and him crying, it's a picture I'll never forget.

Like worms crawling

I think the OCD started coming around those years as well, ten-, eleven-years old. I'd sit in the front seat of my parents' Cadillac and stare at the thermostat knob, you know with red to blue lines, hotter, colder. I'd fixate on that switch, trying in my mind to get it to look just right. It bothered me like heck. What am I *doing*? This is crazy. I wanted to stop doing it, but I had to do it. If I didn't do it I wouldn't feel good, you know?

Later on, after medical school, I was reading about the physiology of Tourette's and saw it's like a braking mechanism that's not working. For example, when I reach for a cup of coffee, the motor neurons in my brain operate like a brake and a release pedal. So certain neurons release when I reach for the coffee. But that braking mechanism, the serotonin, which has an inhibitory effect on dopamine, is not working. It's misfiring, so you do a tic instead. There's no brake. So it's like you lose your free will. It's definitely uncomfortable.

What bothers me the most is the feeling before the tic, the growing urge that's like worms crawling under your skin. It's very unpleasant. Sometimes, in secret, I'll punch my stomach really hard to get rid of the sensation. That works a little bit, displacing the tic. In my late twenties, I was in an airplane, so I decided to try not to tic, sort of using mind over matter [*he chuckles*]. You know motor memory? The sensation of riding a bike, you can remember what that feels like. My arm was jerking at that time, so instead of giving in to that buildup of tension, I remembered the feeling of relief when I do the tic. I tricked my mind into not ticcing. I skipped right to the feeling of release. I think for a good half an hour I was suppressing, but once I got off the plane I went like crazy [*he laughs*]. It takes lots of concentration. After a while, I was thinking, "Oh, man, this is getting tough to do."

That's where she was

Oh, yes, I was on all the meds. Orap, Buspar, Haldol, Clonidine. I think I was nine years old when I started. For the last ten years, I haven't been on anything. For depression and OCD, I was on SSRIs. But as soon as I got married, I no longer needed them because [*he chuckles*] I think finding your match through life, it definitely helps depression. It took me a lot to find her, but I finally did.

I met Shalynn at my cousin's bible study home meeting. I was doing my residency in Loma Linda and was looking for a way to get out of my funk. That's where she was. I think God had a dual purpose there. It wasn't Hollywood-style love at first sight. I saw her playing with my cousin's son, jumping on the trampoline with him. I thought she was really young, a teenager. She was getting her masters [*he laughs*]. At the second home meeting, she was playing the guitar and really enjoying the Lord, and I said, "Hey, you play guitar pretty well." And she said, "Thanks." That was the extent of our first conversation [*he chuckles*]. And then later that evening, I was looking at a painting, and she was looking at it too, and I said, "That's a pretty cool painting, huh?" She smiled and she said, "Yup, it is." And that was our second conversation [*he laughs*].

I told my cousin I was interested in her and he said, "You should pray on it." So I did for about two months, and finally God opened the door for us to have our first date. And I don't think I ticced at all, I was so at ease, enjoying the moment.

Having Tourette's has been a struggle in my marriage at times too. My wife, Shalynn, she's my best friend, and thank God I found her and she found me. But I would say, ninety-five percent of the arguments we have, I instigate. I guess guys mess up most of the time, anyway [*he chuckles*]. I would say my Tourette's, my anger, is probably the biggest issue right now. There's like this explosive temper that comes out. Yeah [*he sighs*]. God's working with my temper, but it's been really bad.

I praise Him every day

Tourette's was why I became a child neurologist. But that didn't answer my question of why me? Genetics makes sense, medically, but why did *I* have Tourette's? Why was I chosen to have this disease? No doctor can answer that question. Only God knows. His purpose for everyone is mysterious. I finally came to the conclusion that He loves me, but gave this to me for a reason. Whatever disability we have in our life, ultimately giving it to the Lord is the answer. That's what's helped me get through this disorder. Besides having a loving family, my wife and children.

So why did he put this on me? I came to the conclusion that if I didn't have Tourette's, I don't know if I'd have turned to God. We turn to God for comfort in our desperation. He allowed me to have Tourette's so I would know Him. I found God because I had Tourette's. And I thank Him for doing that. I praise Him every day.

Unconditional acceptance is ultimately the best thing to help a child succeed with overcoming their Tourette's

I went to medical school at Wayne State University. That was pretty tough with Tourette's [*he chuckles*]. I was able to get accommodations, extra time, but it was stressful. I ticced a lot. Medical school and residency were the most stressful years of my life. Even more than being a dad right now [*he laughs*]. Such a volume of things to memorize, long hours studying, not getting enough sleep, all that made my tics worse. In school, you go through all the rotations of internal medicine, surgery, ob-gyn, but I always loved kids. I wanted to be a teacher if I hadn't been a doctor. So child neurology.

Now, seeing kids as a doctor, I almost can't keep myself from shedding a tear when I see a child with their parents. I say, "I know exactly what you're going through. It really sucks. But you can do anything you want to do in life."

It's important for parents to accept their child and allow them to flourish and grow into their own. And a large majority of the kids I see have true friends who stick by them and don't judge them. I want to be hopeful with parents and say how wonderful it would be if their child outgrows Tourette's. But I don't want to paint a false picture, either. So I tell them, "Accept that your child has TS, and realize that it could be a source of strength." With OCD, for example, it could help being a musician or an athlete. We've seen that many times. It can be debilitating, of course. I don't want to minimize that. But unconditional acceptance is ultimately the best thing to help a child succeed with overcoming their Tourette's. I also encourage parents to find a TSA support group.

Having that love for yourself is something I need to let permeate

Having a family is always what I wanted to have. So me having Tourette's didn't stop us from having kids. That was never a question. We had Emmanuel after being married eleven months, and he's three-and-a-half now. Enoch is twenty-one months. They're both a joy. But it definitely crosses my mind once in a while. I don't know what I'm going to feel if one of my sons has symptoms of TS. I'm probably going to cry like crazy. [*He suddenly weeps. After a little while, he composes himself.*] But if one of my children does have it, like my wife says, what better scenario to have Tourette syndrome than if his dad has it. It'll probably be the worst day of my life if I find out he has it, but at the same time, God has his plan. Like He gave me Tourette syndrome. But if it happens to one of my sons, I'm going to have some serious discussion with God, and I'll probably be blaming myself, or blaming Him, or I don't know. I don't know what's going to happen. But I know ultimately I'm going to have to turn back to Him for strength and comfort. And just like I'm okay, I think Emmanuel and Enoch will be okay too.

It's so true. If we don't love ourselves fully, how can we then be an example for our children and show them that they can overcome Tourette's? God loves unconditionally and I know His love triumphs over everything. But having that love for yourself is definitely something I need to let permeate. I'm getting there.

To hijack Bette Davis' quote about getting older, "Deep Brain Stimulation surgery is not for sissies." Mori is healthy now, but the ordeal he endured after his DBS surgery was monumental. His faith, his family, and his determination pulled him through. He believes that only he has the power to limit himself; it's a shame to let anyone else's idea of his capabilities slow him down. And he's such a sharp dresser that, although he might not be comfortable with it, he could grace the cover of GQ Magazine.

MORI
44 years old

When you're ignorant, then you'll just be ignorant

My mother observed me walkin' across a parking lot, and I would spin in front of cars and think nothing about it. That's what made her get me in to see a neurologist. He knew exactly what it was. It was November the 4th, 1974, that I was diagnosed with Tourette's. I was four years old.

He started me off with Haldol, and I was on that for years. It helped when I was younger, but as I got older it didn't do anything for me. They tried different medicines, but it got to the point where no medicine was helping me. It would decrease the tics a tad bit, but when you're in high school you got peer pressure, and when you're under stress your tics get worse.

Years back people wanted to say I was demon-possessed. It was a horrible thing to say, but when you're ignorant, then you'll just be ignorant. Elementary school was fine, junior high was okay, high school was where my biggest challenge came. Being teased, being talked about at all times. There wasn't a day went past that I wasn't laughed at.

Because of the way I was raised—in a Christian atmosphere—I didn't have low self-esteem. I looked at it as their ignorance, not mine. But it was hard. I had the strength to hold on in front of people, but when I got by myself I would cry.

I've blackened my eyes. I've broken arms

I had faith in God and I read the Bible at all times. And I would see things be manifested before me. For example, ignorant people. You have ignorant people in the Bible. You have people in the Bible who had to deal with issues, and they found strength in their faith. They were inspiring stories.

I made it through high school and went to IUPUI[118] and studied physical therapy. It caught my interest because it has a lot to do with Tourette's. It taught me anatomy of the body. In the beginning I used some techniques I learned to control tics, but it got to where I wasn't able to. The tics were getting worse. They continued to get worse during college and after. It was a lot of head jerking, blinking, a lot of leg kicking and arm swinging. I've blackened my eyes, I've broken arms.

So I got my associate's degree in physical therapy and I also went to bible college and got my bachelor's degree in theology. I did this because I refuse to let my disorder hold me back from progression of life. And I am an Associate Minister at a local fellowship here. But I don't consider myself a minister, I just consider myself a servant. Bishop Anthony Pippens was my greatest inspiration through it all.

I began to read the Bible more

I was working for Indianapolis Public Schools as a custodian and a Special Education assistant teacher. My tics were getting bad and my doctor impressed upon me that I needed to resign my position and go on disability. I was a risk to the job and myself. I didn't like it. I wanted to be stubborn, but the doctor gave me thirty days and if I didn't do it, he was going to do it for me. I've known him very well. He's always taken a great interest in me, you know? He helped me be a speaker at Tourette's conferences. I did trust him. So I retired at thirty-five.

Once I was home, I tried to adjust to the life of not being able to work. It was a struggle. I was so used to going out and making a living, working from sunup to sundown. I began to read the Bible more. Retirement gave me more intimate time with God. It gave me more time to pray and get to know Him better.

---

118 Indiana University-Purdue University Indianapolis.

You have to develop a relationship

It was 2009, my neurologist recommended brain surgery.[119] But it took me almost three years to say 'yes' to it. I had to study on it. One of my main questions was, what are the side effects?

Of course you have fear, because that's major surgery. Somebody opening up your head, that's your life. It takes a lot of trust in them doctors that are doin' it. You have to develop a relationship. We went to lunch, we went out to dinner—I wanted to get to know them or I wasn't going to do it.

I had side effects normally people don't have. Even the doctors didn't know why it happened. They said they'd never seen it. I had to learn how to walk again, I had to learn how to talk again, I had to learn how to write again. My comprehension was gone. I basically went back to a baby stage. I went through extensive therapy, three-to-four hours a day for a little over a year.

It is nothing but God that has brought me this far. It gave me a greater appreciation for things that we take for granted. Just to get up out the bed and walk. To be able to pick up a pen and write. Now when I do it, I have a greater appreciation being able to do these things. And my tics are about ninety percent better than what they was. I'm very grateful.

I have a great team of support around me and I thank God for it. When you have support it makes things a whole lot easier. It starts with my wife and then my family, my doctors, friends. My circle is very small. I don't deal with a lot of people, because it can bring forth unnecessary things. I only deal with people I can trust.

One thing that got me through it—and I stick to this today—is a quote, "My setbacks are setups for my comeback." That's what I go by. You have to stay humble. You have to.

The worst thing is to believe someone else's idea of what you can do

I became the director of Washington Township Special Olympics and did that for a little over seven years, on up until I did my brain surgery. It's

---

119　Deep Brain Stimulation surgery. See tourette.org for details.

an awesome feeling to be around people that have such positive attitudes, whether they win, lose, or draw. It's very fulfilling. You have individuals who can't do what most people can, because of their disability. But yet and still they feel they can do anything that anybody else can do, and I agree with them. I tell the athletes I work with, "If you put your mind to doin' it, you can do it. Because somebody says you can't, don't mean you can't."

The worst thing is to believe someone else's idea of what you can do. If I did that, it would have lowered my self-esteem. It would have made me less than who I am and who God made me. God did not create me to pity on myself. We all have ups and downs, we all have battles. Everybody's struggles are different. We just got to learn how to deal with them the best way we can.

We each of us

One thing I live by is, "He who lives in the past has no future." If you're living with what happened yesterday, how can you move forward? You can't. It's just like in a vehicle, you have a rearview mirror. There's nothing in that rearview that looks forward. Things that's happened in your past, let it go. It's okay to look in that rearview mirror, as long as you don't stay too long. You look at it to remember where you come from. Use it as motivation to get to where you're going.

Have I ever been depressed? Yes I have. I think we all have. But it's all about how you deal with your depression. How I choose to deal with it is through the word of God. So if you keep your focus on Him, things will go smoothly for you.

I believe your attitude determines the altitude of your life. Stay positive, stay focused. Just because you have Tourette's does not mean you can't do anything you want to do in life. Set goals for yourself. Have dreams. Know how you want to get there and stay focused. Stay the course. The course of confidence.

We all have value. People just have to find it. But it's there. We each of us have to find the purpose and meaning of our life.

CHAPTER TWELVE

WORLDVIEW

In a vibrant sense, the world is what we believe it to be. Of course we can't stop an earthquake. But we *can* control our response to it. We can't rid ourselves of Tourette syndrome, but we can take charge of how we *feel* about it. Who we are is a reflection of who we believe we are. What we believe about ourselves colors and conditions our entire response to life.

I'm filled with admiration for the men, women, and children in this book. Again and again, they showed me their exalted strength and hope and perseverance.

It's no wonder people gravitate to stories that begin, "Against the odds…" These narratives show human nature at its finest: overcoming obstacles, acting selflessly to help others, creatively solving problems, never giving up. So it is with the people you'll find in these pages. And so it is with all humans. Our worldview is who we are and our worldview creates what we can become.

So to all Touretters, I say this is *your* story. Be glad! Live life! Stay hopeful!

Discover and follow your bliss. There is no alternative for finding happiness. And who knows? You may inspire someone else by your example. How you live your life is another way of revealing the truth that we are all connected.

About ten years ago, while researching a movie script in Thailand with the Drug Enforcement Administration, I was given a beautifully-carved, soft-stone opium pipe. I wasn't tempted to use it, but I wrestled with the compulsion to see how hard I could twist it before it broke. Speaking with Stephen, my urge suddenly made sense to me. I like his musical talent and sense of humor, and find a lot of truth in his admonition to resist labels others put on us. We end up defining ourselves, true, but Stephen feels we also have the power not to put ourselves in a box. Look at it this way: you can be a box with a closed lid. But if you open the lid, doesn't the box contain all the world? Keep an open mind.

STEPHEN
57 years old

They surprised me

I first noticed tics at seven. It's Christmastime and I'm holding a Christmas ball and the urge to squeeze it was really intense. So I did this game where I'd squeeze it without breaking it. And yet, I wanted to break it. That was the first ritualistic, OCD-ish thing. I've since met a lot of Tourette people who've had that testing-the-limits thing.

The next tics that showed up were blurting sounds and words. Coprolalia was there. Echolalia was definitely around, and that got me in wads of trouble. My parents wanted me to control myself—but you can't. They treated Tourette's like bad behavior. And the first doctor treated it like childhood disobedience.

Right along with the manifestation of Tourette's came a highly creative drive in the arts and music. I thought it was all part of this ticcing thing. So I got into music at a fairly young age. That set the pace for my family—a mix of excitement about my talent and wanting me to control my tics. "Don't be bad. Oh, that's so good." My mom was very supportive.

My first instrument was drums. Then keyboards, the organ in particular. The first instrument I got was a Magnus Air Organ, a tiny thing. When I got older, they rented an organ and put it in the basement rec room. They surprised me when I got home from school. I ticced all over the place I was so excited. I would bang on the keys, testing how far I could go without breaking them. So I'd end up breaking them and having to repair them. Yeah, the keys.

I had tics on it

School life was challenging [*a nervous chuckle*]. Sometimes I'd get in fights because kids thought I was saying something to them. The blurting thing. The word 'Tourette's' never came up. I had some great teachers, I had some who were very difficult. One instrumental piece I wrote was about my science teacher. He wasn't mean, but he thought I was just fooling around.

There are two sides to this. There's the difficulty of not being able to control tics. And there's the shared space, kids who are trying to study. I wasn't blurting a lot of curses in class, but I would do physical stuff. I would give teachers the finger. I wrote a song called "Obscenity." The chorus is, "I'm strangely attracted to obscenity [*he laughs*]." I learned to laugh about it.

My music studies got more and more serious and teachers were very supportive. They saw I was excelling. So I had a cocoon to fall into, music and creating, and surrounding myself with other musicians, who were strange in one way or another.

I was about sixteen when my uncle gave me a guitar. It was great timing because I was interested in writing songs. It was a Harmony guitar, half-size. It didn't last very long. I had tics on it and it broke [*he chuckles*]. Over time I got a decent guitar.

I thought of myself in two ways

At sixteen I went with my mom to a neurologist, who was the first person to say, "This looks like Tourette syndrome." This began the process of exploring support groups and medicine. First we tried behavioral therapy. I got into Transcendental Meditation. I definitely found peace in that. I found some stillness.

At this time I thought of myself in two ways. One was artistic expression. A whole slew of creativity and possibility that was just wonderful. And in public, I wanted to get away and be alone. So my self-image was a mix of 'I don't fit in' and 'I love this thing I can do, music.' You feel awful about yourself and yet have these experiences that other people *want* to have. It's ironic.

A year after my diagnosis I started medication and it messed me up, so I swore off it for twenty-five years. I'd meditate or take walks. I had enough control of my tics to live and do things, but not enough control to be incognito. When I went back to medication in my 40s, I had an awful experience again. That was Paxil and Risperdal, the cocktail. This was with a Tourette specialist, who had a son with Tourette's. He wasn't listening to what I was experiencing. I got a new doctor, a psychiatrist, and she got me on Zoloft and a little bit of Xanax. Within three days I had sixty percent less anxiety. Eventually I quit the Xanax and stayed on Zoloft.

Things that are very human

I'm often asked how does Tourette's affect my creativity. To answer, I decided a visual presentation was more effective than a verbal one. So I created a piece that's a cutaway into my mind and my experience. I play this piano piece and then I turn to a table with lots of other things that represent me being distracted. There is movement and clanging of things. I would describe it as multitasking [*he laughs*]. In managing the Tourette brain, the OCD brain, you are also having to multitask. It's sort of the business management of Tourette's and OCD.

I call it MGD—Multiple-Genre Disorder. The piece was intended to give a taste of the weird elements that make creativity interesting. I have coprolalia flash cards. You hold up the curse word instead of saying it.

It's how you take what you have and what you make of it. I made a film called *The SynapTic Adventure.*[120] My intention is to connect this experience to a universal theme. Tourette's was a question of urges, desires, compulsions—things that are very human. It's just that Tourette's amplifies it.

I was musical director for Sutie Madison's *Band of Artists.*[121] We were on the same page as far as how Tourette's manifests itself and how, when it's redirected, it becomes an art form. I think it's a habit of moving in a creative direction to… see the lemons, see the lemonade.

---

120   synapticadventure.com. The film won "Best Emerging Documentary" at the 2013 Bucks Fever Film Fest.
121   bandofartists.org. See Sutie's interview in Chapter Eight.

Be kind to yourself

I travel in spiritual circles 'cause there was an epiphany I had. I started out with Transcendental Meditation, then got into fundamentalist Christianity, and from there I moved through different forms of Christianity to Quakerism and then Buddhism. All through these, there were various attitudes regarding self-kindness. Be kind to yourself. What I found is it's best to listen to myself. I was listening to the guru or the priest, the minister, a book—everything but me.

So over time I guess I became a sort of 'selfist' [*he chuckles*]. I focused internally. The Zen stuff really helped me get still. So did Quakerism. I'd say I'm just living in the now. When you do a number of things over time, you absorb them into your being. Paying attention and caring about myself became a definite presence in my life.

I have a relationship now. With the ticcing, it has to be a negotiation. If I'm making loud noises or flailing my arms, I have to deal with the people around me. So my girl's response is, "That noise hurts my ear." Then I've got to decide where to go or aim my voice so it's not hurting her ear. It's more practical things she's saying rather than judging me for strange behavior.

You come to recognize the power within your own being that is shared by everyone, to create and see your world

One of the important things I've proved to myself is that engaging in something you love, that's constructive and creative, is utterly important to how you work with Tourette's. With Tourette's or without it, there's still that need to find one's place. I think it's important that you find a thing that you love to do. Maybe you've been more inclined to take care of other people, but haven't paid attention to your own thing. That's crucial.

I would think, "I must be doing this because I'm a bad person." We put descriptions in the way—we've been *given* definitions. "I must be crazy." It's not a reflection of who you are. "Oh, there's that guy who kicks around and talks to himself. He's weird. He's nuts." You're surrounded with it. You come to recognize the power within your own being that is shared by everyone, to create and see your world.

It gets down to, if you're dealing with tics, then find a way to deal with them. Acknowledge it and try to find a solution. The words tend to stop you and you put yourself in a box. "I'm stupid. I'm this or I'm that." But if you don't label yourself, and just look at what's happening, you are better able to come up with a solution.

Maybe the most graphic thing would be, "Ow! I cut my finger. I must be a bad person because I was careless." You can do those things and bleed. Or you can go, "I need a Band-Aid [*he laughs*]." I think it's important to get a handle on what's going on—and we're talking tics—and so we're talking about behavioral stuff that has nothing to do with who you are.

As a child with TS, every day bullies piled the weight of their own pain on me. Open hostility, contempt, ridicule, shunning, shaming—how many techniques are there to wither a kid's self-image? Lauren knows this all too well, both from personal experience and in her work. This is why she emphasizes hope as a pillar of strength for those who are disempowered.

LAUREN
33 years old

Every situation is different

I'm a social worker with the foster care system. I'm now training to teach people how to become foster parents. I think people with Tourette's make pretty good foster parents or social workers because we come from ... well, life isn't always easy [*she chuckles*]. For myself, having Tourette's, I experienced a lot of adversity, so I can relate to some of the experiences of the children I work with. Especially in regards to bullying because many of our kids get bullied a lot.

What do I tell them? Hang in there. It's interesting, coming from a social work standpoint, because I know all the right things to say to these kids, like, "This is how you should react." In reality, when you're faced with that experience, there's no right way to react. Every situation is different.

Emergency confession

For kids who are bullied, what we do is support them. And teachers absolutely need to become involved. I had this situation when I was growing up, third grade and just starting my tics, so I had a lot of overwhelming emotion. I had terrible coordination, so no one would let me bat at softball. It went on like this and I finally had enough and I said, "Please, just one time let me bat the ball." And a girl said, "You're not going to bat. You're too slow." And I just ran over and I bit her [*she laughs*].

But the teacher saw *me* as the aggressor. Girls are good at being secretive about their bullying. So the teachers didn't realize how much I had been emotionally bullied by that point. I knew, "This is never going to stop unless I take matters into my own hands." That whole situation could have been avoided had the teachers done something about it. It was wrong that I bit her [*she laughs*]. It was a Catholic school, so I got marched directly to an emergency confession.

I looked crazy because people made me feel crazy

I tell parents not to ignore bullying if it's happening to their child. A lot of parents, their first reaction is to say, "Oh, just ignore it. Don't feed into it." That's hard to do for a child. I tried that so many times as a kid. I would ignore it for a week, and it kept getting worse and worse and then I would lash out.

I was a mess. I looked crazy because people made me feel crazy. And I didn't know what to do. If parents were to pick a more active stance against bullying and get the teachers involved, that would help so much. Just support their child.

I grew up in a pretty interesting family. My parents fought constantly. They threatened divorce every other day. It was a very chaotic environment. I'm not saying I had a bad upbringing, it just could have been calmer [*she chuckles*]. It elevated my stress, which probably increased my tics.

I spent quite a lot of time with my paternal grandmother, which is probably the only reason that I... she was a respite for me, you know? A break in all the chaos. And bless her heart, she put up with a lot from me. You know, I was a very sweet child, but when my anger got the better of me, I was very violent. She was the only person who could calm me down.

She just held me. She'd wrap her arms around me and she held me until I was done kicking and screaming.

This would have been handy news

I was diagnosed when I was sixteen. I remember my first tics, probably around eight. I've written a book[122] about my experience, and as I wrote the book I realized I had lots of symptoms before anyone realized they were symptoms. My mom said, "Ignore it. It'll go away." My dad didn't really say *anything*, which was fine. I went to a neurologist when I was thirteen because I had seizures. He told my mom he thought I had Tourette's. So when I told my mom I had Tourette's she said, "I know." And I was like, "You've *known*? For how long?" She said since I was thirteen, and here I am almost seventeen. I was like, "This would have been handy news. At least I could have given people an explanation."

So I was placed on meds, which I still take today. They helped calm my tics. I've never taken it as prescribed because it causes me to be sleepy. I take them as they work for me. I'm supposed to take one in the morning and one in the afternoon, and one at night. I take two at night and that does fine, 800 mg of Neurontin.

The day after my high school graduation, I went to Europe for two weeks. That was my graduation present. Then I came back and the next morning we packed my bags and headed to my college. I didn't tell people about the TS right away. A lot of people can't tell, because I've learned to suppress my tics, or disguise them. It took me a while to become open about it because I found that when I did open up to people, they... it's a mixture of shock and, like, "Why are you telling me this?" It's almost as if I said I had AIDS or something. Or they'll say, "That's really cool!" and two days later they'll stop talking to me because they don't know what to do with that information. If I got to know someone better, I would tell because I knew it would affect our friendship if I didn't.

Have a little hope

One thing I want to impart to people who are disempowered—have hope.

---

122   *Tic Talk Around The Clock* by Lauren Ashley. For professional reasons 'Lauren' is a pseudonym. Her book is available on amazon.com for Kindle. You can download the Kindle app on any digital device.

Find that little piece of hope, because it is not as desperate as people think it is. I was involved with a Facebook group that I discontinued because so many parents would complain about their children with Tourette's. How their child wasn't going to be the same, or mourning the loss. Which is… I understand it, but then, have a little hope. It's not a desperate situation. If I have hope, *anyone* can do it [*she chuckles*].

I don't have children yet, but it does make me nervous. It's not because I don't think they would have a successful life. But I know how mean kids can be. So I think that would be my only sadness for my child. And that's the motivation for writing my book and speaking out about Tourette's.[123] I want my child to be raised in a more Tourette-tolerant society.

I see myself as very successful. I mean, I don't make boatloads of money, but I am successful in my own way. I have a master's degree. I help people for a living. When I was in secondary school, people didn't think I was going to go to college, they didn't think I was going to do anything with my life. They thought I was going to hole up at my parents' house, I guess. Well, I have a house, I have a husband, we have a life. To me that's success. And I'm very competitive at work. The biggest motivator is for someone to tell me I can't do something. I'm like, "I *dare* you to tell me that [*she laughs*]." It's like, "Please do." Because I'm going to do it. I'm very stubborn, in a good way. Probably a bad way too, but…

See from a different angle

Healing my self-image, that has taken a lot of support, mainly by my husband. He has always been the biggest support to me. It was funny, because I had a tic for a period of time where I would bark. So my husband, he was on the phone with his mom—and this was a brand-new relationship, maybe three months in—and his mom asks, "Do you have a dog?" And he's like, "No, that's my girlfriend [*a big laugh*]." That was embarrassing. And then he explained, "She has Tourette's," and she's like, "Uh… okay." She's very accepting of me, my mother-in-law.

I think also the process of writing my memoir, that *really* helped to heal me. There were some painful experiences I had to sit down with and see from a different perspective. I think that was *the* biggest thing that helped with my self-image. And there is some comfort in the fact that I

123 She also has a motivational Facebook page, *Lauren Ashley's Intuitive Healing.*

got nothin' to hide anymore [*she laughs*]. If you want to know about me, read my book. There were maybe one or two things I didn't talk about, but there are some things everyone will go to their grave with [*she chuckles*].

Life is not all about high school.
It gets better after high school. Thank God

You know, there's been a lot of gravel. A lot of mountains to climb. But I learned to appreciate the present moment. I don't know what tomorrow is going to hold. And frankly, I'm not worried about it. I mean, of course I worry. What if I never have children? But I have faith that eventually it's going to work out for the better.

My biggest thing is just have hope, you know? Because it does get better. It's going to be hard, but you will get through it. And life is not all about high school. It gets better after high school. Thank God.

David's not the first person in these pages to benefit from growing up in a small town, where everyone knows him. How clearly this illustrates that disability is a social construct. It's society's responsibility to accept and admire those who begin each day with a resolve few people comprehend. David credits his parents with accommodating his needs without treating him differently than his siblings. His sense of humor, perspective, and a little riding around in the mud help him maintain a positive attitude. In Mexico I saw a tattoo parlor with the name, "Perdoname Madre" (Forgive Me Mother). It reminded me of David, who finally got his mother to accept his tattoos.

DAVID
25 years old

It's not like there are in-between days

Right when I was twelve, my tics started. I had no idea what was going on. I couldn't stop it. I was making a noise, like clearing my throat, and it got worse. I got diagnosed with Tourette's around fourteen years old, after we found a good doctor.

I went to a private school, so there were only about ten kids in my class. We all grew up together. When I got older, the tics were getting worse, so I was homeschooled throughout high school because of it. I lost my social life. There was none. There were a few friends I knew from kindergarten and we stayed in touch, but making new friends, meeting new people, it didn't happen.

I wasn't doing a whole lot of anything, the tics were so bad. Real bad twitching, I was grinding my teeth, shaking, swinging my arms, screaming different words. I was swearing. There are people who understand it, but if there are a lot of people around, you have to explain yourself. To me it wasn't worth going anywhere. The swearing went away, then came back a couple of years after high school, but I haven't had any problem with that tic for a while.

I have to say I have milder tics now, but when I have a bad day, I have a really bad day. It's not like there are in-between days. I'll do constant twitching, I'll crunch over, jerk real hard, and it hurts after doing it so much. And it gets frustrating because it won't stop and I can't control it. That puts more stress on me and makes 'em worse.

I never wanted special attention

I was blessed with my parents because I feel they understood. They tried to make it easygoing without babying me, not treating me any different than my brother and sister. I'm thankful for that. I never wanted special attention. I never wanted to take from my brother and sister and put it all on me. My dad's real good with that. He knows I don't want to be treated any different, so growing up with TS, my dad didn't treat me no different. I believe it worked out.

After high school, I worked with my dad and my uncle. They had a construction company and I would go on good days. If it was a bad day, there was somebody with me to make sure nothing happened. I fell down the steps one time. I sat down to fix my sock, I twitched and rolled back, and I guess it forced me over and I fell down the steps.

My dad retired, so now I have a good friend who has a landscaping company. Whenever I have a good day, he'll take me with him. I've been having a lot more good days than bad lately. I can work about half-time.

I live at home with my parents still. If it's not too bad, I'll go do what I have to do. But if it's a bad day, I'd rather stay home. My social life is way better. It's because I live in a small town. Everybody knows me, knows I have Tourette's, so no one questions it. I'm pretty free to do what I want and not worry about people not knowing what it is.

I like to ride in the mud

With my friends, I go fishing. There's a couple of ponds and lakes by my house. If I have a good day, I'll go quad riding with my friend. A quad is like a motorcycle with four wheels, and you can ride it off-road. I like to ride in the mud. I like the sense of freedom I get from it. I do tic when I go on the quad and I have had a wreck from it. So I won't go riding if I'm a little twitchy.

I accept that I have Tourette's and this is what I have to deal with, and I'm going to make the best out of it. But it's hard to not let it win. I have my good days dealing with it and my bad days. Usually I'm pretty positive. I've met a lot of good people from having it. I met some good doctors and they've showed me things I never would have looked at about life.

I have a psychiatrist and I've helped her, she told me, help people deal with TS. She used stuff she found out about me to help a little boy better understand it and deal with it. That makes me feel good. I haven't met him, but if I did I'd tell him to keep his head up and stay positive. Don't let it bring you down.

That's the hardest thing to do, to stay positive. If you can make that happen, you'll be with no problem. And try to make the best out of everything, and try to be laughing and having fun. Having a sense of humor. If I'm not thinking positive, then I tend to get depressed quite easily.

I could relate so much

I posted on Facebook[124] something that, when I saw it... I had a therapist, a long time ago, and he was dead set on I needed to make friends. So I went out and made all these friends that ended up not being friends. All

---

124 "There comes a time in life when you walk away from all the drama and the people who create it and you surround yourself with people who make you laugh. Falling down is part of life, getting up is living."

it did was start drama in my life, a bunch of crazy stuff I didn't need. I elected to stop hanging out with them because they were getting into drugs and alcohol, and I didn't want to do that. And I realized I had no friends again [*he chuckles*]. But I was like, "Man, I got rid of all these people and I'm still smiling." I hear about them and they're either hooked on drugs or in jail.

I felt alone up until I saw the Facebook group. I had no one I could talk to who truly understood. I have my doctors. I have my dad. He's been right by my side since day one with it. He knows me better than anybody. But it's hard to talk even to him about some things. Talking to someone with it, it's healing to me because I've never been able to do that. I could relate *so* much to these people. This is a true blessing because I have somewhere to go if I need to vent or I want to talk. I can message one of these people, and they'll understand. It's been great.

She liked those three words

My best friend is a tattoo artist. I've got tattoos, full sleeves, both arms. I was twenty or twenty-one when I got my first one. I have tattoos of band logos, I've got a couple of Tourette tattoos, I've got some stars and flames, and everything's tied together with clouds. If I'm having a good day I can sit and get tattooed.

I don't know if it sounds crazy, but getting tattooed, I believe it helps keep me focused. I'm focusing on the tattoo and sitting still and not moving. I don't think about anything else but what's going on right now. It seems to make me a lot calmer. When I'm in that zone, everything's good. My Tourette's is better because I'm so focused on not moving. I think a good bit of it is the pain, because they do hurt, *a lot*. So I think the pain has a lot to do with it. I'm focusing on not moving *in* that pain.

My mom wasn't too fond about the tattoos at all for the longest time. And then she got to accepting them after so long of me going and getting them. She likes them now. Across my chest I have written 'Respect Trust Loyalty' and my mom actually helped me pick that out. I was going through different words and phrases and she liked those three words. You have to respect yourself, you have to trust yourself, and you have to be loyal to yourself. I feel that to live life you have to go by those words. I try to be that and do that every day. I think it helps me be true.

Giving up was a mistake

At first, knowing Tourette's is hereditary, I didn't want to have kids.[125] Now, I don't want it to stop me. If my kid was diagnosed with it, I'd be able to help the kid a lot more than maybe my parents did at first. You know, try to show them a positive life with it. I'd say, "We're not going to let this get the best of us. We're going to handle it. We're going to get through it. We're going to stay positive. I've been dealing with it for a while now and I'm doing pretty good, and I'm gonna make sure you do the best you can do."

It took me 'til recently to love myself again, basically. I'm not gonna let anything get me down no more. I'm gonna learn from everything and make the best out of it. Even if it is a real bad day, I'm gonna make the best out of that day. When I was around eighteen, my tics were really, really bad. I was sitting at home all day, miserable, just hating life. I tried to commit suicide because I was so miserable and didn't want to take it no more.

My psychiatrist helped me a good bit. And my dad. And realizing, "Why would I do that? What I'm going through sucks, but it could be so much worse." I'm blessed that I wake up every day, and I *am* smiling and happy, to an extent. But let's be happy and let's smile all the time regardless. I've got to work on it myself, mentally, try to be positive. I know I have this problem, but I can't let it get the best of me. So I kinda got a reality check from all that. And I was thinking, "I'm letting it win. That's not right."

Giving up was a mistake. It really was. I'm not gonna say I've never been depressed, but I've never been that low again, to where I gave up. After all was said and done, I was blessed. It's still a work in progress, being able to make sure I stay positive. But giving up was a mistake, absolutely. There's so much more to life than to let something like this win. It wasn't right.

---

125   David became a father in 2015.

Like many in this book, I understand isolation and the unwelcome urge to hide. For these interviews, everyone introduced themselves to me by name, although many changed their name for publication. Bob is the only person who used a pseudonym when he first contacted me; nor does he want a copy of this book. Yet he felt compelled to be interviewed. How difficult is it to emerge once we have withdrawn?

BOB
67 years old

Nods head frequently

I grew up in Trenton, New Jersey. Onset must have been at six or seven because my parents took me to a doctor and I saw he had written on a pad, 'Nods head frequently.' The doctor told my parents I would outgrow it. Of course, I didn't. I think I have a case that is minor, because I don't have outbursts of obscenities or things like that. If I have to control it for a couple of hours, I can do that. My major tic is with my head. I also have echolalia but I can control all these things, and when I'm with other people, I do. But if I'm by myself I just let it out.

I also have the ADHD and whatever else goes along with it. It made it hard for me to function in school. I wasn't much interested in school, but that didn't help. I have a hard time absorbing a lot of information. Like if someone's telling me directions, after a little while my mind kinda shuts down and I don't understand what they're telling me. I can concentrate when I'm doing something I want to do. But receiving a lot of information at once, I just can't process it.

I feel I'm isolated, but I've come to accept it

It's hard to say the impact of Tourette's because I can't remember anybody teasing me about it. I've always had problems making friends. I have no male friends, only female friends now. I'm not sure how much TS contributed to my inability to interact with other people. It's possible people just avoided me because of TS. The older I got, the harder it became for me to have male friends, and I've pretty much stopped trying. I don't spend a lot of time with my female friends anyway. I feel I'm isolated but I've come to accept it. At my age what am I gonna do about it? I am who I am.

I'm not saying there was no impact on my life as a kid. Why didn't kids in my neighborhood want to play with me? I don't know how much the Tourette's was responsible, or how much just my personality was responsible. My parents, there was some sense of embarrassment when we were in public, I'll say that. As far as my relationship with my parents, that's a whole other deal that I'm sure the Tourette's affected, but it's so complicated I don't even want to go into it.

That was supposed to be my career

Okay... I'm a musician, okay? When I say musician, I have been obsessed with music since I can remember. That was my sole focus in life. And for a long time, when I got to be a teenager, my parents suspected that I was gay. I'm not. But they suspected I was gay because I would rather listen to a concert than go to a baseball game. And they were not people who would accept that. That generation, that's how they were. I don't know how much of that played into my having a problem with kids in the neighborhood. They played with me but I could tell they were tolerating me. I also happen to be Jewish and the kids in my neighborhood were not, for the most part.

I was a singer. I also wrote music and played keyboards and later guitar, when I started to perform in public. I picked up the trombone seven years ago. But my main instrument is voice. That was supposed to be my career. I was a singer/songwriter. I sang in rock bands, pickup bands, whatever. I had no problem on stage because, you know, nodding my head in time with the music. It wasn't like I was doing anything out of the ordinary.

But my ex-wife made it very, very difficult to pursue this, so after a while I just stopped. I stopped trying to be a professional and went on to other things. My voice is pretty well shot at this point. I'll sing sometimes for myself, but it's way past the point where my voice is going to be displayed in public. I continued in an amateur fashion, but not as I was supposed to do, not what I was meant to do. But I've come to terms with that. That's how my life has worked out. I'm not unduly bitter, that's just the way things are. What am I gonna do about it?

I wouldn't have any escape

I never got a Tourette syndrome diagnosis, but the more research I did... I've been to a couple of shrinks and they've brought up medication. The first one, I was about fifty years old, he said, "You've had this for fifty years, why bother now?" And I didn't want to be medicated. I know some of that stuff, it just makes you lethargic. It's not something I want to get involved with. Tourette's is part of me and people who know me know that it exists, and if they can't deal with it, then they can't deal with it. What can I tell ya?

My symptoms are not that severe. People will look at me and maybe see that I'm doing something that's not exactly right, but it's not a huge movement. I don't make noises in public. So if people see me with a head movement, they think it's a nervous habit. But I've never had anybody stare at me or approach me and say, "What are you doing?" And if they did, I don't think I would be forthcoming. That's not something that I discuss or deal with, with anybody. It's always been a source of embarrass-ment for me. I know some people handle it much better than that and are more honest, but that's not me. I prefer to ignore it or pretend it's not there rather than deal with it with somebody.

Tourette's has affected my self-image. I think it's prevented me from doing things I would like to do, career changes. I think, "If I do that, I'll be observed constantly." I don't want to be in that kind of a situation. I realize it would be difficult for me to function without undue pressure to deal with it. I feel I have to hide my symptoms. I do.

There are things I thought about doing with my life but did not, because I would not want to be under that scrutiny. A long time ago I thought that court reporter would be something I'd like to do. I didn't pursue it, mainly because I would be sitting in front of the courtroom and people maybe would look at me as a source of interest, or maybe even amusement. And I wouldn't have any escape.

Going from place to place

I was an optician for thirty years and I had to work with the public. I would work with somebody for maybe fifteen or twenty minutes, then they would leave. So I could control things for the amount of time that I had to deal with the public. And with my coworkers, I didn't bother.

When I would first go to work in a new place, it took me a while to be comfortable. I control things until I am comfortable. Then I start to be myself and they notice it, but nobody's ever said anything about it. Everyone I've ever worked with can see it, but no one's ever asked me about it.

I would typically have a job for three years, maybe less, and move on. So I was never stable as far as that goes. So after thirty years of going from place to place doing the same thing, I'd had enough. I needed to do something else. I saw an ad in the paper and I got a job with this national commercial cleaning company, cleaning people's homes. I worked to learn the business, and after three or four months I opened my own business and did that for seven years. This was easy because ninety-five percent of the time I was by myself. If I wanted to let myself go and be myself, it didn't matter. So that was very comfortable for me.

I've never admitted I have Tourette's or discussed it with anyone, other than a couple of shrinks

Now I'm retired, but I'm a driving instructor part-time. I'm with a student three hours at a time, but I have to talk a lot. I'm animated when I talk, I use my hands and I can move my head in an acceptable manner, so it's not obvious. This allows me to have some kind of motor release. I'm there for three hours but I control myself best I can.

My second wife and I have been married for twenty years. She sees me do these things but I don't know what she thinks. She's said to me a couple of times when she's seen me really get excited, she'll say, "Do you have Tourette's?" And I'll say, "Not that I know of." This is a woman who is very well educated, very intelligent, yet she doesn't know what she's looking at. I don't know why she doesn't understand what's going on. Even with her, I don't wish to discuss it. If she guessed, I'd probably say, "You're probably right." I mean, I couldn't deny it. And she's a very tolerant, supportive person. So it wouldn't be a problem, really, but I have not come face-to-face with that.

What am I afraid of? That's hard to say. I've never admitted I have Tourette's or discussed it with anyone, other than a couple of shrinks. If I ever discussed it with my wife, she'd probably research it and decide what her role should be as far as helping me or not dealing with it or whatever. That would be her decision how she wanted to handle it. It's just a very uncomfortable topic for me. If I found myself sitting next to a kid who had tics, I would just ignore it. Yeah. I wouldn't say, "Hey, guess what? Me too." I'd just ignore it. I have no advice. What am I gonna say? I mean, "Kindred spirit," maybe, but no, I would not say anything.

The medical profession, like any other, has both skilled and inept practitioners. Ken's experience, never being warned of Haldol's side effects, underscores the importance of educating oneself in interactions with doctors. I'm also moved by his open-hearted relationship with his son. True love and insight into character have nothing to do with appearance.

KEN
43 years old

Why do you feel you have to do that?

I think most people with Tourette's, especially adults, find that when they were younger they weren't believed, or they were disciplined for things they could not control because nothing was known about TS. At fourteen, when I started my first vocal tics, my parents kept saying, "It's a habit. It's a habit."

They took me to an ear, nose, and throat doctor who said, "He has a deviated septum." Mind you, my grunting comes from my throat, not my nose. And now I have a hard time smelling, he hacked up my nose so much. That was an unnecessary operation and after, my tics continued.

My first memory of a tic was a vocal tic. Oh, my God, I felt like all eyes were upon me. I felt like the black sheep of the family. And to be honest, to this day I feel like the black sheep. I'm the only one with Tourette's.

I had an abusive father, okay? So with that, it didn't help. He would yell, he would threaten. My mother was more caring but she'd say, "Why do you feel you have to do that?" And I couldn't give her any answers.

School was difficult, but I engrossed myself in sports. The grunts didn't matter there, but in class they were disruptive. I would be sent to the principal's office. Kids would make fun of me. I'm not saying I didn't have friends or was an outcast, but there was teasing that would escalate to fights.

My rock through all this

I had low self-esteem. I didn't feel normal, whatever normalcy is. I wasn't like other kids. I *knew* I was different. I still have a low self-esteem. I still do. I have to tell you—my wife has been my rock through all this. I moved to Florida roughly twenty years ago. I felt the only way I was going to grow up was to be where I didn't have support. So I drove down I-95 and something drew me to Tampa.

I found a job at a restaurant and within a week Michelle starts. We got married in '97... or was it '96? Oh, shit [*he laughs*]. We have one child together and he'll be eighteen soon, and I raised her three children. With my Tourette's, they've always accepted me. I'm not saying they didn't harass me every now and then, "Dad, you're being too loud." But I take it all in humor.

We moved up to Rhode Island for a year because the kids wanted to see snow. So, lo and behold, April first, April Fools Day, we got a three-foot snow storm. So they saw their snow, and they were ready to go back to Florida [*he chuckles*].

Doing what I do best

My tics started getting worse. I started having more motor tics. The vocal tic never changed, but it got more forceful to the point that, years later, a tic popped one of my ribs out of place. Michelle did research, printed out a list of tics and we found a dozen that I did. She said, "You need to see a neurologist." So I'm sitting in his office, grunting up a storm, flailing my arms, you know, doing what I do best. And he comes in and says, "Hi, Ken. Are you here to be treated for Tourette's?" I said, "I'm here to be diagnosed for something." He said, "Great. You have Tourette's. Now let's treat it [*he laughs*]." I was twenty-seven.

No one ever told me any side effects of any of the meds I've been on

I've been a guinea pig on all types of medicines and the one I've been on longest is Haldol. Just recently I decided I want off of it because I've gained a lot of weight. I'm two-hundred-seventy-five pounds. I began thinking, what is Haldol doing to my body? I went to my neurologist, and he diagnosed me with tardive dyskinesia,[126] which is permanent damage. I asked, "What caused it?" And he said, "Being on Haldol."

No one ever told me any side effects of any of the meds I've been on. This is partly my fault. I should have done my research prior to taking any meds. So now my concern is, what do I take next? My choice is to try Orap. But that can cause tardive dyskinesia also. The way I look at it is, "I already got it, so what does it matter?"

Haldol and Orap are pretty much similar, except Orap can give you a heart condition. So before you go on Orap the doctor's supposed to order an EKG to check out your heart, and do an EKG every time there's a dosage increase. It's kind of scary because there's also a low chance of seizures.

I take other medications too. I take Clonidine once a day, I take Clonazepam[127] three times a day, I take Ambien for sleep, I take Remeron for depression. I take a muscle relaxer because I don't want to get addicted to pain pills. So even though I need 'em, I just deal with the pain from my motor tics.

My two doctors don't coordinate personally, but they coordinate with each other through me. I tell each one what the other is doing or wants to do. I think each doctor needs to know what I'm on.

I do want to be medicated but I don't like big pharmaceutical medications. What are my alternatives? In Florida, we are voting on medicinal marijuana.[128] I don't use it now because it's illegal and I would be the person to get busted [*he laughs*]. But I have talked to people with movement disorders and they tell me it helps them drastically.

---

126 A difficult-to-treat and often incurable disorder resulting in involuntary, repetitive body movements.
127 Klonopin.
128 Legal use of medical marijuana was narrowly defeated in Florida in 2014.

Don't let Tourette's stand in your way

When Michelle and I decided to have a child, we never discussed Tourette's because I wasn't diagnosed. Even if I had a diagnosis, we would have had children. With Tourette's and heredity, nothing's a sure thing. I wanted a family and I wouldn't let it get in the way.

Brett, my biological son, is showing signs of a tic disorder. If he were to be diagnosed with Tourette's, I would tell him to embrace life to the fullest. Don't let Tourette's stand in your way. I let it hold me back a lot growing up.

I would tell him to be himself. If a friend doesn't like your actions or they're embarrassed, then they're not your friend. Your friends are going to stick by you no matter what race, gender, sexuality, or disorder you have.

I would hate to be a teen these days. Not necessarily a teen with a disorder, but just a *teen*. Take Brett, for instance. It turns out he is bisexual. So, not only does he have a tic disorder that he's been made fun of for, but he is attracted to both girls and guys. He's accepted it. We've accepted it. We believe in equal rights for all. If you love somebody, it shouldn't matter what race or what sex they are.

Brett's been bullied most of his life. He was small, thin, easy to pick on, wouldn't speak up for himself. Once, bullies threatened they were going to send gang members to his house to kill his family. He fought back and the school was going to suspend him because he started a fight. Michelle said, "There is no way you're suspending my son because I'm withdrawing him immediately." This was seventh grade and he's been homeschooled since.

If you can't make fun of yourself, then how can you live?

My tics come out more when I'm in a crowd. I get anxious. If Michelle sees somebody staring at me, she'll stare right back [*he laughs*]. She stares them down. I'm a non-confrontational guy. I want to help. I'm a caring person. When somebody asks me if I'm okay, or they ask if I have a disorder, I will tell them all about Tourette's.

I use humor to deal with Tourette's. I have to. If you can't make fun of yourself, then how can you live? I have Tourette's, I accept it, and I laugh at it.

I've got my tattoo artist designing my first Tourette's tattoo. You know the national Tourette syndrome guy, that little bubble guy?[129] It's him, but the artist is putting her own creativity into it. I haven't seen it yet, but it's gonna go on my right forearm. I've had a tattoo on my left forearm for a few years and part of my OCD is I have to balance out, you know [*he laughs*]? So I have to have one on my right forearm.

I would sway towards Buddhism

Yesterday I came out of my psychiatrist's office with the most positive attitude I've ever had. We talked about having a positive self-image. If you're not having a good day, think positive thoughts and turn that day around. Make a list of positive things in my life and when I start to feel down, look at that list and remind myself that these things are in my life and they're not negative.

I posted a quote by the Dalai Lama on Facebook.[130] I love the Dalai Lama. I mean, he is a very funny guy. I would love to see him in person. He is such a peaceful guy. I would love to live my life like him. I don't believe in an organized religion, but if I were to sway one way or another, I would sway towards Buddhism. It's the way you live your life, through peace and harmony.

---

129 The TAA logo is a stylized human form with its arms raised.

130 The Dalai Lama said that, although we cannot know the future, we live in hope of something better. He goes on to say that hope means perseverance, it brings self-confidence, and the thought, "I can do this."

———————————————— ☙ ————————————————

If you don't have Tourette's, you can't imagine how frightening and demoralizing it is not to control your mind/body. Without a diagnosis, you're forced to draw your own conclusions, and Alma is one of many who mistakenly ascribed their tics to an unhealthy mental condition. I like her story because it shows how resilient we can be. She speaks English with a slight Spanish accent and in that voice she speaks for all of us who recognize our need for tenderness and love.

ALMA
40 years old

I started to feel like it was my fault

I'm having a lot of tics, lately. I don't know why. I work at the same place, but I changed departments last year because it was hell [*she laughs*]. I'm a *funcionario,*[131] you know? Even with Tourette's I managed to pass a very competitive exam to become an employee of the European Union.[132] There were twenty-six hundred applicants for eighty openings. There were eight different tests and interviews. I was among the top three percent with the highest grades.

I was born and raised in Spain. When I was ten, my family moved to Manhattan. My little brother was born and that's when my tics started, when I was ten. The whole thing with my parents was, they thought the tics were because I was jealous of my little brother and I had developed this horrible attitude. Before my tics, I was the perfect daughter. After that, it just went to hell.

In my teens, I developed really bad tics. My mom would tell me to stop, every day, every meal, pretty much all the time. And she would imitate me. She would imitate my tics, right? Of course, this made me tic more. I'd get angry, curse, spit, slam doors.

I started to feel like it's my fault. Everything is my fault because I'm jealous of my brother and I want more attention. But it was the

---

131   Bureaucrat.

132   The subway stop where Alma gets off for work was bombed in the March 2016 terrorist attack in Brussels.

exact opposite. I wanted the *least* attention possible. I wanted to disappear.

That's how I got my tenderness

I cried every night for years because we never talked about TS at home. A lot of times with TS, people are cool around family because they can be themselves, but with me it's not like that. Being around family is super-stressful, so that's why I tend to be always alone. Alone is where I can be myself. I'd rather be alone. Basically.

When I graduated high school, I went to business school, where I was bullied a lot. I was just twenty. I was behind socially because I'd been overprotected. I didn't know anything about life. I didn't know I had Tourette's, but I had tics.

I wanted to be a model, so I met a lot of guys. We used to go to parties and dance samba all night. That's how I let go because dancing was amazing. These people didn't judge me. But that's also because they used me. I met a lot of men, especially older men. That's how I got my tenderness. I wanted acceptance so bad, I wasn't picky. I hated the sex, but I loved the cuddling. I just needed to be hugged. I did that for years. I didn't like the sex. No, no, no. Now I do. I'm all grown up and normal [*she laughs*].

The job wasn't really a job

In my second year of business school I got to study abroad. I traveled the world thanks to this school. In the third year, we had to find an internship. And this is when my life got a little crazy.

In Bangkok, I met two Mexican guys. I spoke Spanish, so I told them I needed an internship the next year, and they said I could work for their company in Cuernavaca. They said, "We'll send you the ticket." So I convinced my parents, and they let me go to Mexico by myself. But *resulta que...*[133] the job wasn't really a job. The internship never came through.

I worked in coffee shops, modeling jobs in trade shows, as a presenter on a TV cooking show. I got my certificate to teach ESL.[134] I was one of the invited jury members at a small town beauty contest—that was

---

133 It turns out that…
134 English as a Second Language.

awesome. I even got a singing contract. And the guys I met in Bangkok, they were actually *narcotraficantes.*[135]

I grew up like ten years in one year. I lived a lot of intense things. I was in dangerous situations, but I was very lucky that I never got into trouble. I dated this Mexican politician. He was also *narcotraficante.* Little by little I realized that. Last year I was looking him up online, out of curiosity. I found a newspaper article explaining the gang wars between *narcotraficantes* in Cuernavaca, and there he was, among the list of the *asesinatos.*[136]

But I also had great friends. I hung out a lot with the gay community. I used to go out to a gay bar every night and they had a transvestite show. I was the cute little Spanish girl that everybody liked. How come I don't remember my tics? I think because I was super busy. I was kind of in a bliss state. I had tics, but people loved me anyway.

To know I wasn't crazy

And then my visa expired. I went to Manhattan and in the next three years I worked for some financial firms. I got my own apartment. I dated this guy who said to me, "There's something wrong with you. You have to go to the doctor." So I go to the psychiatrist, and this intern said, "You have Tourette syndrome." I had no idea what it was.

Okay, this is a life defining moment. I went to the library and took a book on Tourette's and every page I read, I was like, "They're writing about me. This is *me.*" I couldn't believe it. I wanted to cry because I realized so much pain could have been avoided, everything we went through at home. Finally I wanted it to be about me. To know I wasn't crazy. That I didn't have an attitude problem. That I wasn't jealous of anyone.

But I was so ashamed. I was ashamed until I was in my late thirties. I didn't talk about it. I would hide it. It's only been a few years since I casually say I have Tourette syndrome. Just with time, I guess, it made me accept it. I suffered so much shame and guilt. I've had people, out of nowhere, asking me, "Why do you look guilty?" Like I have this guilty look on my face. For me it's been hard being okay with it. You know?

---

135 Drug traffickers.
136 Murdered.

I curse a lot—in three languages

For years, even at work, I would have my headphones on. I have to have music. It's my way of coping. I have hypersensitivity to sound. There was a guy, when I worked for the department of public health in Manhattan, he cleared his throat all the time. It's hard to explain to non-Touretters. Other people might be annoyed by a sound, but to *you*, you can only hear this. And it takes your whole world. You cannot focus on anything else. It makes you enraged. When I couldn't stand it anymore, I would go to the bathroom and cry. And you feel so embarrassed and stupid. It's the worst part of Tourette's, this rage you get.

I have tons of OCD. At work today, I had two meetings and I had to take minutes, which is hell [*she laughs*]. It's really hard because I catch one sentence and then I disconnect, and miss the beginning of the next one. Even when I focus hard. I'm amazed I worked in an office for twenty years and was really good. But still, I have these things that make it harder for me. And it's tiring. That's why you're tired as fuck when you get home, you know?

I have so many symptoms that are associated with Tourette's. I shout racial slurs sometimes. I curse a lot—in three languages [*she laughs*]. I do a lot of jerking. I make noises quietly. I curse quietly. One of my tics, I used to do it all the time, I tell myself to shut up. Out loud. If I started ticcing or cursing or calling myself names, I'd interrupt myself to shut myself up. For years I did that. I learned to control myself because I was told to stop so much. I don't want people to look at me or stare at me or hear me. So I internalize everything and my body is in a horrible state. Since last year I felt my body just aged. I feel so tired. Sometimes I just want to sit in my chair and not move.

The whole point is to know I'm a good person

I guess the hardest thing for me is not to focus so much on love. In the last ten years, I've only had one boyfriend, and he died. I only want one thing—I want love. It's hard to talk about because I get super emotional. That's the only thing I feel I need. I have everything else. I don't understand why it's not happening. It's not because of my Tourette's. It's just not happening to me.

I grew up Catholic. When we were kids, our parents would tell

us—when we fell or something—they'd say "Es el niño Jesus."[137] It was
Jesus punishing you. For me there was always that bad conscience, that
guilt. It always followed me.

In my early thirties I got really depressed. I was praying and praying
and asking God to help me, but it never helped. Then I had to have surgery.
After, I remember waking up and thinking, "Religion is ridiculous. There
is no God, of course." And that was it. I became a 'good' person. A person
with a clean conscience. I was always scared before.

And from the time I stopped believing in God, I've been a good
person. I have nothing to feel guilty about. I understand religion and
I respect it, but it's not for me. I guess my God is my conscience. The
whole point is to know I'm a good person. Not to feel guilty. That was the
hardest thing for me, that I don't need a third party to judge me. I can be
a good person. I am.

137   "It's baby Jesus."

This is a truncated version of a conversation filled with Jonathon's rapid-fire speech and dense with his ideas. Ever since his playground epiphany, Jonathon has seen life through a 'realistic lens.' His starting point was accepting his difference. This freed him to discover his imagination, enthusiasm, and resilience. Years later, he became an entrepreneur whose high-tech business helps people in dire need. He believes each of us can live in the same manner. Crucial to this life view is recognizing that Tourette's does not impede our ability to be who we are—not unless we allow it. Finding and following our passions. Building strength in the face of opposition. This is how we develop independence and a robust self-image. By accepting Tourette syndrome, Jonathon believes each of us can tap into a power that frees our potential to be happy, creative beings.

JONATHON
34 years old

Pick up your head

There's a growing sensitivity to over-medication. There seems to be a *zeitgeist* shift, where folks are saying, "When you see kids who can't seem to sit still, instead of thinking first that they may have various three-letter acronym disorders, let's focus on the conditions that are real, that can be demonstrated by evidence. Let's acknowledge the ones that may be a response to the rapid-fire, always-on pace of movies and video games, versus the inherent energy of a kid being a kid. How much of their restlessness has to do with giving kids too much corn syrup?"

We may find that a child *is* ill and needs medication or behavioral therapy. But what if a kid is just imaginative, and by giving him or her meds, you've stolen the child's imagination?

Medications had a very bad effect on me. I remember being very unhappy at times because I was this twitchy, chubby kid walking around the playground. Then one day a friend saw me shuffling during recess, looking at my feet, and I'll never forget that he said, "Pick your head up. You'll feel better, and you don't have anything to be ashamed of." That day I picked my head up and started walking straight. You find the inner strength to recognize that everybody's got their *thing* that makes them "different." That's not only okay—it's good.

In hindsight, that may have been the day I became an entrepreneur. Not the day I put it into practice; I was just a kid, and didn't start building businesses until college. But you figure out how to propel yourself forward because everybody else is figuring out how to do so with *their* thing, whatever it is. Growing up is about recognizing there's only so much I can do about that *thing*, so if it's going to be around a while, then I'm going to harness it to maximum benefit. Disability becomes a gift, and an obsolete word. 'Difference' and 'disability' have diametrically different meanings, yet we interchange them too often, which doesn't do anyone any good.

There is no human being on this planet who doesn't have something 'wrong with them'

Societies develop an idea of the 'normal,' when in reality there is no such thing. There is the concept in western civilization of the Adonis, the idealized form, or the Hollywood leading man or woman, and the storybook romance. These were fantasies and models at one point, not meant to be real. But they have blended with our daily existence in a way that isn't necessarily healthy. There is no human being on this planet who doesn't have something 'wrong with them,' especially when compared with an archetype that was meant to be aspirational and even divine, but most likely adopted pieces of this person and that person, not a single individual.

The question is, how well do men and women and boys and girls incorporate uniqueness it into their daily lives? I love my country dearly, but one thing we do horribly here is promote the individual's gifts. The British system of education does a much better job. They are constantly on the lookout for individual children's talents, instead of seeking a lowest common educational denominator, which these days may be called pursuing a Common Core instead of a 'Best Possible You.' In my graduate thesis I referred to the latter as 'Educational Darwinism.' Why don't we let our strengths shine, instead of repressing them by chasing the mean, pedagogically speaking? Just because you don't sit well in a classroom because you're physically constrained or your mind wanders—whatever one might classify as a sign or symptom of some underlying 'disorder'— does not mean you, as a child or an adult, don't have a commensurate gift that isn't being observed. Consider—I have a rather profound nose [*he chuckles*], which has been the source of amusement for some people, shall we say. But at some point during my upbringing I realized that pronounced proboscis is also an evolutionary adaptation. If there's a fire, I'm going to smell it before you, buddy. I'm on my way out before you are, and my genes are more likely to be passed on. Let's say you're a twitchy person. You probably have a higher correlation of fast-twitch muscles, and you may turn out to be a kickass athlete.[138] Put another way, someone who is obese might not do well on the savannah, running away from lions, but this same person is far more likely than a svelte and skinny person to survive an ice age.

We don't look at people through such a diverse lens now. The prevalence of media doesn't help. We look at people against some benchmark 'normal.' But when one says that we have to change society to achieve such a universal embrace, I say hooray! If we stop looking at people against artificial benchmarks, but instead observed our world through realistic lenses, we would be in a much happier place, able to engage both the good and the bad as they *are*, promoting one while correcting the other.

Who does that?

I hope I can be a good parent, but one of the most nerve wracking things about deciding to have a child was knowing that, if he's a boy, there's something like a twenty-five percent chance he'll have this condition.[139] That I may potentially pass on what has not been the easiest part of my life is guilt-inspiring. My wife and I have always said we will deal with whatever comes, but it is nerve-racking.

My parents and my family, they certainly meant well, they tried hard, and my schools were supportive *conceptually*, but the problem was that the execution was often flawed. Some members of my family thought that imitating my tics would make me aware of what I was doing, as if I could stop if I wanted to. It was never from a bad place, but I remember thinking, "I can't help what I'm doing and you're not making me feel any better."

Part of that I chalk down to parents'—mine and anyone's—desperation for an answer. No parent wants to be told that his or her child has

138 For example, star soccer goalie Tim Howard holds a world-record-setting sixteen saves in one game in World Cup competition. He credits Tourette syndrome for giving him faster responses than his opponents.

139 Boys are three times more likely to have TS than girls.

a problem that can't be solved, or that he or she is destined to a life of challenge, beyond those that he or she chooses to take on. I remember being disruptive in classes, but at the same time I was smart. I didn't need Special Ed, but my behavior was inexplicable, so I was put on a range of medications, from Clonidine to Ritalin, all this while I was in elementary and junior high. I remember asking the psychiatrist, a *quack* who should have been *arrested*, why he was giving me these drugs. He told he was testing out a theory involving serotonin reuptake. Experimenting with me?! What the hell are you doing? Who does that? My parents were completely unaware because my 'therapy' sessions were one-on-one. I understand now, in hindsight, how people can find themselves being abused in one way or another when the power dynamic is such that one party is perceived as the expert, and given wide latitude, if not *carte blanche*.

This does not hinder my ability to be who I am

I studied the brain for a long time, and hold a master's degree in psychology, religion, and conflict resolution. Neuropsychology was a particular interest, given my own condition, and there are scholars—if you look back across history—who have attributed all sorts of syndromes to some of the people who have changed the world. They were seen as *weird* at the time, for whatever reasons, and they also happened to be at the fulcrum of many of history's major events.

This 'coincidence' led me to study Tourette syndrome, schizophrenia, religious experience, epilepsy, those sorts of things. I ended up getting an internship at Johns Hopkins University during the summer after my freshman year at college. I'll never forget, one day I was walking through the hallway, and the doctor who worked in the next lab over says, "You have Tourette syndrome." To say I was taken aback would be an understatement. Shocked, dismayed, flabbergasted—more like it.

I had *studied* Tourette syndrome, even though I never thought of myself as having it. Once he pointed out the obvious, however, everything aligned. I was distraught, thinking that I'm not ever getting rid of this condition. I was already past puberty, when the hormone-induced neural realignment can essentially do away with many of TS's symptoms, if not 'cure' the condition. The most reputed doctor for pediatric Tourette's syndrome, Dr. Harvey Singer, happened to be at Johns Hopkins, and my internship mentor fast-tracked me for an appointment. Fifteen minutes in he said, "You know the diagnosis as well as I do." I remember walking out of that office feeling relieved, even happy. It was the most bizarre feeling. I finally had a name for what had been going on with me, a freeing quality that said, "This is who I am. Tourette's is a part of me."

Tourette syndrome is not the biggest deal in the world, if it's not debilitating. I'm not going to die of it, so I thought, "Okay, I can deal with that." Recognizing that this condition will not hinder my ability to be fundamentally who I am was one of the most powerful feelings I ever had in my life. At the same time, it's dangerous to use Tourette's as the foundational basis of your personality, or an excuse on which to blame all manner of misbehaviors or laziness. It is a condition that can easily lend itself to hiding, but it doesn't have to—indeed, I have managed to harness this condition in ways I never would have expected. Getting an article written about me in *Inc. Magazine*[140] has been just one nicely unexpected reward.

Dr. Singer prescribed me Tenex, but the pills diminished my ability to think quickly. I've been off medications now for 18 years.

We all need to thicken our skins a bit

I can be frustrating for people in the disability community because I don't hold a lot of patience for folks using their condition as a crutch. If you're talking about someone who is completely incapacitated, that's a very different story. But the number of folks with Tourette syndrome who are rendered incapable of surviving—even thriving—in society is small. That's not to say that every person should do every job, and TS is just one factor that should be weighed before selecting one's life path. For example, Tourettics with coprolalia might not make excellent librarians. But we all need to thicken our skins a bit. I tell people, especially children, that it gets better. Kids are *mean*, but you can be proud. It gets better. The most interesting shift in my life was when people stopped caring about the unusual movements and sounds. I'm not sure when it happened—high school or after? At some point, people stopped noticing my tics, maybe because I wasn't calling as much attention to them by being overly self-conscious.

On the other hand, speaking of social oppression, I'll never forget sitting down with the admissions director of a major California university when I was preparing to take post-baccalaureate courses when I thought I

---

140 See *Inc. Magazine*, July 14, 2014. *"Life as a Startup CEO with Tourette's."*

might go to med school. I already had my first masters degree, and I had run a business for years. I was sitting in the professor's office in a jacket and tie, overviewing my career and aspirations, when she stops me, five, ten minutes into the interview. She asked, "Are you high?" [*He laughs.*] I said, "Do I *seem* high?" She pointed out I couldn't keep my eyes focused and that I was twitchy. I told her I had Tourette syndrome. The professor felt pretty horrible, and I got into the program.

We did a run through the woods with bayonets

On September 11, 2001, I enlisted in the United States Army Reserve. Let me tell you, getting a Tourettic into the Army is not an easy feat [*he laughs*]! I had to get special waivers from very high up in the medical staff. But I ended up leaving the military because of my condition. My last day was the day we did a run through the woods with bayonets on our rifles. I realized that if my eyes twitched and I missed a step and tripped on a rock, I could knife the person in front of me in the back of the neck. I wasn't willing to risk that, and I requested a transfer out. I never wanted to make Tourette's a crutch, and even less to have it be the cause of harm to a fellow soldier. Certainly you have to be aware of your limitations, but I don't think there have to be many of them. Still, the fact that I'm not destined to run through the woods with a bayonet is probably okay [*he laughs*].

This gets me to where I am today with Beyond Lucid Technologies, the company I co-founded in 2009. The idea of serving those who serve was always very important to me. The work I do now with emergency responders originally came from my military experience. I was slated to become a field medic, but I came to understand what field medics out in the suck[141] *don't* have in terms of technology. It's still very austere medicine, as they say, much like it was fifty, sixty or more years ago.

I met my business partner, who came out of Boeing, at Carnegie Mellon Univeristy, in the business school. Chris is a technical genius, and shortly after we started working together, we pitched the Department of Defense the concept of a field deployable therapeutics tool for post-traumatic stress and traumatic brain injury. DoD asked us instead to focus on diagnostics because they weren't getting enough information to provide therapeutics in the field. This is how we got into Emergency Medical Services. If I'm not going to be the guy on the ground with the

---

141 The battlefield.

bayonet, there is another way I can harness the gifts, strengths, and skills I do have.

You cannot hold us down

I often tell students when I speak with them, "Find what you're good at. Find your passion, and if somebody tries to hold you down, you just keep doin' what you're doin', man." I'm going to tell my son the same thing. I call this freedom the joy of being independent. You cannot hold the independents down. We will find a way. There are always going to be people who try to stop you. This may stem from people needing to put others down to get ahead, or to feel better about themselves. It has to do with competition, and people's perception that life is a zero-sum game.

But it has nothing to do with Tourette syndrome. I see Tourette's as an unlikely gift, a source of strength and power. Society's response to so much difference—and what is too often called 'disability' or 'handicap'—compresses the self. It puts the self into a box and squeezes. But what happens when you push down on something that doesn't want to be compressed, when you apply pressure to something that resists it? The thing in the box gets hot, and it gets hard. That's just physics. So imagine the self—Tourettic or not—as lump of coal being compressed by the externalities of society. That piece of coal eventually turns into a diamond. You don't have a choice. I mean, I guess you do—you could stop living, but that doesn't work out so well.

You gotta get to tomorrow

Shortly after I graduated from business school, Ramin, a dear old friend, called me to get lunch one day at Los Angeles's Century City Mall. I was standing in line at a restaurant, and behind me was a woman in a trench coat and sunglasses, indoors, in July. So I turned to her and said, "If we put a fedora on you, you'd look like an old school detective." I ended up seeing Mabel again outside, and I was simply-tongue tied. *Me, tongue-tied!* I would have said *anything* to keep her there.

A few days later we went on a date to the beach for coffee. While we were there, I got a call from some business school buddies, asking us to join them at the Getty Center. Mabel was game, but the Getty was closed, so this motley crew of ten people—all strangers to her—wanted to go to dinner. About *ten* hours later, I drove her back to her car, at the end of one of the oddest first dates I had ever had. It turned out to be the last one.

A month later, to the day, I asked her to marry me. We got married a year later. But I ask myself, what if I hadn't gone to lunch that day? What if we'd gone somewhere else, or if I hadn't said something? I often tell people, especially kids having a tough time with whatever makes them different, "Don't do anything rash, and don't count yourself out. You've got to get to tomorrow, because tomorrow is *interesting*. You don't know if it's going to be good or horrible compared to today. But isn't that interesting? Suspenseful? And the thing that seems really awful right now may turn out to be the saving grace later." You've got to keep your head up and keep moving forward, like I learned on the playground so many years ago.

APPENDIX A

A list of Tourette syndrome camps in the United States.

Tourette Syndrome Camp USA, Illinois

The Tourette Syndrome Camp USA in Illinois is a residential camping program designed for girls and boys ages eight-to-sixteen-plus whose primary diagnosis is TS, and to a lesser degree, OCD and ADD/ADHD. Find them at tourettecamp.org.

Camp Twitch And Shout, Georgia

Camp Twitch and Shout is a one-week overnight camp for children ages eight-to-seventeen who have been diagnosed with Tourette syndrome. It is organized and managed by T.I.C.S. of Georgia, in partnership with Camp Twin Lakes, and is located at Camp Will-A-Way in Winder, Georgia. Find them at camptwitchandshout.org.

Camp George, Southern California

Camp George in Southern California is named after Georges Gilles de la Tourette. Its mission is to provide an annual family summer camp experience to children and families dealing with Tourette syndrome. Find them at tsa-socal.org/camp-george.

Joshua Center Camp, Missouri

Joshua Center Camp is available to children with a primary diagnosis of Tourette syndrome, Asperger syndrome, or obsessive-compulsive disorder. Find them at joshuacenter.com/summer-camp.

Camp Connect TS, West Virginia

Camp Connect TS offers children and teens with Tourette syndrome, ages seven-to-seventeen, seven days and six nights of summer fun and social connections. Children experience all the fun and adventure of a sleepaway camp with medical staff close at hand. Find them at brainycamps.com/camps/camp-connect-t.

Camp Bernie, New Jersey

The NJCTS Family Retreat Weekend at YMCA Camp Bernie. The weekend allows children and families to meet others with Tourette syndrome, learn more about their diagnosis, and engage with peer mentors in a fun, safe environment. Find them at njcts.org/camp_bernie.php. Telephone: 908.575.7350.

Camp Excel, Bergen County, New Jersey

Day camp program throughout the summer for children ages five-to-seventeen diagnosed with ADHD, Asperger syndrome, Tourette syndrome, obsessive-compulsive disorder, anxiety, depression, central auditory processing disorder, and mild learning disabilities. There are also Saturday programs offered throughout the school year. Find them at: campexcel. com. Telephone: 732.282.0150. FAX: 732.282.0151.

Camp du Ballon Rouge, Texas

Weekend camp for children with a primary diagnosis of Tourette syndrome ages six-to-eighteen, and related conditions such as obsessive compulsive-disorder and attention deficit disorder. Find them at: TouretteTexas. org/camp. Telephone: 866.896.8484. Alternate Phone: 281.238.8096. FAX: 281.238.0468.

Camp Ticapalooza, New York

A weekend camp at the YMCA Camp on Keuka Lake in Penn Yan, NY. Tourette Association of Greater New York. Find them at: tsa-gnys.org.

Camp Carton, New York

Camp Carton is a week-long sleepaway camp, serving children ages ten-to-thirteen diagnosed with Tourette syndrome who reside in the Northeast, primarily the Tri-State Area (New York, New Jersey, and Connecticut). Find them at campcarton.com.

Family Camp, Minnesota

A weekend of hope, acceptance, and FUN for Minnesota children ages six-through-seventeen with a primary diagnosis of Tourette syndrome and their families. At least one parent must accompany every family group. Find them at tsa-mn.org.

Family Camp, Pennsylvania

The PA Tourette Syndrome Alliance sponsors a two-day summer camp and one-day retreat in autumn in the Appalachian Mountains. Find them at patsainc.org. Telephone: 717.337.1134. Alternate telephone: 800.990.3300.

Family Weekend, Florida

Kids with Tourette's and their siblings engage in camp activities like canoeing, archery, arts and crafts, and a bonfire. All day Saturday parents and other adult family members take part in educational sessions hosted by members of TSA Florida and guest speakers from the medical and education fields knowledgeable about Tourette's. Find them at tsa-fl.org/events/family-weekend. Telephone: 727.418.0240.

Camp Tanager, Iowa

A weekend camp for youth ages six-through-seventeen with Tourette syndrome and their parents and siblings. Find them at camptanager.org. Telephone: 319.363.0681.

For camps in Canada check Tourette Canada at tourette.ca. Telephone: 800.361.3120. FAX: 800-387-0120.

APPENDIX B

USEFUL INFORMATION FROM
THE INTERVIEWS

This list is by no means exhaustive. I made an effort to collect a representative sample of good ideas people shared. As with the interviews themselves, any medical advice is the opinion of the interviewees and not my own. Quotes are taken directly from the interviews.

GENERAL

Find the Tourette Association of America chapter in your area. They may still be listed under Tourette Syndrome Association. Also check tourette. org.

Accept Tourette syndrome. Believe it's going to be okay and this is just how it is for now. Things change.

Advocate for yourself.

At school, speak to your teachers, administrators, and classmates to educate them about Tourette's. Get the accommodations you need.

In public, speak up if appropriate. An educated public is less judgmental.

At work, perhaps you can get some accommodations.

The law is on your side.

By creating awareness about Tourette syndrome, you are making life easier for future generations of Touretters.

Don't suppress tics, if possible. Sometimes it's necessary to suppress, but try becoming more comfortable with ticcing. Suppressing hurts you and causes more stress. Suppressing can make you feel that you are not being yourself.

OCD can be helpful in detail-oriented activities and careers.

Treat Tourette's by treating society. "Disability" is a disorder of society's response to people's differences. This fundamental ignorance is why educating individuals and society is so important.

"If you educate someone about TS, you give them the chance to be compassionate."

"We don't need to 'fix' kids with Tourette's. Touretters and their families need to learn coping strategies, get accommodations in school and at work, and be in supportive environments."

When meeting new people, see how they respond to your TS. If they accept it, good. If they have difficulties, educate them. If they still can't accept it, learn to leave them behind.

Try not to cause your own isolation. Teasing and bullying hurt a lot. But when you *assume* people are going to hurt you, you push them away before they have a chance to demonstrate if they're good people or not.

Don't hang out with people just because they accept your tics. Judge them by their qualities.

Find support groups.

Go to a Tourette camp as a camper or counselor.

"We all have to thicken our skins a little bit."

"Okay, we have this. Now how are we going to survive? How are we going to do well *anyway*?"

Being idle can often increase tension and anxiety because you tend to think too much about problems. And because you're idle, you tend to feel helpless.

Get out and do something!

Be active and creative. Find your interests, your passions, and follow them. See where they lead.

If you're fully engaged in what you love, that path leads away from stress and tics.

If you're trying to make what seem like large changes, don't attempt them all at once. Break the change process down into smaller steps. You can have success with each small step and build to the large change, gaining confidence as you go.

Be compassionate, be caring, love one another. Be generous with your time and resources, whatever they might be. Help others less fortunate.

"Judging yourself negatively for ticcing is like accidentally cutting yourself and saying, 'I must be a bad person because I'm careless.' You wouldn't do this—instead you'd get a Band Aid. Be aware how you think about yourself when you tic. Try not to put yourself in a box by thinking, 'I'm stupid, I'm weird.' It's not so."

Find a practical way to deal with your tics. That begins with accepting your Tourette syndrome.

Find other people with Tourette's and talk with them. TS camps are good for this and so is Facebook and other support groups. Having someone who understands what you're going through is some of the best therapy. Even loving, well-intentioned parents and friends don't know exactly what it's like. Find someone who also has TS and talk with them.

"One of the biggest lessons in my life I've learned—absolutely no fear. I've let fear in my life overrule everything."

"Once you've made it through a dark period, you know you can face with confidence another dark period, if one appears."

"You have a choice. Are you going to let Tourette's ruin your life or are you going to figure out how to live with it and have a happy, productive life?"

"Everyone has a cross to bear. Tourette's is ours."

Being honest about your tics and emotions is important for you to stay healthy. Talking with trusted loved ones and friends helps bring problems to light; you can think about them and find solutions. If you're not voicing your difficulties, your support network can't help you with them.

"Tourette's just happened to me. Why should I be ashamed of it?"

"We all have limitations. What's important is how we deal with them. Disability is, in some important ways, a point of view and not a physical condition."

"Don't count yourself out. You've got to get to tomorrow, because tomorrow is interesting. You don't know what it contains, good or bad."

For women, tics seem to worsen during menstruation.

PARENTS

It's important to know your child can have a satisfying life with TS.

Put things in perspective. There are parents out there whose children have worse problems, and those parents would switch with you if they could.

There is a natural grieving process when you get the Tourette syndrome diagnosis. Understand this, feel it, and let it pass.

You'll make mistakes, but don't blame yourself. Learn from your errors and keep going. Be patient and forgiving with yourself.

Parents need to be patient with each other, especially at the end of a long day.

Find a way to rest and rejuvenate yourself. Take time alone for yourself. And don't forget your relationship with your spouse!

Find and encourage your child's interests. Support talents and help him or her find happiness in this way.

You have to speak up for your child and never quit. Don't stay quiet about your child's diagnosis. Learn, talk, advocate.

Listen to, believe, and validate your child's feelings and statements about TS.

Help them deal with their emotions and problems regarding TS.

Talk about Tourette's with them and the family.

Treat all your children the same, though this sometimes is difficult, depending on the severity of Tourette's or other comorbid conditions. Don't expend so much energy on one child that you inadvertently neglect your others.

Be aware of what your kids are eating and how it affects their symptoms. Avoid caffeine, sugar, high fructose corn syrup, food dyes, and junk foods. Send your own snacks to school and be careful with school lunches.

Punishment is not the answer for many kids. See your child as *having* a problem, not *being* the problem.

It's sometimes difficult to distinguish between what is the child's bad behavior and what is a symptom of TS and comorbid conditions. Don't be harsh on yourself if you can't always tell the difference.

If your child has rage issues, it's good to take a deep breath, and stay calm. Maintaining your cool can help de-escalate the situation.

Getting angry with a child is often counterproductive, especially if the child has rage issues. Parents can monitor each other, and when one becomes impatient or angry, the other can take over.

If a child is yelling or expressing uncontrollable rage, try whispering to them. A low, calm voice can change the dynamic of a moment. Quietly speaking breaks the child's focus from their behavior to what you're saying.

When in public, pick your battles about responding to people's reactions.

You have a unique ability to spot other parents with kids with special issues, and if you see someone having a difficult time, you can offer to help. You understand like no one else.

Stay open to information from all sources. Sometimes talking about Tourette's can bring a valuable comment from someone you know, or even a stranger.

Some people will blame you for Tourette's, either as parent or one who has it. Let that blame bounce off you.

Depending on your child's needs, find other children like him or her with whom to create relationships.

Investigate the new 529-Able tax-free savings accounts that are a simpler, less expensive way for families to save money for members with disabilities.

FAMILY

Keep the family calm.

The whole family needs to learn about Tourette's and comorbid conditions.

Support groups, conferences, seminars, and reading materials related to the subject are good sources.

Everyone's feelings are important.

You can get through this difficult time by working together.

Sometimes anything that's a disruption of schedule for a TS kid makes stress and tics worse.

Break chores into parts; reward each completed part. Have your child repeat the instructions back to you.

Go over new chores or expectations clearly.

Check with state and county offices for programs that will benefit your child and your family. Services offered by departments of rehabilitation or disability services, for example, can be fruitful.

Find groups that support you, your child, and your family such as the Tourette Association of America at tourette.org.

For military families, check out the Exceptional Family Member Program for your branch of service.

Some families go to therapy together, or with one particular child.

Try adapting family customs to accommodate your TS child's needs and what it takes to maintain peace in the home. All within reason, naturally.

People with Tourette's and parents of kids with TS tend to feel isolated, and think they are the only family experiencing this difficulty. Take heart—you're not alone. Find others, talk to them for inspiration, courage, and comfort. Also realize how good it feels to use your knowledge to help someone else.

SUPPORT

Reinforce the idea that your child is okay just as he or she is.

Support your child's strengths. Encourage your child to find interests.

Teach children that they can do what they set their mind to. Teach them to believe in their own powers and efforts.

It's important for parents to show love and support for their kids with TS, even when applying discipline or pressure to accomplish something.

Give your child love and support, but don't let them use TS as an excuse for avoiding responsibilities.

Learn and teach coping skills.

CHILDREN

Children have to learn to live with their tics, at least for a while. The good news is about seventy percent of kids outgrow their tics as they get older, especially when they reach their early twenties, due to brain maturation.

Try different activities because you never know what's going to interest you; you never know what you're going to be good at.

Go to a Tourette syndrome camp!

Find role models and use their examples to bolster your spirits and motivate your activities.

Superheroes such as Spiderman, the Hulk, and the X-Men are like people with Tourette's. They are struggling to overcome the social consequences of being different. They haven't chosen to be this way. They are reluctant heroes making the most of the special gifts they've been given.

DEALING WITH DOCTORS

Do your research and know about Tourette's, so when you are with a doctor they will take you more seriously. You will also be able to judge the quality of a doctor's Tourette syndrome knowledge.

Find a doctor who understands and believes what you're saying about your child and Tourette's.

Don't do something just because a doctor says so. Decisions about treatment are yours to make.

Investigate, think, and feel about what your doctor is saying and recommending.

What's best for your child? What's best for the family?

Your doctors must believe you when you describe symptoms and responses to drugs. You must be your own advocate.

If you feel the doctor doesn't accept your information, find a new doctor.

Sometimes it's difficult to know if positive changes are from medications or maturation. This is a normal quandary.

Keep good records of your child's symptoms and behaviors and note what you've done in response.

Keep close track of medications, their results, and side effects.

Learn your or your child's sensitivity level to drugs.

Video record your child ticcing so you can show the doctor. Sometimes children will suppress in a doctor's office.

Medicine is not always the best option for someone with Tourette syndrome.

Sometimes social interventions, school accommodations, alternative therapies, and coping strategies are more effective.

Monitor what drugs you're being given, especially in emergency situations. You know what drugs you can't tolerate. You must be proactive about this because the medical community sometimes makes mistakes.

Most experts in the field would agree that PANDAS (Pediatric Autoimmune Neuropsychiatric Disorders Associated with Strep) is an actual condition and can cause tics in children exposed to strep. The recommendation is to treat strep throat immediately.

SCHOOL

Advocate for yourself (or your child) in class and in the schoolyard. Enlist your friends.

Use your own research and TAA materials.

Perhaps invite a TAA Youth Ambassador to your school.

Accommodations in school: IEPs and 401s.

Think about having your child with you in school meetings to express his or her needs. This can give them confidence to speak up and advocate for themselves.

Don't schedule difficult classes close together. Space them out during the day.

Try making arrangements for your child to do homework at school because bringing schoolwork home, the safe place, may cause tension.

See tourette.org for more information about your rights.

Schools and school districts will respond differently to your requests for accommodations.

If the schools resist, keep at it, find new ways to present material.

Be polite but firm.

The law is on your side.

With substitute teachers, the TS child should immediately introduce himself or herself, and tell the teacher about Tourette's.

Deal with bullying right away when it's happening to your child.

Saying "Just ignore it and it will go away" isn't practical sometimes and is very difficult for a child to do.

Get teachers and school administrators involved immediately.

Life is not all about high school. It may be ugly now, but people's behavior toward you most often will get better after high school.

If grades are an issue for a college-bound student, be sure to mention Tourette syndrome in the personal statement portion of the college application.

Use the resources at Learning Disability Centers or other such offices at colleges and universities.

Homeschooling is a possibility if conventional schooling becomes difficult. You can always mainstream your child again once homeschool isn't necessary.

Remember to maintain your child's social life so he or she doesn't feel isolated.

Small private schools are an option for those who can afford them.

TECHNIQUES FOR DEALING WITH TICS

Maintain a positive attitude. Say to yourself, "I might not like it, but I can accept it."

Make sure you eat well and get plenty of rest. Being overtired makes your tics worse.

Find something creative to do. This can make you feel more connected to yourself and other people. You can create. You are somebody with thoughts, feelings, ideas, and value.

Try writing about yourself and thinking about your story. This might give you a new perspective on Tourette's. Many people said thinking deeply and writing about their life with Tourette's felt good and made them happy.

Acknowledging the mind-body connection, you might explore bodywork, cautiously and appropriately. Feldenkrais, Reiki, and deep tissue massage were mentioned.

Deep breathing and counting slowly backwards from ten are ways to calm down and tic less. Focus on the counting and it will change your focus from tics. Learn to recognize tension as it arises, so you can begin an early counter-measure.

Cognitive Behavioral Intervention for Tics (CBIT), Cognitive Behavioral Therapy (CBT), and habit reversal therapy may help tics. But realize these techniques are not a cure for TS. They only alleviate symptoms.

Isolate the tension surrounding a tic and try to visualize slowly moving it out of your body.

Investigate the new mouth orthotic that has helped some people lessen their tics. See more at Tourette.org.

Stress squeeze balls sometimes help relieve tension.

See if you can find a smaller, less visible movement, or combination of movements, that satisfies the feeling of doing a tic.

With vocal tics, experiment with transforming them into more acceptable noises or words.

If tics interfere with falling asleep, try doing something that relaxes or tires you out before getting ready for bed. For example, go for a walk or exercise.

Biofeedback and meditation help with stress, which helps with tics.

Learn about mindfulness from writers like Jon Kabat-Zinn. Mindfulness helps you take a step back from stressful situations and calm down, which lessens tics. It's about not trying to control the moment and what it contains. Some people and things you can change, but some you cannot. Learn to distinguish between the two.

358   An Unlikely Strength

Humor is sometimes a way to diminish the public tension that tics can cause. It helps others feel less self-conscious and helps them accept your tics. As long as they are laughing *with* you and not at you, naturally. But don't use humor to make fun of yourself in a self-deprecating manner. Don't diminish yourself.

Self-medicating with alcohol and drugs is not an answer for TS. You have to deal with your symptoms and emotions, not run away from them.

Nicotine patches have given some people relief from tics. However DO NOT use any other nicotine products in any form. No cigarettes, no chewing tobacco, and no vaping. Vaping is *not* a safe alternative to cigarettes, despite what tobacco companies want you to believe.

Some people find swimming is relaxing for their tics.

Accupressure, massage and self-massage, and compression help some people with their tics.

Ice packs and Tiger Balm can help with the pain caused by tics.

Tai chi and yoga are good forms of relaxation.

Try listening to mantra music and gong baths which create relaxing sounds and environments. Find them on the internet.

Investigate Deep Brain Stimulation surgery if your TS is severe. But keep in mind that it is expensive, can be risky, and doesn't always work. Even if DBS works for you, it isn't an immediate solution to tics. It requires fine tuning of the device and this can take some time. Be patient.

If you have health insurance, check your policy to see if the procedure is covered.

Ask your doctor and/or surgeon to help meeting DBS insurance requirements.

Service dogs can be of great help to severe Touretters.

A weighted blanket sometimes helps relieve severe body tics.

Noise-cancelling headphones help if you have sensitivity to sound. Contoured earplugs also help dampen sound.

Sunglasses, outdoors and indoors, can help with light sensitivity.

Some Touretters say herbs like valerian root, hops, chamomile, and lemon balm have given them relief from panic attacks.

Aconite for panic attacks helps some people. Neuroflam from Apex Energetics helps one person with stress and nervousness that cause increased tics.

Homeopathic tinctures help some people with tics and other symptoms. For example, you can try nervines with kava, skullcap, and valerian for severe tics or panic disorder.

Zentangle, crossword puzzles, and other close work can grab your attention, focus your mind, and lessen tics.

Try controlling your environment to eliminate or lessen the effects of people, places, or things that trigger stress and tics.

If your tics are bothering someone, it's helpful to find positive actions you can take. How might you modify a tic for the moment to make conditions better for the other person?

APPENDIX C

This is by no means a complete list. Search on your own (amazon.com is a good resource) because materials continue to appear both by the medical and scientific community and from within the Tourette community itself.

As always, there is the Tourette Association of America (tourette.org), 42-40 Bell Boulevard, Suite 205, Bayside, New York 11361. Telephone: 718.224.2999. Their website is filled with information about Tourette syndrome, the medical community and treatments, meetings and support groups, and educational materials.

Books

<u>Non-Fiction</u>

Touretties, Chris Mason. Available on amazon.com.

What Makes Me Tic, Chris Mason. Available on amazon.com.

How God Saved Me: My Inspirational Story by Christopher Fox. Available on amazon.com.

Tic Talk Around The Clock by Lauren Ashley. Available on amazon.com.

A Family's Quest for Rhythm: Living with Tourette, ADD, OCD & Challenging Behaviors by Kathy Giordano and Matt Giordano. Available at afamilysquest.com and on amazon.com.

Front of the Class: How Tourette Syndrome Made Me the Teacher I Never Had, by Brad Cohen and Lisa Wysocky. The book was made into the Hallmark Hall of Fame TV movie *Front of the Class*. Also see bradcohentourettefoundation.com.

Man's Search For Meaning, Viktor Frankl.

The Explosive Child, Dr. Ross Greene.

The Cursing Brain, Howard I. Kushner.

Tourette's Syndrome—Tics, Obsessions, Compulsions, edited by James F. Leckman and Donald J. Cohen.

A Family's Guide to Tourette Syndrome, edited by John T. Walkup, M.D., Jonathan W. Mink, M.D., Ph.D., and Kevin St.P. McNaught, Ph.D.

Children with Tourette Syndrome—A Parents' Guide, edited by Tracy Haerle.

Ticked: A Medical Miracle, a Friendship, and the Weird World of Tourette Syndrome by James A. Fussell and Jeff Matovik.

Living with Tourette Syndrome, Elaine Fantle Shimberg.

Fiction and Poetry

from a dungeon of dawn by Michael C. Mahan. Available on amazon.com.

Motherless Brooklyn, Jonathan Lethem.

On youtube.com search: Jamie Sanders, This Time, Tourettes.

Videos and Other Creative Outlets

I Have Tourette's, But Tourette's Doesn't Have Me. This HBO documentary can help children not feel so alone because they see others like them dealing with TS. The documentary is also useful for explaining TS to school administrators and classmates. You can order copies at tourette.org. Also check HBO On Demand or HBOGO.com to see if you can stream the documentary.

Information about the upcoming documentary *My Life, My Story, My Tourette's* can be found at primodiostudios.com/my-life-my-story-my-tourettes.html.

See a documentary about Tourette camp at missionmanmedia.com.

For Tourette-inspired dance see bandofartists.com.

Another documentary by a Touretter can be found at synapticadventure.com.

For artistic expressions for advocacy and education about Tourette syndrome see andrewfrueh.com.

A blog about Tourette's is at writingmyemotions.wordpress.com.

A blog about Tourette's is at totestourettes.blogspot.com.